INTRODUCTION TO HEALTH ECONOMICS

Dr. Kavita Ramanathan

ALLIED HEALTH PRESS

Introduction to Health Economics

Author: **Dr. Kavita Ramanathan**

Allied Health Press
4164 Lakeshore Road
Burlington ON L7L 1A4
Canada
www.alliedhealthpress.com
Email: orders@arclereducation.com

ISBN: 978-1-77956-256-2

Word Roots, Prefixes, and Suffixes by Chapter

Chapter 1 Understanding Health Economics

Micro/small-scale: or individual level

chron/o-: time

norm-: normal

eco-: home

-nomos: account

Patient, patiens: to suffer or bear

Chapter 2 Demand for Health and Healthcare

anti-: against

bio-: life

psych/o-: mind

hetero: different

micro-: small

op-, opt-: vision

Chapter 3 Supply in Healthcare

Cardi(o)-: (related to the heart)

Hypo-: (below, deficient)

-itis: (inflammation)

Derm(a)-: (related to the skin)

Hyper-: (excessive, above normal)

-ectomy: (surgical removal)

Hepat(o)-: (related to the liver)

Chapter 4 Equity and Health

Equi-: Denotes equality or fairness, as in equidistant (equal distance).

In-: Indicates negation or absence, as in injustice (lack of justice).

Well-: Denotes good or healthy, as in well-being.

-ity: Forms abstract nouns indicating a state or quality, as in equity (state of being fair).

-ness: Forms abstract nouns indicating a state or condition, as in wellness (state of being well).

-ity: Forms abstract nouns indicating a state or condition, as in inequality (state of being unequal).

-th: Forms nouns indicating a state or condition, as in health (state of being free from illness or injury).

Chapter 5 Financing and Insurance in Healthcare

cardi/o: heart

chem/o: drug; chemical

contra-: against; opposite

-ia: condition

iatr/o: physician; treatment

-ician: specialist

immun/o: immune; protection; safe

-ist: specialist

path/o: disease

Chapter 6 Role of Government in Health

Im-: Mortal

Un-: Manage

In-: Equal

-ity: Inequality

-ly: Illegally

-sion: (conversion, invasion)

Chapter 7 Technology Transfer in Healthcare

arteri-: arteries

cardi-, coron-: the heart

cerebr-: the brain

col-: the colon/large intestine

neuro-: nerves and the nervous system

epi-: over, above, on top

fore-: before or ahead

fron-: about the forehead

Chapter 8 Theory and Principles of Economic Evaluation

infra-: below

inter-: between, among

pre-, pro-: before

super-, supra-: above, over, superior to

trans-: across

micr-: small

Chapter 9 Health Efficiency

bio- : life (e.g., biology, bioengineering)

-therapy: treatment (e.g., chemotherapy, physiotherapy)

cardio-: heart (e.g., cardiovascular, cardiology)

-genic: producing, causing (e.g., pathogenic, biogenic)

hemo- : blood (e.g., hemoglobin, hemostasis)

-lysis: breakdown, destruction (e.g., dialysis, hemolysis)

Chapter 10 Public Health and Policies

Inter-: Among, between, or connecting.

Pre-: Before or in advance of.

Epi-: Upon, on, over, or among

Bio-: life or living organisms

Multi-:Multiple.

-logy (or -ology): subject or field.

Table of Contents

LIST OF FIGURES

LIST OF TABLES

PREFACE

The application of economic principles in the healthcare sector represents a relatively recent development. Historically, the field of public health has not fully appreciated the potential impact that established economic concepts could have within its domain. However, there has been a notable shift in this perspective, with a growing recognition of the significance of introducing economics into the realm of healthcare. This recognition has led to the emergence of health economics as a crucial field of study.

While various disciplines contribute to our understanding of the factors influencing individual health outcomes, health economics offers unique insights into the behavioral aspects that underpin these outcomes. Health economists examine how individuals make decisions by weighing current health status, as well as the associated time and financial costs, against the anticipated future benefits in terms of improved health and reduced risk of disease or mortality. This approach provides a valuable framework for understanding and predicting healthcare-related behaviors.

The central challenge facing the field of health economics is the elucidation of these decision-making processes, along with numerous other issues related to its application in healthcare settings. By addressing these challenges, health economics has the potential to enhance our understanding of healthcare systems, improve decision-making processes, and ultimately contribute to better health outcomes for individuals and populations alike.

"Introduction to Health Economics" aims to provide a comprehensive overview of the key concepts and principles in health economics, with a focus on their application in healthcare systems worldwide. The book is designed for students and professionals in healthcare management, economics, and policy, as well as healthcare practitioners seeking to understand the economic aspects of healthcare delivery.

The book begins by introducing the fundamental concepts of health economics, such as supply and demand, efficiency, equity, and market failure. It then explores how these concepts are applied to the healthcare sector, examining issues such as healthcare financing, insurance, and the role of government in healthcare markets.

This book is to help readers understand the unique challenges facing healthcare systems, including rising costs, limited resources, and the need to improve quality and access to care. It also aims to provide readers with the tools and frameworks needed to analyze and address these challenges, such as cost-effectiveness analysis, economic evaluation, and health policy analysis. Against a background of increasing demands on limited resources, health economics is exerting an influence on decision-making at all levels of healthcare. Health economics seeks to facilitate decision-making by offering an explicit decision-making framework based on the principle of efficiency. It is not the only consideration, but it is an important one, and practitioners will need to have an understanding of its basic principles and how it can impact on clinical decision-making. This book covers some of the basic principles of health economics and, in particular, economic evaluation. Finally, this book equips readers with a solid foundation in health economics theory and practice, enabling them to critically evaluate healthcare systems and policies, and to contribute to the development of more efficient, equitable, and sustainable healthcare systems.

Chapter

UNDERSTANDING HEALTH ECONOMICS

1

Contents

Introduction

Economics is the study of how individuals and society ultimately decide, with or without the use of money, to make use of limited productive resources that have potential use to produce a variety of goods and distribute them for consumption, either now or in the future, among different individuals and social groups. It examines the advantages and disadvantages of enhancing resource allocation patterns. Such a definition treats economics as the study of scarcity and choice in the context of health as a commodity or service; for example, it addresses how to allocate a given amount of resources among various alternatives to improve health or determine the optimal combination of resources to deliver in-patient care. Economics is not limited by the definition to any particular category of human endeavor. Economics applies to any activity in which there is choice and scarcity.

Treating health economics as a separate scientific field and giving particular attention to issues pertaining to the economics of the healthcare industry have grown in popularity over the past 30 years or so. Nowadays, health economics is a well-established field that is taught in most university curricula. Although the majority of health economists work in medical departments, the field's links to economics as a whole are being strengthened, and the approaches used are becoming more sophisticated.

The study of health economics focuses on the distribution of health, health-related services, and health among individuals and groups in society. It also examines how limited resources are distributed among alternative uses for the treatment of illness and the promotion, maintenance, and improvement of health. In general, it can be described as "the application of economic theories, concepts, and techniques to the health sector." Thus, it is concerned with things like how resources are distributed among different health-promoting initiatives, how many resources are used to deliver health services, how health service institutions are organized and funded, how effectively resources are distributed and used for health, and how preventive, curative, and rehabilitative health services affect people individually as well as society as a whole.

Because of this, health economics has emerged as a unique area of study, focusing on how economic theory can be applied to real-world issues involving better resource allocation to provide effective and efficient healthcare. The main topics covered by health economics include the financial aspects of healthcare services, the economic aspects of the relationship between productivity and health, the planning of health development, the financial aspects of health and medical care institutions, and other related aspects. Health and medical care as economic goods, health as a private or public good, health measurement, health stock, investment aspects of health, loss due to illness, resource costs of various diseases, effects of health and medical care provision, planning of health and medical care, technology choice in the healthcare system, are some prominent features of health economics.

There are two perspectives on the issue in health economics: normative and positive. The normative concerns, among other things, the proper budgetary allocation for HIV/AIDS control. All contemporary microeconomic theory is applied to health and medical care by the positive branch of health economics. Positive health economics studies healthcare demand that is influenced by an individual's income, preferences, access to public and private healthcare, and other factors.

The relationship between an individual's (or the population's) health status and the use of medical services establishes the connection between the "economics of health" and the "economics of healthcare." Any service that affects a person's health status and is rendered by professionals or paraprofessionals is referred to as healthcare. The healthcare system is a formal framework for a specific population, with laws and regulations defining its administration, finances, scope, and content. It stipulates that services must be provided to individuals to support their health, and that these services must be provided in specified locations, including homes, workplaces, schools, public spaces, communities, hospitals, clinics, and so on.

Orientation and Directional Terms:

Term	Definition	Illustration
Economics	Economics is a social science that focuses on the production, distribution, and consumption of goods and services. The study of economics is primarily concerned with analyzing the choices that individuals, businesses, governments, and nations make to allocate limited resources.	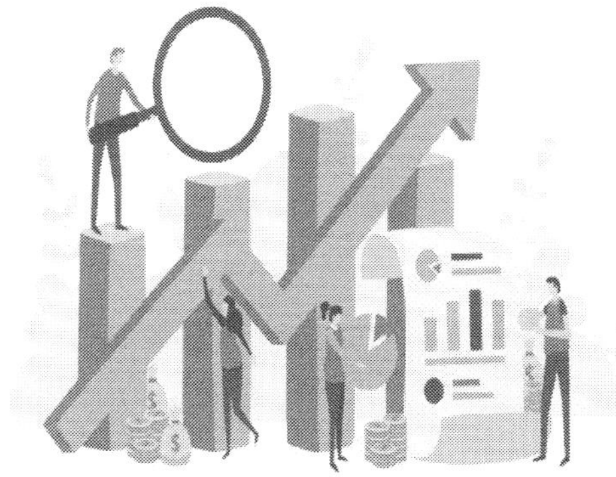
Healthcare	Healthcare is the improvement of health via the prevention, diagnosis, treatment, amelioration or cure of disease, illness, injury, and other physical and mental impairments in people.	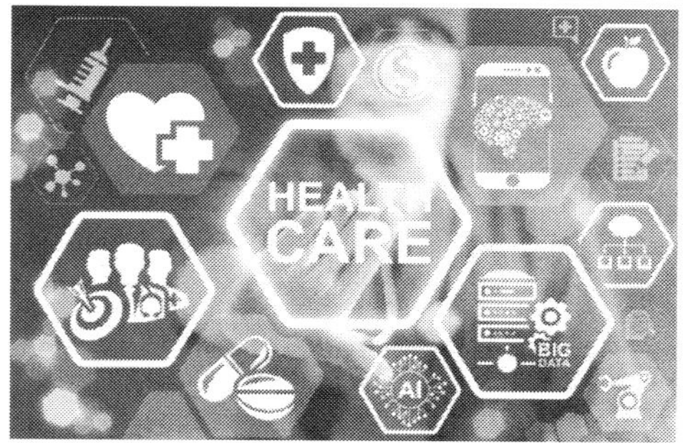
Gross domestic product	Gross domestic product is the monetary value of all finished goods and services made within a country during a specific period.	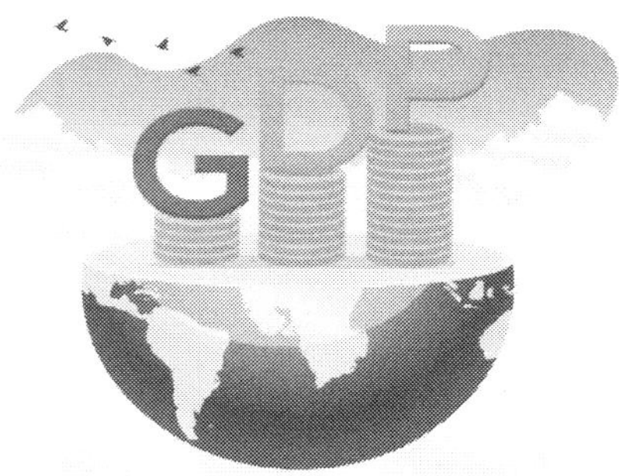
World Health Organization (WHO)	The World Health Organization (WHO) is a specialized agency of the United Nations responsible for international public health. It is headquartered in Geneva, Switzerland, and has six regional offices and 150 field offices worldwide.	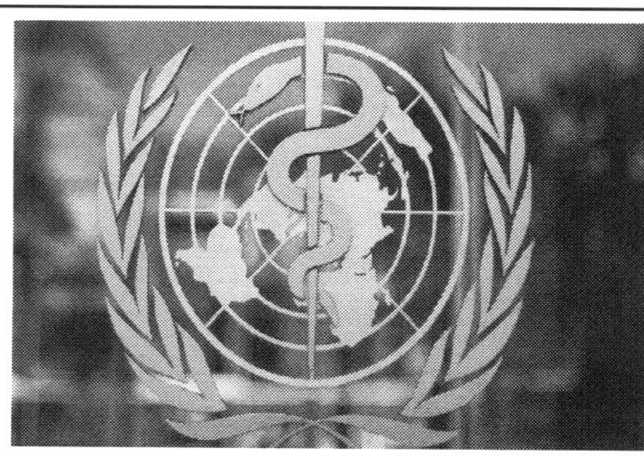

1.1. History of Health Economics

The ancient Greek philosopher Aristotle once discussed the production and exchange relationship between physicians and farmers in the third century BC. British classical economist William Petty noted in the 17th century that worker health and medical costs would have a positive economic impact.

With its many sub-disciplines and research domains, modern health economics is currently a well-known interdisciplinary field that links economic theory with healthcare practice. This knowledge's scholarly origins can typically be found in the U.S. custom.

The American Medical Association (AMA) was founded in 1848 with the primary objectives of advancing science, establishing medical education standards, initiating a medical ethics program, and achieving better public health. However, it wasn't until 1931 that the AMA Bureau of Medical Economics was founded, tasked with researching all financial issues about the medical field, that economic concerns were given more weight.

Medical and health expenses increased significantly after World War II due to several factors, including the aging of the population, the sharp rise in chronic diseases, the improvement in people's demand for healthcare, the rapid advancement of medical research technology, the modernization of diagnosis and treatment methods, and health facilities and equipment. For instance, the total U.S. The importance that society placed on healthcare in comparison to other non-health goods and services is demonstrated by the steady increase in health expenditures as a percentage of GDP. Health spending as a percentage of GDP grew from 5% to 17% between 1960 and 2013. While nominal GDP growth was 6.7% during the same period, the average annual growth in nominal national health expenditures was 9.2%. Concurrently, many European nations saw a rise in healthcare spending, which by the end of the 1970s accounted for 8% of GDP, up from 4% in the 1950s. Growth-wise, many countries saw increases in the percentage of healthcare spending in GNP (gross national product) of 1% in the 1950s, 1% in the 1960s, and 2% in the 1970s. The government, business owners, employees, and families were all heavily impacted financially by the high cost of healthcare, so there was a need to find a way to slow its rise.

In addition, the scope of health services expanded, technological tools improved, and specialization and division of labor increased. The healthcare sector, which now accounts for a sizeable portion of labor and capital and plays a significant role in both social and economic life, emerged from the medical and health services sector. Research on the financial issues facing the healthcare industry has grown in importance within the field of economics.

Following the 1960s, health economics research continued to grow, and in the United States, a third and a second academic seminar on the subject were held in 1968 and 1962, respectively. The World Health Organization convened its inaugural global health economics symposium in Moscow in 1968. The three meetings' calling demonstrated that health economics had joined an academic forum as a separate field. Following the 1970s, the health economy began to grow quickly, and nursing economics started to take shape. The field of nursing economics began to take shape in 1979 when renowned American health economist Paul Feldstein applied economic principles to the discussion of long-term care, registered markets, and other nursing economy issues.

Nursing Economics Magazine was established in the United States in 1983. Topics covered in its research included nursing economic management, nursing cost accounting, nursing market development, and policies about nursing services. The formal establishment of nursing economics was marked by the magazine's publication. The University of Iowa Cost Research Center carried out the NIC System, a systematic nursing cost study, in 1993. The specific practice involved classifying the nursing cost accounting content, creating a dedicated research facility with full-time researchers, and ultimately identifying 433 items in 6 categories. To conduct nursing cost management, including cost assessment, reasonable budgeting, decision-making, and other tasks, the Center adopted computer technology at the same time. This helped to alleviate the nursing management crisis and improve nursing management efficiency, and it also marked the official formation of the health economy.

1.2. Relationship Between Healthcare and Economy

We must go back to the fundamental principles of economic science and its operations to comprehend the role of economics in the context of healthcare. The study of economics aims to explain how various people and organizations interact concerning the production and consumption of goods and services. Explaining how the institutional framework and the behavioral norms established for individuals and organizations affect the outcome is the primary goal of the study of these interrelationships. The market mechanism is studied by classical economics disciplines such as welfare theory and price theory. The consequences of imperfect competition for incomes, welfare, and prices are the main focus of industrial organization. The theory of international trade looks into how various regulations governing international commodity exchanges, trade profits, and similar matters operate.

At this point, it shouldn't be shocking to learn that the field of health economics can be defined as the study of the relationships between institutions and regulations, the population's ensuing health, and the institutional frameworks for healthcare (consumption, provision, and financing). The field is still only partially described, and it appears impossible to do so in a few succinct sentences. It should be noted that benefit-cost ratio analyses and cost-effectiveness analyses of health management are not always the focus of health economists. That is not, however, the sole responsibility of a health economist. Instead, cost-effectiveness is arguably viewed as the least significant contribution that a health economist can make. Economists are generally interested in making better decisions, especially when it comes to maximizing the use of already-existing resources and expanding their availability. The field of health economics developed as economists began to study issues in the healthcare industry. The distribution of resources among conflicting demands is a concern shared by economists across industries. It is assumed that there is no limit to demands and that needs for consumption are infinite. On the other hand, resources (labor, raw materials, manufacturing equipment, land, etc.) are never in sufficient supply. The core issue that economists try to solve is the scarcity of resources—not in the sense of "rarity," but rather in the sense of resource availability concerning demand. Health-related economists also attempt to specifically address the same in the context of competing ends and limited health resources.

Society has two options for deciding how to distribute the services that are produced among those who desire them and how to allocate resources to the health sector's production. A society can either plan, usually by assigning its government the responsibility of gathering resources from the populace, allocating those to define production activities, and distributing the produced services among the populace, or it can leave these decisions to the market, letting demand, supply, and prices determine resource allocation. Throughout the last century, the plan-market dichotomy has persisted as a source of concern for academics and others. Its scope includes health economics as well.

Health economics is becoming a subject of increasing significance, particularly in developing countries primarily because of:

- An economic climate where resources are extremely scarce and decisions on priorities are crucial but difficult;
- A growing appreciation among health professionals and policy-makers that health economics and economists can help them formulate policies and make decisions;
- The increasing maturity of the sub-disciplines of health economics; and
- The growing interest among economists and others in applying their economic skills to health issues.

Economists are currently tasked with extracting valuations that could help develop health services policy. Initially, it could take the shape of demand studies or an effort to ascertain the preferences of decision-makers. Second, it's important to determine the actual costs of providing healthcare or to make an estimate of all of the true costs, including lost productivity from other parts of the system and patient time. Thirdly, it is imperative to assess the comparative advantages and disadvantages of specific policy alternatives. Fourth, the consequences of specific economic factors such as user fees, accessibility costs in terms of both time and distance, etc., on the use of medical services could be approximated. Fifth, adjustments to the healthcare delivery system's planning, budgeting, and potential modifications thereto must be made.

Though it covers a larger area, the economics of health is by no means insignificant. The healthcare industry is not the same as the financial services, industrial, or agricultural sectors. Although its results are a little elusive, they unquestionably exceed what can be valued in monetary terms. The main reason for this is that the ultimate result in this case is individual health, or more precisely, improvements in individual health conditions, quantities that are difficult to compare between people and are not quantifiable in terms of money. Due to the sector's unique characteristics, numerous basic issues arise, each of which poses a challenge to economic theory. The use of economic principles in the field of health may present several additional unique challenges. Perhaps there is no adequate way to quantify the benefits of health services to society or the health outputs they produce; as a result, there are no standards for evaluating productivity or allocating resources in a way that upholds the equality principle.

As a result, a health economist faces numerous and difficult tasks. Although applying the fundamentals of economics to health economics may help address some of the industry's current issues, the subjective nature of healthcare may necessitate the use of different approaches. In any event, since health is still the most important need for humans, health economics may continue to grow in significance (Birch et al., 2015; Gafni et al., 2015).

1.3. The Relevance of Health Economics

The study of health economics is important and interesting in three related ways:

- The size of the contribution of the health sector to the overall economy;
- The national policy concerns resulting from the importance many people attach to the economic problems they face in pursuing and maintaining their health; and
- The many health issues that have a substantial economic element.

1.3.1. The Size and Scope of the Health Economy

The size of the health economy, which accounts for a sizable portion of GDP in both the US and other nations, calls for attention. It also signifies a sizable and expanding portion of the labor force as well as a significant capital investment.

1.3.2. Healthcare's Share of GDP in the United States

In the US economy, the health sector accounted for more than $1 of every $6 spent on final goods and services by the second decade of the 21st century. The market value of final goods and services produced within a nation's borders in a given year is called GDP, and as recently as 1980, the share of GDP allocated to healthcare was $1 in $11, compared to just $1 in $20 in 1960. Our economy's largest and fastest-growing sector is the healthcare industry.

In calculating the share of GDP spent on healthcare, we net out the effects of general inflation. Therefore, only three major possibilities exist to explain the substantially increased ratios:

- Perhaps more people are purchasing health services. It's possible that more tests are being ordered, more drugs are being prescribed, or patients are seeing medical professionals more frequently.
- Higher-quality healthcare services, including ones that weren't previously offered, might be purchased by consumers. Measles vaccinations, laser surgery, organ transplants, and novel burn victim treatments—all unheard of in 1960—have improved the standard of care. According to economic theory, consumers are prepared to pay more for superior products.
- There's a chance that the inflation rate in healthcare will be higher than overall. Over time, rising incomes and the prevalence of insurance, including major government programs may have contributed to rising healthcare costs.

Our goal is to comprehend these occurrences and how they affect overall spending. This challenge will be met in part by research on labor supply, technology, production, insurance, and demand.

1.3.3. Healthcare Spending in Other Countries

We can better understand the US health economy by looking at the health economies of other nations. Numerous nations with sizable healthcare sectors deal with the same main problems. We show how, in the majority of countries, healthcare spending increased rapidly between 1960 and 1980 as a percentage of GDP. After 1980, the picture becomes more ambiguous. The data also show how big the US health economy is compared to other nations' economies. For instance, the United States' GDP share of healthcare is almost twice that of the United Kingdom, a nation that offers universal health insurance.

1.3.4. Importance of the Health Economy in Personal Spending

Other important indicators also show the size of the health economy because it represents a significant portion of the country's GDP. Two of these are especially easy to relate to at the personal level: (i) the share of income spent on medical care; and (ii) the number of jobs in the health economy.

1.3.5. Time – The Ultimate Resource

Only a portion of the resources used by people to produce health is reflected in data on healthcare costs and labor and capital inputs. Important inputs are not purchased and sold on the open market. These include the time and effort that individuals personally put into providing healthcare and have actual financial costs to society.

For instance, the value of the leisure that people give up when they use their own time to care for loved ones or improve their own health comes at a cost to both society and the individuals involved. The two hours of care that adults give their aging parents every day, seven days a week, replaces the $15 per hour or more that would otherwise need to be paid for outside of their home. In this straightforward example, the care providers furnish services valued at more than $10,500 annually. These time costs need to be included in addition to our measured healthcare costs, even though these examples may not be typical of the population.

Although we have focused on inputs, the value of health as an output—or health itself—is ultimately what determines how much health resources contribute to the economy. We quantify the benefits of better health in terms of both production and consumption. We appreciate health for its own sake and for the way it helps to produce other things. In the end, the intrinsic value of health comes down to the value we place on life and limb, which is often described as infinite in some situations and at least significant in others. Not only do lower absenteeism rates demonstrate the importance of health in the production of other goods, but they also demonstrate the productivity of each worker on the job. The health sector's output significantly boosts the economy in both its production and consumption facets.

1.3.6. The Importance Attached to Economic Problems of Healthcare Delivery

Policymakers pay attention to the health sector because of the widespread perception of its issues. The average amount of money spent on healthcare across the country provides a more meaningful reflection of the significant resources allocated to this field.

1.3.7. Inflation

Healthcare costs have historically increased more quickly than the overall cost, even though we have deflated the spending values using the CPI. Keep in mind that the cost of hospital and physician care has increased far more quickly than the CPI; this is a common occurrence for other healthcare services and goods as well.

Medical price inflation is a common issue that arises when trying to maintain health programs, and it has led to multiple government initiatives aimed at cost containment. Comprehending and assessing the consequences of said measures are crucial duties for the health economist.

1.3.8. Access

The growing costs severely limit many people's accesses to healthcare. Demand for the majority of goods and services is influenced by financial affordability, and there are numerous explanations for why some individuals lack health insurance. Fewer people lack insurance as a result of the Affordable Care Act of 2010. The number of Americans without health insurance decreased by 20 million between 2010 and 2016. One type of federal health insurance is provided by the ACA.

1.3.9. Quality

Spending increases are partly attributable to improvements in care quality. The emphasis is frequently on assuring quality through professional certification and licensure as well as, particularly for hospitals, through quality assurance initiatives. Simultaneously, worries about receiving high-quality care arise, and they don't just affect people with little or no insurance. However, some observers worry that American healthcare is frequently overpriced, particularly for certain "high-tech" procedures. The costs of resources for these treatments might outweigh the benefits for the patients. Economists are particularly interested in how insurance, technology, and consumption interact.

1.3.10. The Economic Side of Other Health Issues

Economics naturally plays a role in production, costs, and insurance, but economic concerns also play a significant role in many other health-related issues, despite their apparent medical focus. A few examples help to clarify this.

Many people believe that choosing a medical treatment is solely a matter of personal preference, though doctors and other healthcare professionals are beginning to consider the financial aspects of alternative treatments when making decisions. The costs of alternative methods must be investigated. Additionally, doctors are becoming more aware of the financial aspects of the patient-physician relationship. When assessing whether a particular treatment is appropriate, the patient's preferences are taken into consideration.

We also need to investigate why people make the health decisions they do. Sometimes people take good care of themselves, and other times they don't. One way to think of people's desired health status is as an important economic decision. When considered as a potentially sensible economic decision, addiction to any drug—even one as dangerous as methamphetamine or one as relatively benign as caffeine—becomes easier to understand. Other health-related concerns, such as whether or not the government should be involved in healthcare, what investments a developing nation should make in healthcare, and whether or not tobacco advertising should be outlawed, are undoubtedly economic.

1.4. Features of Economic Analysis

Many distinctive features of economics might be exhaustively identified, but we emphasize four:

1. Scarcity of societal resources;
2. Assumption of rational decision making;
3. Concept of marginal analysis; and
4. Use of economic models.

1.4.1. Scarcity of Resources

The foundation of economic analysis is the idea that people have to give up some of one resource in order to obtain some of another. This implies that, on a national scale, higher GDP proportions allocated to healthcare eventually translate into lower GDP proportions available for other purposes. The "opportunity cost" associated with receiving healthcare could be high.

Economists consider time to be the most scarce resource, even though most people are aware of the monetary costs of goods and services. People trade their time for money, and even if offered more than their regular pay rate, many people will turn down overtime work because they believe it isn't worthwhile. Likewise, a lot of people will turn down "free" medical care because the costs associated with travel and waiting are too great.

1.4.2. Rational Decision Making

When tackling issues related to human economic behavior, economists generally begin by presuming that the decision-maker is a reasonable individual. "Making decisions that best further one's ends given one's resource constraints" is our definition of rationality. Certain actions could seem illogical. But when disagreements about rationality emerge, economists frequently try to point out—possibly with a hint of amusement—that so-called irrational behavior frequently makes sense when the incentives that a decision-maker must weigh are properly understood.

1.4.3. Marginal Analysis

Marginal reasoning is a feature of mainstream economic analysis. Decision-makers need to be aware of both the advantages and disadvantages of the subsequent, or marginal, unit to make an informed decision. Trading off the incremental costs against the incremental benefits at the margin is a common mental exercise in marginal analysis.

An excellent illustration is the purchase of name-brand medications. When it comes to elective treatments in particular, patients' decisions to purchase name-brand medications may be heavily influenced by whether they have to pay \$2 or \$3 per pill or only a portion of those amounts if prescription drug insurance is offered.

1.4.4. Use of Models

Lastly, economics creates models to illustrate its subject matter as is customary. Words, graphs, or mathematical descriptions of the models are all possible. There are graphs and words in this text. Every model has its limits and needs to be checked against reality first and then the facts. Still, we can draw lessons from them and they can be relevant. Economic models are frequently figurative. In both economics and daily life, abstract models are useful for making sense of the world. When a young child asks what the solar system is like, they will most likely be shown the abstract model, which is the well-known drawing of the Sun and planets in their orbits. Although everyone quickly understands the drawing, nobody believes that this is how the sky actually looks (Tilley et al., 2006; Chalkley et al., 2018).

1.5. The Special Characteristics of the Market for Healthcare

That model has several notable features:

- The main interested parties are the buyers and sellers in the market.
- Buyers are good judges of what they get from sellers.
- Buyers pay sellers directly for the goods and services being exchanged.
- Market prices are the primary mechanism for coordinating the decisions of market participants.
- The invisible hand, left to its own devices, leads to an efficient allocation of resources.

This model provides a fairly accurate description of a large number of goods and services within the economy. However, none of these five standard model features capture the dynamics of the healthcare market. The healthcare market has producers (doctors, nurses, etc.) and consumers (patients), just like other markets. However, several aspects of this market make it more difficult to analyze how they interact:

1. Third parties—insurers, governments, and unwitting bystanders—often have an interest in healthcare outcomes.
2. Patients often don't know what they need and cannot evaluate the treatment they are getting.
3. Healthcare providers are often paid not by the patients but by private or government health insurance.
4. The rules established by these insurers, more than market prices, determine the allocation of resources.
5. In light of the foregoing four points, the invisible hand can't work its magic, and so the allocation of resources in the healthcare market can end up highly inefficient.

There are other goods and services in the economy besides healthcare that deviate from the conventional understanding of supply, demand, and the invisible hand. However, the most significant good or service that deviates from this standard so drastically may be healthcare. Analyzing the unique characteristics of this market is a good place to start when trying to figure out why the government is heavily involved in healthcare provision and why health policy is frequently difficult to understand.

1.5.1. The Prevalence of Externalities

Externalities can lead to inefficient market outcomes. When someone does something that affects a bystander's well-being without being compensated for it, that action is considered an externality. An adverse effect on a bystander is referred to as a negative externality. It is referred to as a positive externality if it is advantageous. When externalities exist, society's interest in the result of the market goes beyond the welfare of participants in the market, such as buyers and sellers, to encompass the welfare of onlookers who are indirectly impacted. When determining how much to supply or demand, buyers and sellers often overlook the external consequences of their decisions, which can lead to an inefficient unregulated market outcome.

This broad conclusion is essential to comprehending healthcare due to the high prevalence of externalities in the market. To address the market failure, these externalities may necessitate government intervention.

Consider vaccines as an example. A person is less likely to contract an illness if she vaccinates herself against it. However, she is less likely to become a carrier and spread the infection to others because she is less likely to contract it. Therefore, receiving a vaccination communicates a benefit to society. Too few people will decide to get vaccinated if doing so comes with a cost, whether it be in terms of money, time, or the possibility of unfavorable side effects. This is because they will probably weigh the benefits of vaccination against the costs and decide not to pursue it. The government could mandate vaccination or subsidize the research, production, and distribution of vaccines to address this issue.

Medical research is an example of an externality within the healthcare system. A doctor's discovery of a new treatment for a disease contributes to society's medical knowledge base. It is a positive externality that benefits patients and other doctors. Without government intervention, there would be insufficient research.

Governments take various actions to address this externality. For example, in the case of new pharmaceutical drugs, the government may grant the researcher a patent for the innovative product. The patent allows the holder to benefit from a temporary monopoly, which encourages further research. It is argued that the patent internalizes the externality. However, because the monopoly price is higher than the marginal cost of production, this approach is not perfect. The patented treatment may be used less due to the high monopoly price, leading to inefficiency and deadweight loss. Additionally, patients with lower incomes may struggle with the high costs.

Another way the government addresses this issue is by subsidizing medical research. The National Institutes of Health, for instance, receives over $30 billion in annual funding, which amounts to roughly $100 per person, for medical research. Funding for these policies comes from taxes, which also have deadweight losses. However, overall welfare can increase if the benefits of the funded research outweigh the costs, including deadweight losses.

1.5.2. The Difficulty of Monitoring Quality

In most markets, buyers are aware of what they want and are able to assess their satisfaction with the final product after it has been purchased. The healthcare industry is unique. You might not be aware of the best course of action when you become ill. You trust a doctor's opinion, as they have received years of specialized training. Furthermore, you cannot always determine for yourself whether the course of treatment the doctor recommended for you was the best one, even in retrospect. Modern medicine can occasionally fall short of improving a patient's condition. Furthermore, the incorrect course of treatment may occasionally seem effective due to the body's innate ability to heal itself.

Regulations are a result of healthcare consumers' incapacity to keep an eye on the quality of the products they purchase. Above all, doctors, dentists, nurses, and other health professionals must obtain licenses from the government. Only after completing demanding coursework and attending an authorized school are these licenses awarded. If found practicing without a license, one faces jail time. Similar to this, the Food and Drug Administration (FDA) ensures new pharmaceutical drugs are safe and effective by supervising their testing and release.

Apart from governmental regulations, the medical field also keeps an eye on itself through the accreditation of medical schools, the promotion of best practices, and the establishment of professional standards of conduct. Advice from doctors should always be given with the patient's best interests in mind, not their own. Patients rely on a certain level of trust—which is frequently fostered by long-term relationships between doctor and patient—when they accept the advice.

The preponderance of nonprofit hospitals may be explained by misgivings regarding the role of trust in healthcare relationships and the standard economic motive of self-interest. Hospitals and hotels are similar in certain aspects, but unlike hotels, which are typically operated by for-profit companies, hospitals are typically government-run or nonprofit organizations. In situations where buyers lack the ability to assess the quality of the goods they are purchasing, they might be more inclined to put their trust in an organization whose main goal is not to enrich its founders.

There are, of course, those who oppose the public and private healthcare regulations. For instance, some economists contend that opening new medical schools is too difficult. They contend that the medical industry functions like a monopoly, driving up healthcare costs for patients and physician salaries by limiting the number of doctors in the field. The FDA approves new drugs too slowly, according to other economists. Some patients are compelled to forgo experimental treatments even though they might have been beneficial. There is constant discussion about how to strike the right balance between preserving public safety and granting individuals the autonomy to choose their own healthcare providers.

1.5.3. The Insurance Market and Its Imperfections

Healthcare costs are unpredictable because people never know when they will become ill or what kind of treatments they will require. The fact that we have the health institutions that we do is largely due to this uncertainty and how people react to it.

1.5.3.1. The Value of Insurance Most People Are Risk-Averse

Put another way, they detest uncertainty. Let's say you have to choose between earning a fixed $1,00,000 and having a 50% chance of earning $50,000 or $15,000. The average income from the two options is the same, but the second is riskier. Your preference for the certain $1,00,000 indicates risk aversion.

The variability in healthcare costs leads to the same kind of behavior. Assume that everyone has the same chance of contracting a disease that affects 2% of the population. The cost of treatment is $30,000. In this instance, the anticipated medical expenses come to $600, or 2% of $30,000. Risk-averse individuals would rather pay $600 with assurance than take a 2% chance of having to pay $30,000.

The whole point of insurance is to give people this choice. A person facing a risk pays an insurance company a sum of money, known as a premium, and the insurance company agrees to accept all or part of the risk in exchange. This is the general feature of insurance contracts. Numerous kinds of insurance exist. Health insurance protects against the possibility that you will require costly medical care, fire insurance against the possibility that your home will burn down, and auto insurance against the risk of being in an automobile accident. In our scenario, a health insurance provider agrees to pay the $30,000 treatment for the 2% of its clients who contract the illness in exchange for a $600 premium (or a little bit more to turn a profit). Insurance markets can help lower risk, but two issues prevent them from doing so completely and effectively.

1.5.3.2. Moral Hazard

The first issue that prevents insurance markets from functioning properly is moral hazard: people are less likely to behave in a way that will limit their healthcare spending when they have insurance to cover their expenses. For instance, if patients are not required to pay for each visit to the doctor, they might schedule appointments too soon for minor ailments like a sore finger or runny nose. In a similar vein, doctors might order questionable tests more frequently if they are aware that their insurance will pay for them.

1.5.4. Adverse Selection

Adverse selection is the second issue impeding the functioning of insurance markets. In cases where customers have known differences in pertinent attributes (like having a chronic illness), but insurers are unable to observe these differences, the mix of individuals choosing to purchase insurance may make it particularly costly to insure. Specifically, compared to healthy individuals, those with more hidden health issues are more likely to purchase health insurance. Therefore, the cost of health insurance must be commensurate with the expense of an individual who is sicker than usual for the insurance company to make a profit. Even those in average health might choose not to have insurance after seeing the high cost. The insurance market falls short of its goal of removing the financial risk associated with illness as more people choose not to carry coverage.

The death spiral is a phenomenon that can result from adverse selection. Assume that insurance companies are required to charge the same rate to all customers because an individual's health profile is considered private information. It might initially seem reasonable for an insurance provider to base an insurance policy's cost on the health characteristics of the general population. However, once it does, the healthiest individuals might decide insurance is not worth the price and leave the pool of people who are insured. The business must increase insurance prices due to increased costs stemming from an unexpectedly sicker customer base. The next healthiest group of people decide not to purchase insurance as a result of the increased cost, which raises the price even further. As a result of this process, more people cease having insurance, the insured population becomes less robust, and costs continue to climb. The insurance market might eventually vanish.

In the discussion of health policy, adverse selection has been a major issue. For instance, the Affordable Care Act forbade health insurance providers from raising premiums for those who already had a medical condition. Adverse selection was guaranteed by this rule, which was implemented to aid those with persistent medical issues. Those with pre-existing conditions would perceive insurance as a better deal than those without it, increasing their likelihood of purchasing health insurance. There would be an incentive for healthy people to put off getting insurance until they became ill.

Lawmakers knew about this issue. The Affordable Care Act mandated that all Americans obtain health insurance and penalized those who did not comply. It also provided subsidies to lower-income households so they could afford insurance. The purpose of the mandate was to lower insurance costs and lessen the issue of adverse selection by encouraging more healthy individuals to purchase insurance. Healthy individuals would essentially subsidize those with pre-existing conditions as more of them joined the insurance market.

Regarding how well the Affordable Care Act has improved the healthcare market, analysts have differing opinions. Many (presumably healthy) people decided to forgo insurance and pay the fine. This finding can be explained by the fact that there was insufficient penalty for not getting insurance to deter a significant amount of adverse selection. However, one of the law's primary objectives—to increase the number of people with health insurance—has been achieved. Between 2010 and 2015, the percentage of people without insurance decreased from 16 to 9%.

1.5.5. Healthcare as a Right

Generally, it is not a big deal for society when some people choose not to purchase a good or service—possibly because they believe the cost is too high given their income. Assume that the cost of a ticket to a popular Broadway production increase and that people with lesser incomes opt for alternative entertainment options. Though few would contend that this amounts to a major injustice, we can bemoan the fact that excellent theater is not appreciated by more people.

The medical field is unique. It seems unfair to refuse medical care to someone who becomes ill because of their financial situation. Compared to Broadway show tickets, healthcare can be considered a human right. This judgment goes beyond the scope of economics and is best left to political philosophers, but we should acknowledge this belief as we study the economics of healthcare.

Healthcare is similar to food in that it is essential for survival, and society works to ensure everyone has access to these resources. The Supplemental Nutrition Assistance Program (SNAP) is designed to help provide essential food resources to those in need. However, there is a distinct difference between food and healthcare. The cost of food has historically increased at a slower rate than incomes, making it easier for households to afford an adequate diet. On the other hand, the cost of healthcare has risen rapidly, making it increasingly difficult for households to afford state-of-the-art healthcare services.

The growing cost of healthcare and the belief that it is a right have made the government play a major role in providing it. Many countries, including Canada and England, have government-run healthcare systems that are primarily funded by taxes. Because the government's health service is the only organization that covers all costs, this system is sometimes referred to as single-payer.

In contrast, the majority of people in the United States have private health insurance, frequently provided by their employers, but the government is still very much in place. The Affordable Care Act regulates the market for private health insurance and provides insurance subsidies to many lower-income households. Medicare provides health insurance for those 65 and older. Medicaid provides health insurance for the poor. The Veterans Health Administration provides healthcare to former military personnel. There is ongoing discussion about whether and how these programs can be made better. However, there is little question that the government will continue to have a significant influence over the healthcare system because it is frequently seen as a human right.

1.5.6. The Rules Governing the Healthcare Marketplace

Because health insurance is so important, the healthcare market must function differently from most other markets in the economy, regardless of whether it is offered by the government or private sector. There are buyers and sellers in the market. A seller charges a fee for an item or service. A buyer needs to secure the item and make the appropriate financial offer.

The provider (the seller of medical services) is not paid directly by the patient (the buyer). Instead, the patient pays money to an insurer in the form of either a premium (if the insurer is a private company) or taxes (if the insurer is the government). The insurer uses this money to compensate the provider, who in turn provides medical services to the patient.

Three sets of rules are needed to direct behavior in this process. The financing, or who pays for the insurance and how much they pay, is decided by the first group. Paying for healthcare becomes a component of creating the tax system if the government serves as the insurer. Healthcare is funded by the premiums that customers of health insurance pay for their coverage if the insurer is a private business. In the insurance market, prices are determined by costs, just like in other markets. Nonetheless, state and federal governments frequently control the private insurance industry. They might, for instance, restrict how much businesses can charge with age, sex, and pre-existing conditions. Therefore, public policy continues to influence healthcare financing even in situations where it happens between a patient and a private insurer.

A patient's eligibility for healthcare is decided by the second set of regulations. As we've talked about, overuse is a possibility because insured patients do not pay the full cost of every medical service they use. The insurer (whether a public or private organization) is subject to regulations that restrict access when it makes sense in order to reduce the issue of moral hazard. To put it another way, these regulations restrict the use of medical services with projected costs and benefits. For instance, a patient might only be able to see a general practitioner for a referral before scheduling an appointment with a more costly specialist, or they might only be able to see a small number of doctors for routine checkups once a year. These kinds of access restrictions are required because market prices no longer provide people with the appropriate signals about how to distribute limited resources once they have insurance to cover the expenses.

The payments made by insurers to providers are governed by the third set of regulations. These regulations specify what an insurer will cover as well as the maximum amount that will be paid. The cost of care has an impact on the treatments that doctors recommend to their patients. Certain treatments may be deemed by insurers to be too costly, too experimental, or not worth enough to warrant payment at all. When this occurs, providers frequently decline to provide the services to patients. But occasionally, as is frequently the case with cosmetic procedures, providers will serve if the patient covers the entire cost of the treatment. In this instance, the healthcare market returns to the more typical market shown in panel (a) from panel (b) in Figure 1.1.

The laws governing access, payment, and financing are interconnected and collectively influence the type of healthcare system that a country has. Public policy establishes these regulations for countries with government-run systems. These guidelines are established by insurance companies as they compete for clients in countries with higher rates of private insurance, like the United States, and are subject to different government regulations.

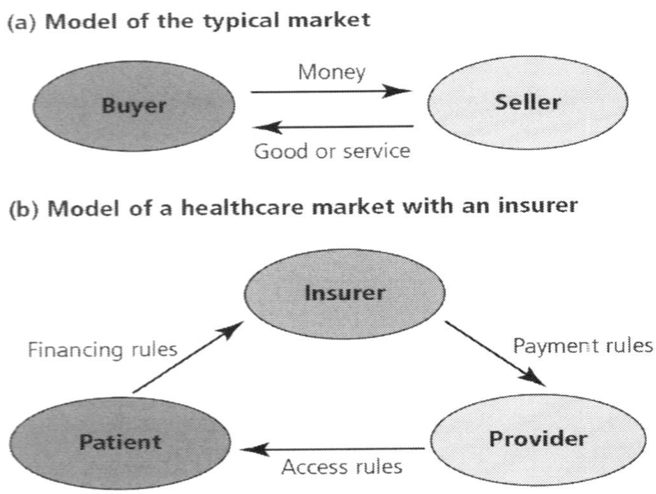

Figure 1.1. *How an insurer changes a market?*

Source: https://scholar.harvard.edu/files/mankiw/files/economics_of_healthcare.pdf.

1.6. Trends Related to Increased Healthcare Costs

Compared to other nations, the United States has the highest healthcare costs, with a substantial financial impact on our economy. U.S. spending on healthcare increased by 4% in 2019 to $3 trillion, or $11,582 per person. The entire yearly value of goods produced and services rendered, or GDP, is comprised of 17.07% of spending on healthcare. A graph showing how much the US spends on healthcare as a percentage of GDP as compared to other nations can be found in Figure 1.2.

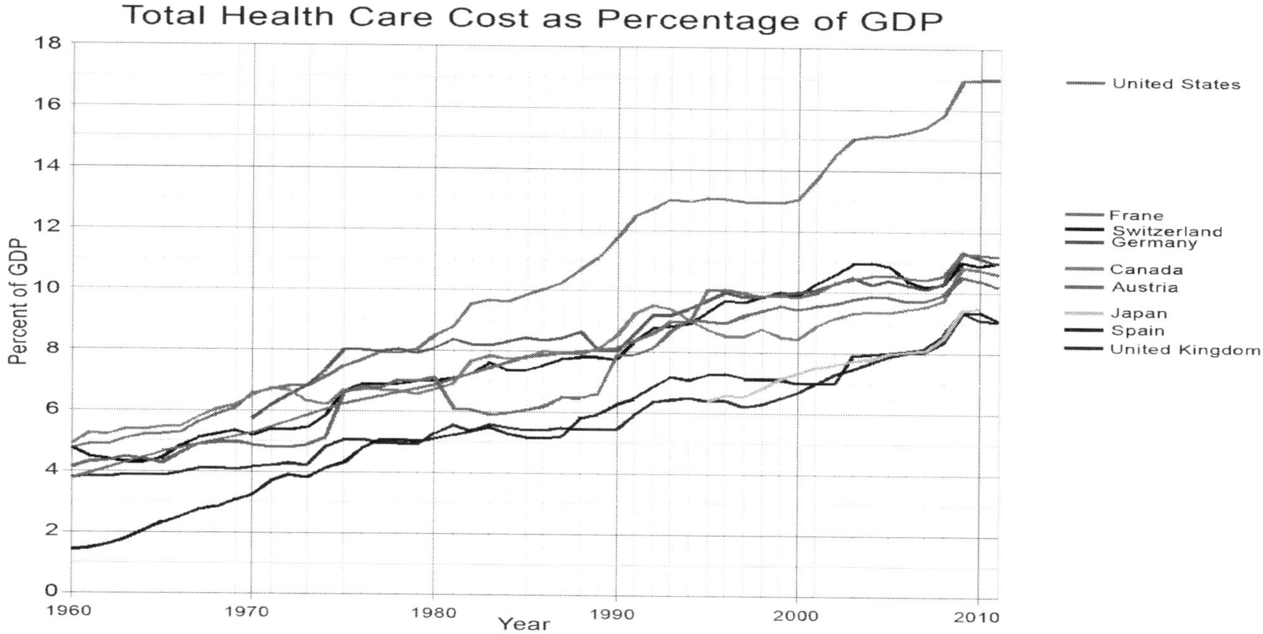

Figure 1.2. *Comparison of healthcare costs.*

Source: https://www.ncbi.nlm.nih.gov/books/NBK598375/.

Even though the United States invests more funds into healthcare compared to other wealthy nations, it consistently experiences subpar health results. This is evidenced by the country having the shortest life expectancy, the highest infant mortality rate, and a greater occurrence of chronic illnesses. The increasing costs of healthcare also have several negative impacts on society, employers, and individuals, including the following effects:

- When the government spends more on healthcare, the national debt increases, and funds available for other programs decrease.
- When people spend more on healthcare, they have less money to spend on other items.
- When health insurance is paid by employers, employees are paid less.
- When employers spend more on healthcare, the costs of their products and services increase. Jobs may be moved to countries with lower healthcare costs.
- An increasing number of people cannot afford healthcare insurance. When people

without healthcare insurance receive healthcare, they often cannot pay for it. As a result of unpaid bills, this care is indirectly paid for by other people paying increased insurance premiums and taxes.

- People without healthcare insurance may not seek preventative care and develop a more costly, serious medical disorder that could have been prevented.
- Medical bills that are not covered by health insurance can cause bankruptcy.

Numerous national trends are influencing the cost of healthcare and its related consequences, such as the aging population, rising expenses of medical technology, escalating costs of prescription medications, the Affordable Care Act, and social determinants of health.

1.6.1. Aging Population

According to the Agency for Healthcare Research and Quality (AHRQ), the United States has a growing number of older adults (age 65 years or older) who are living longer than previous generations. It is anticipated that older adults will make up more than 20 percent of the U.S. population by 2030.

1.6.2. Increased Costs of Medical Technology

Medical technologies that are widely recognized, like organ transplantation, diagnostic imaging systems, and biotechnology products, are subject to both commendation and criticism. While new medical technologies have the potential to save lives and enhance patient outcomes, they are also seen as a major contributor to the ongoing rise in medical expenses. According to research, medical technology is responsible for between 10% and 40% of the long-term rise in healthcare costs. Additional ethical conundrums arise from these expenses when decisions are made about which patients receive what limited resources. See Figure 1.3 for a picture of typical medical technology.

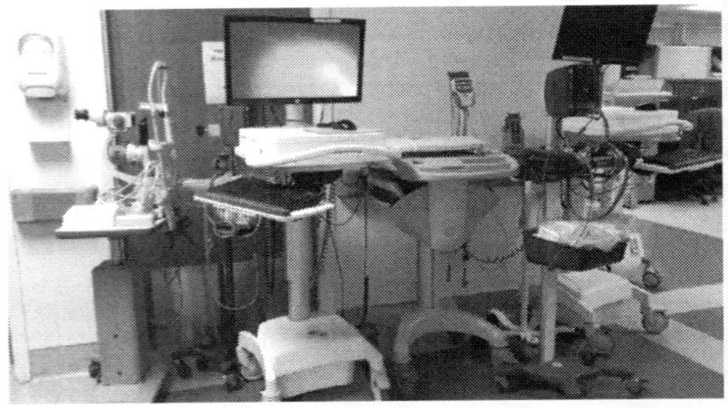

Figure 1.3. *Healthcare technology.*

Source: https://www.ncbi.nlm.nih.gov/books/NBK598375/.

New medical technologies, in particular, have to demonstrate their value in an environment where there are competing demands on scarce resources. The goal of cost-effectiveness in American society guides the distribution of resources: a new technology should be adopted if it can improve health outcomes at a lower cost than its current counterpart. If not, it should not be adopted.

1.6.3. Increased Prescription Medication Costs

Retail prices for frequently used prescription drugs are still rising at a rate twice as fast as inflation, which raises the possibility that many Americans will not be able to afford these life-saving drugs and adds to the expense of healthcare. A recent AARP Rx Price Watch report states that while the overall rate of inflation was 1.3% in 2020, the cost of 260 commonly used medications increased by 2.9%. For instance, the price of the drug Symbicort, which is used to treat COPD and asthma, went up 46% to $4,282 (Figure 1.4).

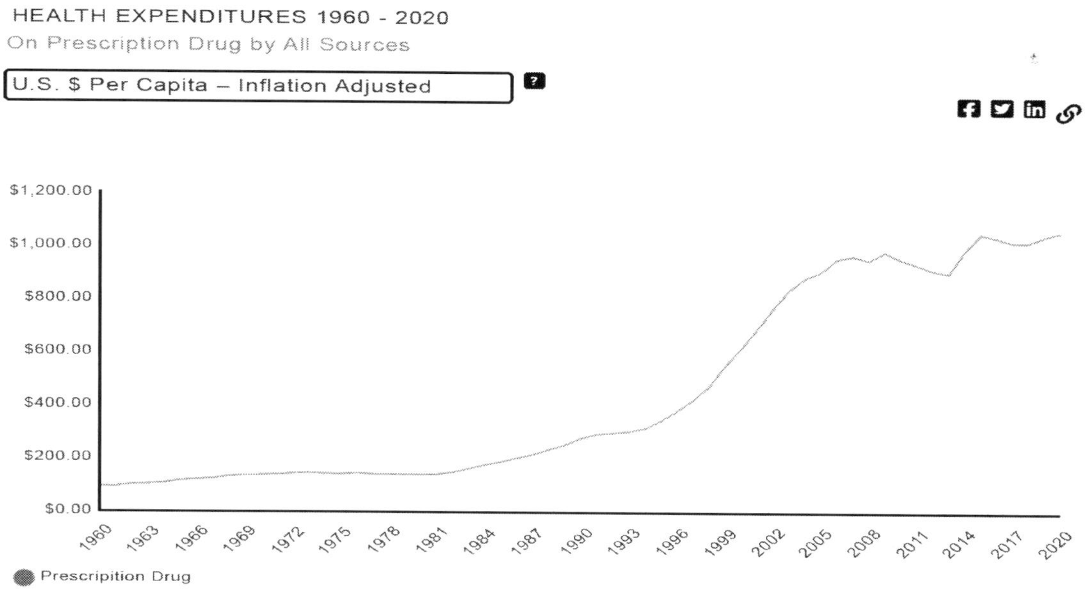

Figure 1.4. *Prescription medication costs.*

Source: https://www.ncbi.nlm.nih.gov/books/NBK598375/.

Although most Americans receive assistance in paying for their prescription drugs from either public or private insurance, rising drug costs translate into higher health insurance premiums and increased government spending on the Medicare and Medicaid programs. Certain insurance companies only pay for drugs on their approved formularies. Consequently, national associations such as the American Association of Retired Persons (AARP) push for changes to national policy, like letting Medicare bargain with drug companies for lower prescription drug prices and making those savings available to private insurance plans.

Many consumers are faced with the tough choice of paying for their families' housing and food while having to choose between buying pricey prescription medication or forgoing it altogether. Nurses frequently get involved in case management when helping patients get prescription drugs that they cannot afford.

1.6.4. Social Determinants of Health

The conditions that influence a variety of outcomes in the settings where people live, learn, work, and play are known as social determinants of health (SDOH). SDOH includes neighborhood and environment, social and community context, economic stability, and access to and quality of education. These influences have a significant effect on people's health and well-being, which in turn impacts the cost of healthcare nationally.

The development of chronic diseases, people's access to regular healthcare, and their health behaviors are all directly impacted by SDOH. However, compared to comparable nations with superior health outcomes, the United States spends a notably smaller portion of its GDP on social services.

The US Department of Health and Human Services created Healthy People (2030), which outlines public health priorities to assist people, groups, and communities nationwide in enhancing health and well-being by addressing SDOH over the next 10 years. "Create social, physical, and economic environments that promote attaining the full potential for health and well-being for everyone" is one of Healthy People 2030's objectives. Nurses advocate for people, families, and communities in a variety of ways, which helps to address these priorities (Eow et al., 2019; Evans et al., 1985).

1.7. Healthcare Reimbursement Models

For services rendered to individuals, hospitals, and healthcare providers are paid by private insurance companies, government insurance programs, or people paying out-of-pocket. Healthcare organizations were traditionally compensated using a "fee-for-service" model. For instance, if a patient was diagnosed with pneumonia and admitted to the hospital, the hospital would bill the patient's insurance company for the necessary treatment.

However, insurance providers have switched to "Pay for Performance" reimbursement models, which are based on overall agency performance and patient outcomes, as part of a recent national strategy to lower healthcare costs.

1.7.1. Pay for Performance

Value-based payment, or pay for performance, is a term used to describe reimbursement schemes that link provider and agency performance to monetary rewards. Pay for Performance models align payment with value and quality by linking higher reimbursement payments to patient satisfaction, best practices, and positive patient outcomes. Based on their documentation of nursing care plans and the attainment of anticipated patient outcomes, nurses advocate for increased reimbursement levels to their employers.

Two Pay-for-performance models exist. According to how well hospitals and providers do on process, quality, and efficiency metrics, the first model pays them more in reimbursement. The second model lowers reimbursement amount to hospitals and providers who perform below expectations. For instance, pressure injuries and urinary tract infections linked to catheter use are examples of preventable conditions for which Medicare no longer pays hospitals to treat patients.

Driven by the Affordable Care Act, the Centers for Medicare and Medicaid Services (CMS) has pioneered value-based payment through a range of payment models. With nearly 40% of all Medicare and Medicaid spending going toward healthcare, CMS is the biggest healthcare funder in the country. Three Pay for Performance models that CMS developed affect Medicare reimbursement to hospitals. The Hospital-Acquired Condition Reduction Program, the Hospital Readmissions Reduction Program, and the Hospital Value-Based Purchasing Program are the names of these models. Performance-based payment models are a commitment shared by private insurers. Value-based care models accounted for nearly half of insurer reimbursements, according to a 2017 Forbes report.

1.7.1.1. Hospital Value-Based Purchasing Program

Through the use of financial incentives that incentivize hospitals to adhere to accepted best clinical practices and raise patient satisfaction levels through patient satisfaction surveys, the Hospital Value-Based Purchasing Program (VBP) was created to enhance the quality of healthcare and the patient experience. Hospital performance on metrics broken down into four quality domains—safety, clinical care, efficiency, and cost-cutting, and patient and caregiver-centered experience—determines reimbursement.

1.7.1.2. Hospital Readmissions Reduction Program

Hospitals that have higher than average rates of patient readmissions are subject to penalties under the Hospital Readmissions Reduction Program (HRRP). Patients with certain conditions, such as heart attacks, heart failure, pneumonia, chronic obstructive pulmonary disease (COPD), hip or knee replacements, and coronary bypass surgery, are eligible for the HRRP, which was created by the Affordable Care Act. Medicare payments to hospitals that perform poorly are reduced by 3%. Congress, however, passed legislation in 2019 that separated hospitals into comparison groups based on the socioeconomic status of their patient populations after it was found that hospitals with higher proportions of low-income patients were penalized the most.

1.7.1.3. Hospital-Acquired Condition Reduction Program

The Affordable Care Act created the Hospital-Acquired Condition Reduction Program (HACRP). Under the Pay for Performance model, hospitals receive a reduction in payments when they perform poorly in terms of patient safety and hospital-acquired conditions like pressure injuries, hip fractures from falls, and surgical site infections. Medicare has saved about $350 million annually thanks to this approach.

Methicillin-resistant *Staphylococcus aureus* (MRSA), *Clostridium difficile* (*C. difficile*), surgical site infections (SSI), catheter-associated urinary tract infections (CAUTI), and central line-associated bloodstream infections (CLABSI) are among the hospital-acquired conditions that the HACRP model tracks. As a result, nurses have observed modifications made to routine procedures in light of these conditions' evidence-based practices. For instance, clients with Foley catheters must now maintain thorough records demonstrating their ongoing need and related infection control procedures.

1.7.1.4. Other CMS Pay for Performance Models

Other value-based payment programs, such as the End-Stage Renal Disease (ESRD) Quality Initiative Program, the Skilled Nursing Facility Value-Based Program (SNFVBP), the Home Health Value-Based Program (HHVBP), and the Value Modifier (VM) Program, were developed by CMS for organizations other than hospitals. Medicare Part B providers who score high, average, or low in comparison to peer agencies on quality and cost metrics are targeted by the VM program.

1.7.2. Impacts of Value-Based Payment

Reward for Performance (i.e., value-based payment (VBP) prioritizes quality over quantity of care and enables payers of healthcare to use payment to support optimal clinical practices and favorable patient outcomes. Through the use of publicly available metrics, it emphasizes transparency and encourages businesses to uphold and enhance their reputations. Pay for Performance models promote responsibility and informed consumer choice in this way.

Both the cost of healthcare and the frequency of unfavorable patient outcomes have decreased thanks to pay-for-performance models. For instance, since 2012, 30-day hospital readmission rates have decreased, suggesting that HRRP and HACRP are having an effect.

Nevertheless, value-based payment has drawbacks as well. As previously mentioned, preliminary studies showed that hospitals with larger percentages of low-income patients were penalized more than others, leading to further legislation that compared hospital performance in groups according to the socioeconomic status of their patients. Nursing leaders are still emphasizing approaches that advance health equity and address socioeconomic determinants of health.

1.7.3. Nursing Considerations

Nurses directly influence both the quality of care provided and the reimbursement rates that their employers receive. Nurses can take a variety of steps to raise patient satisfaction, cut expenses, and increase reimbursement. Nurses can ensure their employer provides the funding they require to deliver high-quality patient care and that resources are distributed to patients fairly by implementing these measures into their daily care.

The following categories of actions to improve the quality of care are based on the Institute of Medicine (IOM) report To Err Is Human: Building a Safer Healthcare System and Crossing the Quality Chasm:

1. **Effectiveness and Efficiency:** Through careful documentation, coordinated care, and individualized nursing care planning, nurses contribute to the effectiveness and efficiency of their institution. Care duplication and waste are decreased with timely and accurate documentation and care coordination. Reducing the likelihood of hospital readmissions is another benefit of care coordination.
2. **Timeliness:** By setting priorities and assigning care, nurses have a positive influence on timeliness. This shortens the time patients must wait for care and delays in it.
3. **Safety:** When a patient's condition changes, nurses are alert to it and make sure the right people on the healthcare team are informed. They raise concerns about client care up the chain of command until they are satisfied.
4. **Patient-Centered Care:** By making sure that each patient's nursing care plan is unique, nurses contribute to this quality measure. Care plans that work well can increase patient compliance, which enhances patient outcomes.
5. **Evidence-based Practice:** Using this approach, nurses deliver care to patients. The American Nurses Association defines Evidence-Based Practice (EBP) as a lifelong approach to problem-solving that incorporates clinical expertise, evidence from assessments of the healthcare consumer's history and condition, as well as evidence from evidence-based theories; and patient, family, group, community, and population preferences and values. Scholarly Inquiry, one of the ANA's Standards of Professional Practice, includes EBP. The application of EBP by nurses guarantees that the right resources are given to the right clients. EBP

encourages effective, efficient, and safe medical care.

6. **Equity:** Medical facilities provide care to all community members, irrespective of client demographics and the social determinants of health (SDOH) that go along with them. Places of residence, education, employment, and recreation that have an impact on a variety of health risks and consequences are referred to as SDOH. In reports, the Agency for Healthcare Research and Quality (AHRQ) has consistently documented health disparities in communities with low SDOH.

To address the negative determinants of health, nurses support policies that lessen health disparities and encourage the provision of resources for equitable access to healthcare. Health disparities refer to the variations in health outcomes brought about by SDOH. Promoting resources that improve quality of life has a big impact on the health results in a community. Safe and affordable housing, education, public safety, the availability of healthful foods, nearby emergency and medical services, and environments free of potentially fatal pollutants are a few examples of resources that support health.

Healthcare disparities, which describe variations in insurance coverage and access to medical care, are related terms. Life expectancy can be shortened, personal expenses can rise, and there can be discrepancies in health and healthcare. In general, these differences also result in higher societal costs, such as the cost of untreated chronic illnesses. Nurse practitioners who treat underprivileged populations in rural communities in accordance with their scope of practice are an example of how nurses are addressing healthcare disparities.

1.8. Budgets and Staffing

The budgets of healthcare institutions are impacted by economics and models of healthcare reimbursement, which in turn affect nurse staffing. An estimate of revenue and expenses for a given period, typically a year, is what makes up a budget. Operating and capital budgets are the two main categories of healthcare spending that have an impact on nursing. Capital budgets are used to schedule upgrades and investments in physical assets that appreciate or depreciate over time. Capital refers to tangible objects like computers and buildings. Personnel expenses and yearly facility operating costs are included in operating budgets. Nursing staffing typically accounts for 40% of healthcare agencies' operating budgets. Nursing is therefore frequently singled out for fewer hours worked and other reductions.

Although nurses are invaluable to the patients, families, and communities they serve, healthcare organizations must determine how much it will cost to provide high-quality, safe nursing care while adhering to budget-friendly staffing models. Every member of the healthcare team must comprehend the interplay between economics, resources, budgeting, and staffing, and how these matters impact their capacity to deliver safe, high-quality patient care.

Many nurses are seeing changes in staffing models as healthcare organizations continue to adjust to "Pay for Performance" reimbursement models and provide cost-effective care to an aging population with complex health needs. Agencies use a variety of tactics, such as acuity-based staffing, team nursing, required overtime, floating, on-call, and off-with-benefits, to enable cost-effective nurse staffing. When there is a shortage of nurses, agencies may also use agency nurses.

1.8.1. Acuity-Based Staffing

In the past, "nurse-to-patient ratios," or the number of patients assigned to each registered nurse during a shift, were the main focus of inpatient staffing patterns. Acuity-based staffing refers to a patient assignment model that considers the degree of care needed for a patient depending on how serious their illness or condition is. The number of patients a nurse attends to during a shift frequently fluctuates due to acuity-based staffing, as patient needs alter. By guaranteeing that nurses have sufficient time to care for complex patients, acuity-based staffing encourages the effective use of resources.

1.8.2. Team Nursing

A popular staffing pattern called "team nursing" involves providing patient care to a group of patients using a mix of Registered Nurses (RNs), Licensed Practical/Vocational Nurses (LPN/VNs), and Assistive Personnel (AP). As the team's leader, the registered nurse (RN) assigns tasks and nursing care to other team members under proper supervision. One sensible use of human resources to deliver high-quality, reasonably priced care is team nursing. Team members must coordinate their shifts as a unit and use effective communication for team nursing to be successful.

1.8.3. Mandatory Overtime

As an agency staffing tool, mandatory overtime for nurses may be required when client numbers and acuity levels surpass the number of staff members scheduled for a shift. When there is a shortage of nursing staff, mandatory overtime forces a nurse to stay and care for patients after their scheduled shift (often referred to as short staffing). Mandatory overtime is recognized by the American Nurses Association as a risky staffing practice due to concerns about patient safety resulting from fatigued staff. Depending on state regulations, nurses who refuse to stay when asked may be held accountable for patient neglect or abandonment. Nurses need to be informed about organizational and state regulations pertaining to required overtime.

1.8.4. Floating

To help cover a shift with a shortage of staff, agencies frequently use the floating staffing strategy, which asks nurses to work temporarily on a different unit. By lowering employee overtime compensation, floating can lower personnel costs. It can also lessen the risk of nurse burnout brought on by working in an understaffed setting.

When asked to float, nurses still have obligations to provide safe patient care under professional standards and their state's Nurse Practice Act. As such, they need to be aware of their rights and responsibilities. Before beginning patient care, nurses should confirm that a floating assignment complements their skill set and that they have received orientation to the new setting. The fact that the nurse was given a floating assignment does not excuse them from responsibility if a mistake is made and they are found guilty. According to the American Nurses Association, nurses are required to decline a floating patient assignment if it poses a risk, in addition to having the option to do so. To help nurses decide which patient assignments to accept, the ANA has created several questions.

1.8.5. On-Call and Off with Benefits

Agencies frequently cut staffing because of operating budget constraints when the number of clients admitted and their acuity exceed the staffing projected for a shift. Agency staffing reductions on a shift-by-shift basis typically take two forms: putting nurses "on call" or "off with benefits."

1.8.5.1. On Call

When a nurse is not immediately needed for their scheduled shift, an agency staffing strategy called "on call" can be used. The nurse may choose to stay at home or report to work and complete work-related education. A nurse's hourly pay is usually lowered and they have a set response time when they are on call. If an on-call nurse is needed later in the shift, they must be able to report and take over patient care within the allotted time frame. This is known as a required response time.

1.8.5.2. Off with Benefits

If a nurse is not required for their scheduled shift, they may be put "off with benefits." When a nurse is laid off with benefits, they usually don't get paid on an hourly basis, and aren't required to show up for work or be available 24/7, but they do still get benefits like paid time off and insurance.

1.8.5.3. Agency Nursing

The healthcare industry's agency nursing sector supplies nurses to hospitals and other healthcare facilities that are short-staffed. Nurse agencies hire nurses on an as-needed basis and assign them to facilities experiencing a staffing deficit.

1.8.6. Advocacy by the ANA for Appropriate Nurse Staffing

The American Nurses Association (ANA) states that substantial data indicates that having the right number of nurses on staff improves patient outcomes and increases staff and client satisfaction.

Appropriate staffing levels have multiple client benefits, including the following:

- Reduced mortality rates;
- Reduced length of client stays;
- Reduced number of preventable events, such as falls and infections.

Adequate staffing has benefits for nurses as well. An appropriate workload relieves nurses of the burden of fatigue and enables them to use their full expertise.

A recent report suggested that staff levels should depend on the following factors:

- Patient complexity, acuity, or stability;
- Number of admissions, discharges, and transfers;
- Professional nurses' and other staff members' skill levels and expertise;
- Physical space and layout of the nursing unit;
- Availability of technical support and other resources.

1.8.7. Cost-Effective Nursing Care

Resource Stewardship is one of the ANA's Standards of Professional Performance. "The registered nurse uses appropriate resources to plan, provide, and sustain evidence-based nursing services that are safe, effective, financially responsible, and used judiciously, according to the Resource Stewardship standard." By standing up for patients and making sure they receive timely care, an appropriate and personalized plan of care, and properly completed documentation, nurses can contribute to the containment of healthcare costs. These actions cut down on waste, prevent repeat testing, and guarantee prompt medical attention that improves patient outcomes and saves money.

Nurses routinely incorporate these practices to provide cost-effective nursing care in their daily practice:

- Keeping supplies near the client's room;

- Preventing waste by only bringing needed supplies into a client's room;
- Avoiding prepackaged kits with unnecessary supplies;
- Avoiding "Admission Bags" with unnecessary supplies;
- Using financially-sound thinking;
- Understanding healthcare costs and reimbursement models;
- Charging out supplies and equipment according to agency policy.

Being productive:

- Organizing and prioritizing;
- Using effective time management;
- Grouping tasks when entering client rooms (i.e., clustering care);
- Assigning and delegating nursing care to the nursing team according to the state Nurse Practice Act and agency policy;
- Using effective team communication to avoid duplication of tasks and request assistance when needed;
- Updating and individualizing clients' nursing care plans according to their current needs;
- Documenting for continuity of client care that avoids duplication and focuses on effective interventions based on identified outcomes and goals (Grembowski et al., 1988; Grytten et al., 2017).

1.9. Special Challenges for Healthcare Manager

Healthcare managers face five issues more than other managers do:

- The central roles of risk and uncertainty;
- The complexities created by insurance;
- The perils produced by information asymmetries;
- The problems posed by not-for-profit organizations;
- The rapid and confusing course of technical and institutional change.

Let us look at each of these challenges in more depth.

1.9.1. Risk and Uncertainty

Healthcare markets and organizations are characterized by risk and uncertainty. Probabilities should be used to describe the prevalence of disease and the efficacy of medical treatment. For instance, there is typically some chance of failure when the proper therapy is administered. A certain percentage of patients will benefit while others will suffer negative side effects. Consequently, managing costs and quality poses challenging issues. It's not always clear why a provider performed poorly—did his colleagues fail him, was he incompetent, careless, or lazy, or was he just unlucky enough to treat a panel of patients who were incredibly sick or for whom standard therapies were ineffective?

1.9.2. Insurance

A large number of consumers have health insurance because risk and uncertainty are inherent in the healthcare industry, and healthcare organizations must deal with the management challenges that insurance brings. First of all, insurance casts doubt on the identity of the client. Consumers use the products, but insurance covers the majority of the cost in most cases. Furthermore, the majority of individuals who possess private medical insurance obtain it via their employer, primarily due to the favorable tax structure. Even though most economists concur that workers eventually pay for insurance through wage reductions, the majority of workers are unaware of the costs of their insurance options and are not particularly interested in learning about them unless they are changing jobs. Because of this, staff members are unwilling to weigh cost and value and are still ignorant of the true costs of healthcare. Most patients select the best, most expensive treatment when insurance bears the cost—a decision they might not make if they were responsible for the entire cost.

Furthermore, insurance complicates even straightforward transactions. The patient, the insurer, and the provider are the three parties involved in the majority of transactions, and many involve more. The majority of providers deal with a broad range of insurance plans and encounter mountains of different claim forms and payment systems, which further contributes to the confusion. Many healthcare providers are left feeling wistful as more insurance plans negotiate their payment plans and rates, leaving them in awe of businesses that merely charge consumers for their services. The intricacy of insurance transactions also raises the risk of fraud and error. Both are rather common.

Many providers still rely on a small number of plans for their revenue despite this confusing array of insurance plans—a situation that most managers try to avoid. For instance, Medicare accounts for at least one-third of the revenue received by most hospitals. Therefore, modifications to Medicare rules or payment procedures have the potential to significantly impact a healthcare organization's future. Reimbursement terms have the power to suddenly turn a profitable market for all players into one where only the strongest, best-led, and best-positioned companies can thrive.

1.9.3. Information Asymmetries

Healthcare markets frequently experience information asymmetries, which lead to a variety of issues. When one party to a transaction knows more than the other, there is an information asymmetry. The person with more information in this scenario has the chance to exploit the person with less information. Acknowledging a disadvantage, the less informed party might start to doubt the other party's intentions and turn down a recommendation that could have been advantageous. For instance, doctors and other healthcare professionals typically have a better understanding of patients' medical options than do patients. Patients may accept treatments that are not cost-effective without realizing their options, or they may reject recommendations made in their best interests because they know they are susceptible to doctors' self-serving advice.

A manager can view asymmetric information as giving providers several leeway in therapy recommendations. Managers must make sure that providers are not incentivized to use their superior knowledge for personal gain, since the operations of insurance plans, hospitals, and group practices are largely defined by the recommendations made by these professionals. On the other hand, in some circumstances, patients are in a better position and can probably predict their healthcare needs more precisely than insurers. Patients are aware of their desire to begin a family, whether they seek medical care at the first sign of illness, and whether any symptoms they may be experiencing could be signs of a possible ailment. Because of this, health plans are susceptible to adverse selection, which increases the likelihood that high-risk customers will seek insurance while healthier people will forego it.

1.9.4. Not-for-Profit Organizations

Although the majority of non-profit organizations have admirable objectives that their managers take seriously, these groups can also cause issues for managers in the healthcare industry. Non-profit organizations, for instance, typically have a variety of stakeholders. Multiple stakeholders equate to multiple goals, making it more difficult to manage organizations and evaluate managers' performance. All organizations have the potential for managers to prioritize their needs over those of their stakeholders, but not-for-profit organizations are more difficult to identify because they lack a clear bottom line. Not-for-profit companies could also be more difficult to manage successfully. They are governed by a complex set of rules that are intended to keep them from being used as tax havens. These rules complicate the process of establishing incentive-based pay plans for supervisors, workers, and contractors—physicians being the most significant group of these. Furthermore, not-for-profit organizations find it more difficult to find other uses for the resources they invested in a failed project when it fails. For instance, to sell or otherwise use the assets of a not-for-profit organization, the trustees may need to obtain permission from the court. Managers of not-for-profit organizations can always argue that poor performance is a reflection of their more complicated environment because of these unique circumstances.

1.9.5. Technological and Institutional Change

The previous four challenges are nothing compared to this fifth one. There is a lot of change in the healthcare system. It seems as though no one knows where the healthcare system is headed, and almost every aspect of the industry is reinventing itself. It is challenging to exercise leadership if you are unsure of your direction. Change is a constant challenge for managers in the healthcare industry (Grytten & Skau, 2017).

The impact of education on the probability of receiving periodontal treatment. Causal effects were measured by the introduction of a school reform in Norway. Social Science and Medicine 188, 128–136 (Harris et al., 2012; Hettiarachchi et al., 2018).

A Closer Look

How the Healthcare Industry Helps Contributing to the Economy:

Despite the economic slowdown, one of the industries with the fastest rate of growth currently is healthcare. The increasing number of hospitals, medical device manufacturers, clinical trial providers, outsourcing firms, telemedicine providers, medical tourists, health insurance providers, and medical equipment manufacturers is driving the growth of this industry globally. Furthermore, public and private doctors are working to maintain the growth surge by increasing investments and enhancing networks, services, and coverage.

A strong healthcare system is critical to easing the burden on families and promoting national development. A robust healthcare system guarantees a robust economy. According to their research, a mere 10% increase in life expectancy guarantees approximately 0.4% annual economic growth. Developing nations are beginning to understand how vital life expectancy and access to healthcare are to economic expansion. Due to the availability of a large pool of highly qualified medical professionals and consistent investments in healthcare infrastructure, some have even grown competitive. In many of these nations, the cost of treatment has drastically decreased in recent years. Whether forcing people to pay for healthcare or providing financial assistance is a good thing is still hotly debated. Hospital stays paid for out of pocket have exposed entire populations to enormous financial burdens in many societies, leading to the rise of poverty. However, many private players have objected to subsidization, citing poor performance, corruption, and a lack of competition. Policymakers must exercise extreme caution when addressing these matters. There are additional difficulties. For example, private entities hardly ever pay attention to state-subsidized insurance. It's time for policymakers to make sure healthcare companies see people as growth partners instead of consumers. This will contribute to the availability, affordability, and accessibility of healthcare. Excellent healthcare is still a luxury that is primarily available in urban areas. In actuality, the vast number of people in developing nations reside in rural areas with limited access to healthcare, yet they nevertheless account for more than half of GDP in their nation. Concerns are still raised by the appalling doctor-to-patient ratio that exists in the majority of developing nations' rural areas. Technology, policy changes, and community involvement are crucial in providing healthcare organizations a different viewpoint.

It is past time for the healthcare industry to view investing in people as the key performance indicator. Since technology has made helping people so much easier, many pharmaceutical companies now have their service agencies to help the vulnerable. In actuality, they have been successful in connecting with the rural populace, enhancing healthcare, and fostering the local economy. By starting their outreach programs, other healthcare companies can learn from these pharmaceutical companies and assist individuals in taking charge of their health and well-being, and contribute to the country's economic growth.

Summary

- Economics is the study of how people and society end up choosing, with or without the use of money, to employ scarce productive resources that could have alternative uses, to produce various commodities and distribute them for consumption, now or in the future, among various persons and groups in society.
- Health economics is the study of how scarce resources are allocated among alternative uses for the care of sickness and the promotion, maintenance, and improvement of health, including the study of how healthcare and health-related services, their costs and benefits, and health itself are distributed among individuals and groups in society.
- Data on healthcare expenses and labor and capital inputs reflect only some of the items used by people to produce health.
- The health sector receives attention from policymakers because of its widely perceived problems. The substantial resources devoted to healthcare are reflected in a more meaningful way through the average level of the nation's spending for healthcare.
- Production, costs, and insurance naturally involve economics, but many other health issues have economic components, even though they may seem to be purely medical concerns.
- The inability of healthcare consumers to monitor the quality of the product they are buying leads to various regulations.
- Research suggests that medical technology accounts for about 10% to 40% of the increase in healthcare expenditures over time. These costs also lead to further ethical dilemmas as decisions regarding what scarce resources are provided to which patients are made.
- Social Determinants of Health (SDOH) are the conditions in the environments where people live, learn, work, and play that affect a wide range of outcomes.
- Pay for Performance refers to reimbursement models that attach financial incentives to the performance of healthcare agencies and providers.
- The hospital value-based purchasing program (VBP) was designed to improve healthcare quality and patient experience by using financial incentives that encourage hospitals to follow established best clinical practices and improve patient satisfaction scores via patient satisfaction surveys.
- The hospital readmissions reduction program (HRRP) penalizes hospitals with higher rates of patient readmissions compared to other hospitals.
- Floating is a common agency staffing strategy that asks nurses to temporarily work on a different unit to help cover a short-staffed shift.

References

1. Birch, S. (1986). Measuring dental health: Improvements on the DMF-Index. *Community Dental Health, 3*(4), 303–311.
2. Birch, S. (1988). The identification of supplier-inducement in a fixed price system of health care provision: The case of dentistry in the United Kingdom. *Journal of Health Economics, 7*(2), 129–150.

3. Birch, S., & Anderson, R. (2005). Financing and delivering oral health care: What can we learn from other countries? *Journal of the Canadian Dental Association, 71*(4), 243–247.
4. Birch, S., & Gafni, A. (1992). Cost-effectiveness/utility analyses: Do current decision rules lead us to where we want to be? *Journal of Health Economics, 11*(3), 279–296.
5. Birch, S., & Gafni, A. (2002). On being NICE in the UK: Guidelines for technology appraisal for the NHS in England and Wales. *Health Economics, 11*(2), 185–191.
6. Birch, S., & Gafni, A. (2003). Economics and the evaluation of health care programs: Generalizability of methods and implications for generalizability of results. *Health Policy, 64*(2), 207–219.
7. Birch, S., & Gafni, A. (2015). On the margins of health economics: A response to 'resolving NICE's nasty dilemma.' *Health Economics Policy and Law, 10*(2), 183–193.
8. Birch, S., Jerrett, M., Wilson, K., Law, M., Elliott, S., & Eyles, J. (2005). Heterogeneities in the production of health: Smoking, health status and place. *Health Policy, 72*(3), 301–310.
9. Birch, S., Kephart, G., Tomblin-Murphy, G., O'Brien-Pallas, L., Alder, R., & MacKenzie, A. (2007). Human resources planning and the production of health: A needs-based analytical framework. *Canadian Public Policy, 33*(Supplement 1), S1–S16.
10. Birch, S., Sohn, W., Ismail, A., Lepkowski, J., & Belli, R. (2004). Willingness to pay for dentin regeneration in a sample of dentate adults. *Community Dentistry and Oral Epidemiology, 32*(3), 210–216.
11. Burt, B. A., & Pai, S. (2001). Sugar consumption and caries risk: A systematic review. *Journal of Dental Education, 65*(10), 1017–1023.
12. Chalkley, M., & Listl, S. (2018). First not harm–The impact of financial incentives on dental X-rays. *Journal of Health Economics, 58*, 1–9.
13. Chalkley, M., & Tilley, C. (2006). Treatment intensity and provider remuneration: Dentists in the British National Health Service. *Health Economics, 15*(9), 933–946.
14. Cleary, S., Mooney, G., & McIntyre, D. (2010). Equity and efficiency in HIV-treatment in South Africa: The contribution of mathematical programming to priority setting. *Health Economics, 19*(10), 1166–1180.
15. De Coster, P. J., Marks, L. A., Martens, L. C., & Huysseune, A. (2009). Dental agenesis: Genetic and clinical perspectives. *Journal of Oral Pathology & Medicine, 38*(1), 1–17.
16. Donaldson, C., Birch, S., & Gafni, A. (2002). The distribution problem in economic evaluation: Income and the valuation of costs and consequences of healthcare programs. *Health Economics, 11*(1), 55–70.
17. Donaldson, C., Thomas, R., & Torgerson, D. (1997). Validity of open-ended and payment scale approaches to eliciting willingness to pay. *Applied Economics, 29*(1), 79–84.
18. Ellis, R., & McGuire, T. (1996). Hospital response to prospective payment: Moral hazard, selection, and practice-style effects. *Journal of Health Economics, 15*(3), 257–277.
19. Eow, J., Duane, B., Solaiman, A., Hussain, U., Lemasney, N., Ang, R., O'Kelly-Lynch, N., Girgis, G., Collazo, L., & Johnston, B. (2019). What evidence do economic evaluations in dental care provide? A scoping review. *Community Dental Health, 36*(2), 118–125.

20. Evans, R. (1985). Illusions of necessity: Evading responsibility for choice in health care. *Journal of Health Politics, Policy and Law, 10*(3), 439–467.
21. Gafni, A., & Birch, S. (1993). Searching for a common currency: Critical appraisal of the scientific basis underlying European harmonization of the measurement of health-related quality of life (EuroQol). *Health Policy, 23*(3), 219–228.
22. Gafni, A., & Birch, S. (2006). Incremental cost-effectiveness ratios (ICERs): The silence of the lambda. *Social Science & Medicine, 62*(9), 2091–2100.
23. Gafni, A., Birch, S., & Mehrez, A. (1993). Economics, health and health economics: HYEs versus QALYs. *Journal of Health Economics, 12*(3), 325–339.
24. Grembowski, D., & Milgrom, P. (1988). The influence of dentist supply on the relationship between fluoridation and restorative care among children. *Medical Care, 26*(9), 907–917.
25. Grytten, J. (2017). Payment systems and incentives in dentistry. *Community Dentistry and Oral Epidemiology, 45*(1), 1–11.
26. Grytten, J., & Holst, D. (2013). Perspectives on providing good access to dental services for elderly people: Patient selection, dentists' responsibility and budget management. *Gerodontology, 30*(1), 98–104.
27. Grytten, J., & Skau, I. (2017). The impact of education on the probability of receiving periodontal treatment: Causal effects were measured by introduction of a school reform in Norway. *Social Science & Medicine, 188*, 128–136.
28. Grytten, J., & Skau, I. (2018). Do patients with more education receive more subsidized dental care? Evidence from a natural experiment using the introduction of school reform in Norway as an instrumental variable. *Medical Care, 56*(10), 877–882.
29. Grytten, J., Holst, D., & Skau, I. (2013). Per capita remuneration of dentists and the quality of dental services. *Community Dentistry and Oral Epidemiology, 41*(5), 395–400.
30. Harris, R. V., & Sun, N. (2012). Dental practitioner concepts of efficiency related to the use of dental therapists. *Community Dentistry and Oral Epidemiology, 40*(3), 247–256.
31. Hettiarachchi, R. M., Kularatna, S., Downes, M. J., Byrnes, J., Kroon, J., Lalloo, R., Johnson, N. W., & Scuffham, P. A. (2018). The cost-effectiveness of oral health interventions: A systematic review of cost-utility analyses. *Community Dentistry and Oral Epidemiology, 46*(2), 118–124.

Chapter

DEMAND FOR HEALTH AND HEALTHCARE

2

Contents

Introduction

Many people find it difficult to explain why maintaining one's health is important. This might be the result of their improper self-care practices stemming from their ignorance of the value of health. Although many people still act in ways that indicate their health is not a top priority in their lives, health can generally be considered the foundation of life. They spend their budget on non-essential items and a lot of time on the opportunities they find rather than learning to exercise and maintain good health. But they pay less for a healthier diet.

The World Health Organization defines health as a condition of total physical, mental, and social well-being as opposed to just the absence of illness or disability. Since the UN Summit in Almaty in 1978, greater consideration has been given to this definition of health. The members of this organization were required to provide Primary Healthcare by offering an essential package aimed at reducing the health gap between different countries and with the goal of Health for all by the year 2000 due to the significant differences in health levels across the globe. The lack of resources in light of the population's increasing need for primary healthcare over the years has unquestionably been one of the most important issues and difficulties that various nations have had to deal with.

Therefore, health is viewed as a type of capital that provides services and is a durable good by health economists. Over the course of a person's lifetime, the flow of services generated from the stock of health capital is continuously consumed. It is assumed that each individual is born with a specific stock of health, say a year. The value of health declines with age over time and may be enhanced by investments in healthcare services. When a person's health falls below a crucially low threshold, death results.

Sustainable development revolves around healthy people, and people have always tried to increase their health reserves to maintain and improve their health. In general, improving each person's degree of health is greatly influenced by the use of services or the demand for medical services. The desire for healthcare is a result of the desire for health and is impacted by several variables, such as cost, income, population, etc.

Orientation and Directional Terms:

Term	Definition	Illustration
Healthcare provider	A healthcare provider is a person or entity that provides medical care or treatment. Healthcare providers include doctors, nurse practitioners, midwives, radiologists, labs, hospitals, urgent care clinics, medical supply companies, and other professionals, facilities, and businesses that provide such services.	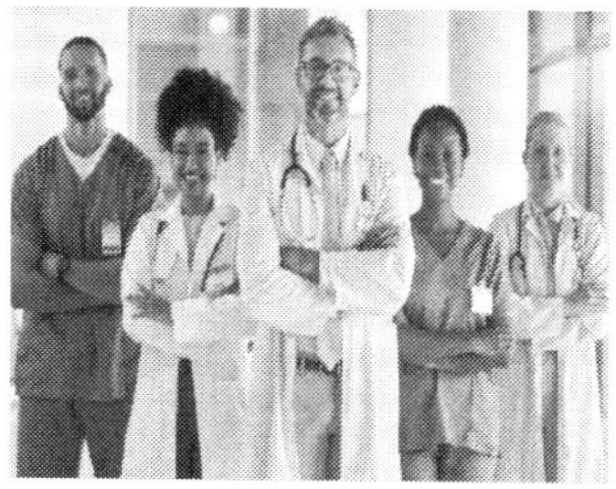
Primary healthcare	Primary healthcare is "essential healthcare" based on scientifically sound and socially acceptable methods and technology. This makes universal healthcare accessible to all individuals and families in a community.	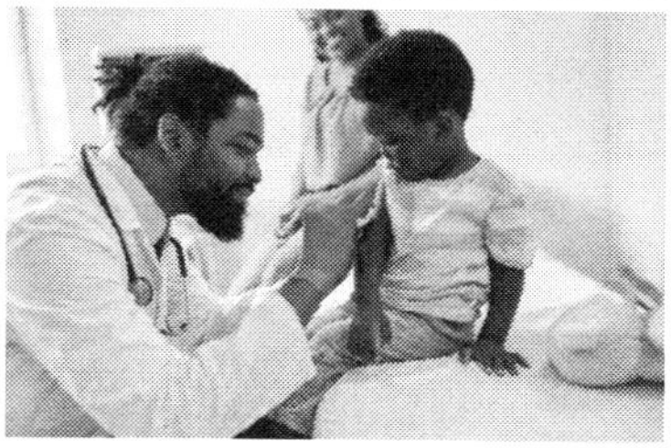
Human capital theory	Human capital theory is about the idea of humans increasing their productivity and efficiency through a greater focus on education and training.	
Competitive market	A competitive market is a term in economics that refers to a marketplace where there are a large amount of buyers and sellers and no single buyer or seller can affect the market.	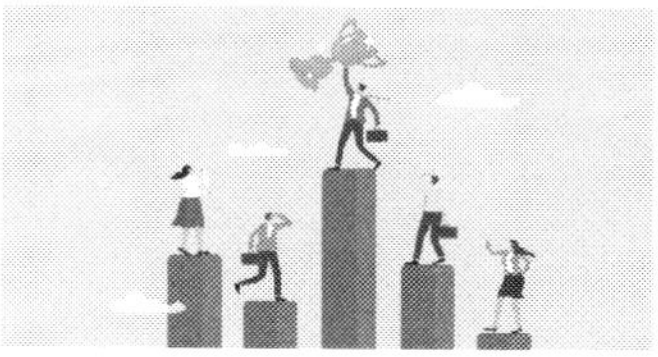

2.1. Demand

You must be able to pay for the item or service you want, be willing to ask for it, and have a clear plan on how you will get it. In actuality, desires are people's boundless inclinations and desires for products and services. If something wasn't so expensive or you could afford it, picture yourself being able to buy it. Scarcity ensures that many of our desires will never be fulfilled when we make decisions. Demand is an expression of our goals and plans for the demands that will be satisfied. The quantity of goods and services a consumer intends to purchase is determined by many variables, including population, advertising, preferences, personal income, commodity prices, and related commodity prices.

First, we need to talk about how price and demand for a good or service are related. The Ceteris Paribus principle, which describes this relationship, requires that all other demand-influencing factors be held constant. The price of an item or service and its demand are inversely correlated; as the price rises, so does the demand.

2.1.1. Demand Curve

The demand curve is a geometric arrangement of points where the price of an item is the independent variable and the rate of use of that good is the dependent variable. Generally speaking, the demand curve indicates the maximum demand for an item at various prices as well as the final price for a specific quantity of an item. Typically, the quantity of goods or services is plotted on the x-axis, and the price variable is displayed on the y-axis (Figure 2.1).

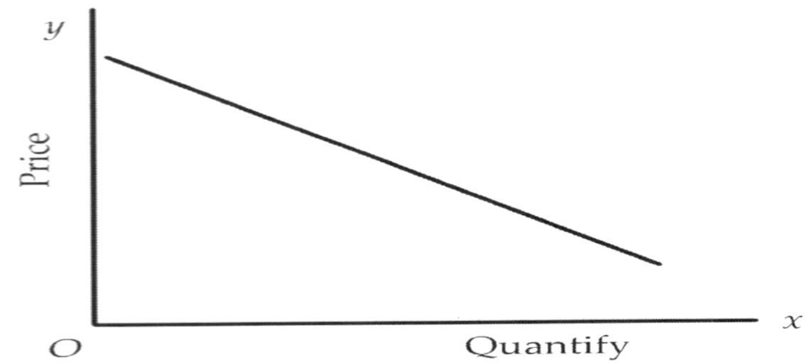

Figure 2.1. *Demand curve.*

Source: *https://www.intechopen.com/chapters/77622.*

This illustrates the willingness of an individual to pay for a slight increase in consumption. It is important to use "demand" accurately, referring not just to a specific price point on the demand curve but to a range of values within the price range. The demand for a good or service is influenced by its price and consumer income. The demand curve visually represents this relationship, with price changes resulting in movement along the curve and shifts in revenue impacting the entire curve. When using the demand curve in healthcare, it is crucial to consider factors such as consumer uncertainty about future illness, treatment effectiveness, and cost, as well as the emotional and physical toll of illness. Additionally, external demand for healthcare services may exist beyond individual needs, and the price paid by consumers may not accurately reflect the actual cost to providers (Figure 2.2).

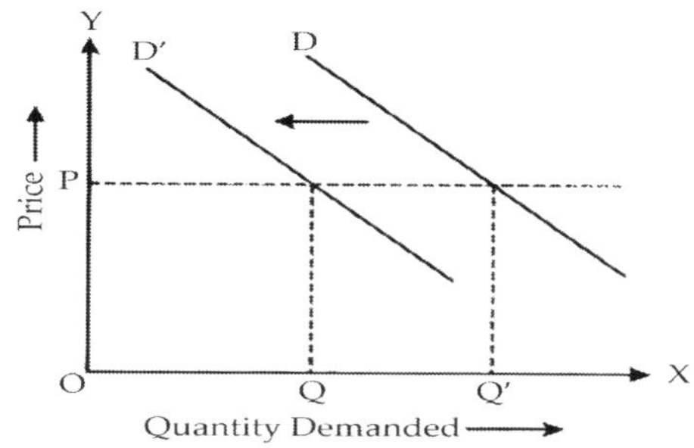

Figure 2.2. *Change in the demand curve.*

Source: *https://www.intechopen.com/chapters/77622.*

The demand curve can also be thought of as a payment ability curve that represents the final benefit. The maximum price a person is willing and able to pay for their most recent purchase is displayed on this curve. The maximum price that a person is willing and able to pay for a larger unit will be higher if there are fewer goods available. However, the ultimate benefit of each extra unit of available goods decreases as their quantity increases and the highest price offered on the demand curve also decreases.

We can look at the relationship between the demand for a product and other factors in the space of the demand curve in addition to the price of the product in question, which is inversely related to the demand for that product.

2.1.1.1. Prices of Other Goods

Customers' plans to purchase quantities of goods and services are influenced by the costs of other goods and services. There are two different kinds of goods in this situation: complementary and substitute goods. One substitute good can be used in place of another, and if the price of one rise, people are more likely to demand a substitute product, and the demand for the original good will decline.

A complementary good is one that is used in conjunction with another commodity, and in the event that the price of one of these commodities rises, there will be a corresponding decrease in demand for the other commodity.

2.1.1.2. Income

When people's incomes rise, they purchase more goods and services, and vice versa, assuming all other variables remain constant. Normal goods are those for which demand rises as income rises; inferior goods are those for which demand falls as income rises. However, generally speaking, income has little bearing on the demand for health-related products and services. People's income cannot significantly affect the demand for medical goods and services since they prioritize their health. Nonetheless, the need for upscale medical care will grow as incomes rise.

2.1.1.3. Population

The size and age distribution of the population also have an impact on demand. Population growth results in higher demand for all goods and services, while lower population growth leads to less demand for products and services. Additionally, when other variables remain constant, the population of a specific age group grows, increasing the demand for the goods and services that members of that age group use.

2.1.1.4. Consumer Preferences

Consumer preferences also influence demand. People's attitudes and tastes toward various products and services are known as preferences. Preferences are influenced by various cultural and social factors, genetics, advertising, past experiences, and religious beliefs.

2.1.2. Medical Goods

Medical care includes numerous products and services that preserve, enhance, or restore a person's health. For example, a young man might need wrist surgery to repair a torn tendon so he can return to work, an elderly woman might need cataract surgery to improve her vision, or a parent might need to take their child to the dentist annually to prevent future issues. Medical supplies consist of items like prescription medications, glasses, and dentures; medical services include surgeries, routine check-ups, and doctor visits. Distinguishing medical care from other products and services is challenging due to the differences between medical and preventive care. Four key features that differentiate medical care services are inventory, consistency, intangibility, and inseparability.

Medical services that are intangible cannot be evaluated by the five senses. Medical services are not something that the consumer can see, taste, or touch, unlike new shoes, a vegetable salad dinner, or a new cell phone. Indivisibility also refers to the simultaneous nature of a medical service's production and consumption. For instance, you use ophthalmic services at the moment of production when you visit an ophthalmologist for an examination. Furthermore, a patient is frequently viewed as a producer as well as a consumer. Inseparability has a direct bearing on inventory. Healthcare providers are unable to store or maintain medical services because they are produced and consumed simultaneously. For instance, in order to accommodate demand during peak hours, a physiotherapist is unable to provide a list of various physiotherapy services. Lastly, inconsistency means that there are significant differences in the range, makeup, and caliber of medical services. There are several reasons to visit a doctor, even though multiple people may do so at the same time. While one person may visit a doctor for a common physical issue, another may do so in the event of a heart attack. Individual differences and temporal variations can result in substantial variations in the combination of prescribed medical care or the frequency of its use.

2.1.2.1. Demand for Healthcare

People must look for a service they can afford and are prepared to pay for to meet demand. The care that physicians deem necessary for an individual to maintain their health is known as healthcare. Patients occasionally feel as though they need medical attention, but doctors don't think they can benefit from it. Sometimes a patient refuses to see their doctor because they would rather not receive treatment or because they do not think there is a medical need, even though the doctor thinks there is one. Patients' demands might not match their needs, even if they are as knowledgeable as doctors.

The following factors affect the demand for healthcare:

- Needs (based on patient perception);
- Patient preferences;
- Price or cost of use;
- Income;
- Transportation cost;
- Waiting time;
- Quality of care (based on patient perception).

Planners may find themselves in a situation where some services are overused and some are underused if they allocate resources based on need rather than demand.

The demand for healthcare differs from the simple demand model, just as the healthcare market does from other commodity markets. One distinction is that healthcare is self-satisfying and thus not required. Ultimately, receiving healthcare by itself does not result in happiness. On the contrary, people are content with their activities when they are well, which is why healthcare is in demand. Thus, there is a derived demand for healthcare.

Medical professionals have a significant impact on patients' perceptions of their need for and ability to benefit from healthcare. Healthcare consumers assign this decision-making authority to healthcare professionals who are more aware of their consumption patterns, even though it is assumed in economics that consumers can make informed decisions about them. This phenomenon can be attributed to the information asymmetry that exists between patients and healthcare providers, which may lead to induced demand on the part of providers to enhance revenue. The extremely diverse nature of healthcare presents another challenge. Every patient experience pain and symptoms in a somewhat unique way. Because of this, each patient must purchase a somewhat unique package of care, the efficacy of which is unknown to both the patient and the doctor.

The fact that many health services are funded in part by outside sources is another significant distinction. Payments from insurance companies or third parties: These sources can raise ethical questions and drive-up demand for unnecessary services for patients, even though they greatly boost people's purchasing power for healthcare.

In the event of illness, an individual's level of consumption determines the demand for healthcare; the amount of consumption varies depending on the factors that influence the demand, including income, service price, education, social norms, and quality. Rather than healthcare, a person's decision to use or not use services is influenced by their status as ill or injured. To meet their international commitments and ensure that everyone has access to healthcare, developing nations are concentrating on promoting healthcare as a critical policy. Nonetheless, rather than emphasizing the demand-side healthcare needs pattern, many policies have concentrated more on enhancing physical access. In low-income nations, the distribution of limited financial resources is determined by precise standards for how investments in the health sector affect the demand for services.

Due to the absence or inadequacy of social security systems in these nations, the occurrence of the disease results in higher medical expenses, lower labor productivity, and a reduction in household welfare. Due to insurance, many health services are used in developed nations with little to no consumer payment; in developing nations, on the other hand, there are worries about a decrease in the use of health services relative to their availability or a poor level of access is linked. Nonetheless, the rate of exploitation is low even in the health services sector because of several demand-side obstacles about the expense of care, travel expenses, and service quality. Furthermore, the social assessment and analysis of an individual's health and social surroundings are linked to the significance of that individual's health status in a clinical setting. Research has indicated that people's perception of how important it is to maintain their health is correlated with their risk of dying.

Improving people's health is one of the top concerns for health policymakers, so it is important to pay closer attention to the many variables that both directly and indirectly influence the demand for healthcare services.

Determining the elements that influence people's decisions to seek medical attention and select from various providers. Thus, assessing the factors that influence the demand for health services will enable the introduction and execution of suitable incentive programs to promote higher-quality healthcare. Being healthy can greatly improve a person's capacity to carry out a variety of tasks, including productive ones, as well as being one of the fundamental elements of human capital and the cornerstone of sustainable development. People are searching for health as a result. Individual health is primarily impacted by a variety of factors, including lifestyle choices, biological factors, non-medical purchases made, medical purchases made, and various socioeconomic traits. People's perceptions and expectations of the quality of healthcare are crucial because health service consumption and behavior are frequently influenced by the perceived quality of the services.

2.1.3. Derived Demand for Healthcare

Grossman explained the demand for healthcare using the theory of human capital. Human capital theory states that people invest in their health and education to earn more money.

Grossman proposed an approach in which many important aspects of the demand for health services differ from the traditional demand approach:

- That consumers are looking for health and demand health services to achieve it.
- To achieve health, consumers buy health services from the market and combine them with their efforts to improve health, such as diet and exercise.
- The health gained lasts more than a period and is not immediately depreciated to be analyzed as a capital good.

Most remarkably, it is possible to view health as a capital good in addition to a consumer good. People see health as a product to be purchased because it improves their quality of life. Because it extends people's healthy days to work and make money, it is a capital good that is beneficial to health. A straightforward diagram that illustrates the idea of health capital is shown in Figure 2.3. One can comprehend the savings of one's health capital, the result of which is "healthy days," in the same way that one thinks of cars or laptops as capital goods that provide their services over time. Outflow can be measured in multiple dimensions related to limited activity, and mental and physical health, or it can be viewed as one aspect of a healthy day. People invest in health savings because they consume a variety of health inputs, such as time, food, exercise, and healthcare. These expenditures give customers healthy days by preserving or enhancing their health reserves. Health reserves have the potential to increase, stay the same, or decline with age as a result of disease or trauma. Figure 2.3 illustrates how consumers make decisions concerning the quantity, timing, and cost of investing in health storage based on the ultimate goal of "healthy days." It will be evident that the costs associated with healthcare, the rate at which people are paid, and their productivity in generating health are what dictate the distribution of resources between health capital and other consumer goods and services. Think about a customer who purchases market inputs (e.g., food, clothing, and medical attention) and combines them with their own time to produce a health capital reserve that raises their usefulness.

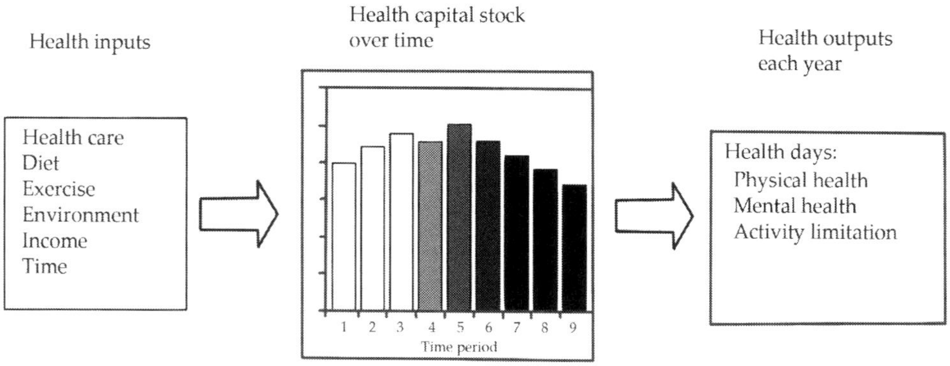

Figure 2.3. *Investing in health.*

Source: https://www.intechopen.com/chapters/77622.

An inverse relationship exists between an item's price and demand in the economy. That is, demand for a good increases with decreasing price, and vice versa for commodities: higher prices correspond to lower demand. A 1% change in a good's price results in a few percent changes in demand, according to price elasticity of demand. For instance, if an automobile's price increases by 1%, demand for it will decrease by a similar amount, and if a vehicle's price decreases by 1%, demand will rise by a similar amount.

Three things can happen when we calculate the price elasticity for a commodity:

- A 1% change in a commodity's price causes a greater than 1% change in demand for that commodity. These products are sensitive to price.
- A product is considered inelastic when a 1% change in its price results in a less than 1% change in demand. There is a modest response in demand for these kinds of goods to price fluctuations.
- The third scenario is when a 1% change in an item's price results in a corresponding 1% change in the good's demand.

Demand elasticity will always be negative if price and demand have an inverse relationship because a negative fraction represents the percentage change in one face or the denominator. Thus, after determining the price elasticity of demand, the good with elasticity is less than one, the commodity without elasticity, if the result, regardless of the negative sign of the number, becomes more than one, and if it is equal to one, the good has a single elasticity.

Certain factors influence this ratio even though the only way to determine a commodity's price elasticity is to gather price data and perform calculations.

2.1.4. Factors Affecting the Price Elasticity of Demand

2.1.4.1. Alternative Goods

The price elasticity of a product increases with the number of substitute goods available. That is, the demand for that product varies more sharply when the price varies. Additionally, a product's price change results in a change in the demand for substitute goods. There are typically few alternatives to a health or medical intervention in the healthcare industry.

2.1.4.2. Complementary Goods

When a product has a complement, the demand for one product changes in response to a change in the price of a complementary product. In the realm of health, maternal, and child care can be considered complementary goods.

2.1.4.3. Commodity Prices

Generally speaking, when a commodity is priced extremely low, demand is not affected by price fluctuations. But expensive goods have an allure. On the other hand, the price at which the demand elasticity is calculated yields varying results. As was first stated, there is an inverse relationship between a product's price and its level of demand. A commodity has one elasticity when its price falls in the middle of its demand curve. Furthermore, the product in that range is unappealing if the price is less than the midpoint.

2.1.4.4. Marginal Modes in Demand Elasticity

Additionally, there are two scenarios where the product is either totally inelastic or elastic. If the price of the good changes slightly, there will be no demand for the fully elastic good. This could apply to a salesman in a market with intense competition. Demand, independent of price range, is a fixed quantity if the good is inelastic.

2.2. Grossman Model of Health Demand

The Grossman model of health demand is a model for studying the demand for health and medical care outlined by Michael Grossman in a monograph in 1972 entitled: The Demand for Health: "A Theoretical and Empirical Investigation." The model-based demand for medical care on the interaction between a demand function for health and a production function for health. Andrew Jones, Nigel Rice, and Paul Contoyannis call the model the "founding father of demand for health models."

2.2.1. Model

According to this model, one's health is a capital good that is durable, inherited, and gradually loses value. Purchases of medical care and other inputs are considered investments in health, and depreciation is understood to be the inevitable decline in health over time. In the model, health is incorporated into the utility function both directly—as something that makes people happy—and indirectly—as an investment that frees up more time for both market and non-market activities.

To maximize utility over gross investment in health over each period, medical care consumption, and time inputs in the gross investment function over each period, the model generates a dynamic system of equations that can be formulated as an optimization problem. The agent's lifespan is therefore partially endogenous to the model.

Comparative statics are frequently used to optimize dynamic optimization problems by setting the partial derivatives of the outcome function of interest—in this case, the utility function—to zero. The investment model is the sub-model that results when the partial derivative of the utility function about health consumption is taken to equal zero. Generally speaking, solutions to these sub-models demonstrate that the opportunity cost of the capital and its rate of return must be equal. As a result, the ideal stock of health declines as the depreciation rate rises over time. Gross investment increases over time if the capital curve's marginal efficiency is inelastic. Thus, in real terms, this model predicts that older people will spend more time improving their health, take more time off from work, and pay more for medical care overall than younger people. Another implication is that as wages rise, the demand for health capital will rise as well, shifting the marginal efficiency of the capital curve to the right and increasing the slope of the curve.

2.2.2. Theoretical Expansions

There were several ways to expand the Grossman model. Maureen Cropper and Charles Phelps were among the first to incorporate uncertainty into the model. The model by Isaac Ehrlich expanded on the connection between health and education. One crucial question concerning the relationship between the demand for medical care and education is whether or not capital elasticity's marginal efficiency about education is greater than or equal to one. The need for medical care will rise in response to education if the curve is elastic (elasticity greater than 1). Conversely, if the curve is not elastic, education will reduce the need for medical care. Jan Acton extended the time restriction to include waiting and travel times for medical services.

2.2.3. Criticisms

Health is not a pure consumption or pure investment good in the model, but health stock helps the agent in two ways: first, by directly increasing utility, and second, by increasing the amount of healthy time that can be spent on other activities. A common objection is that it defies intuition to conceptualize health as a binary concept since it is both simultaneously both and simultaneously provides both options.

Similarly, detractors of Grossman's model have framed the problem from the perspective of preventing illness, which is a disutility in and of itself, rather than the demand for healthcare. In this regard, being ill is viewed as a factor that reduces or interrupts a person's capacity to reach their maximum level of utility, while passing away is viewed as a permanent interruption.

Contrary to Grossman's model, Maureen Cropper, an Economics professor at the University of Maryland, suggests that healthcare demand should be separated into preventative care and treatment of illness. The latter is often linked to end-of-life care and can be more random due to illness occurrence. Preventative care, on the other hand, is more predictable and typically associated with younger individuals in the labor market.

Furthermore, the independence of the model's component variables—such as income, education, and socioeconomic and occupational status—has been called into question by researchers. Riskier occupations have received more attention because they typically pay more due to workplace hazards, which makes this variable co-dependent. Similarly, Dr. Victor Fuchs contends that within the model, gendered and genetic differences function as unobservable, immutable variables (Frankel et al., 1989; Bagust et al., 1999).

2.3. The Elasticity of Demand for Healthcare Services

Detailed information on personal characteristics, use of medical services, and the effective price paid for an additional unit of healthcare would be ideal empirical data for estimating the elasticity of demand for healthcare. Above all, the observed differences in price and subsequent use in the ideal data would be exogenous. But in most cases, the perfect data are not available. As a result, scientists have created a range of approaches that deal with numerous problems brought on by inadequate data. Three broad categories can be used to group the methods that are commonly employed in the literature: observational, quasi-experimental, and experimental. To determine the effects of a specific treatment, experimental studies randomly assign participants to treatment and control groups. As individuals under study are unable to choose whether to receive treatment, the randomization of participants into different treatments prevents selection bias, which is thought to provide estimates from experiments with a "gold standard." On the other hand, experimental research has certain drawbacks. They can be challenging to develop and put into practice. They also take a long time and are very expensive. Before the effects of the experiment can be properly assessed, many years may pass. Most crucially, for this review, it should be noted that experimental study results are not always generalizable. It's possible that the results of effects measured in a strictly regulated environment won't translate to a larger implementation.

Quasi-experiments comprise the second category of studies on the elasticity of demand for healthcare. Although there are treatments and outcome measures in these studies, they differ from experiments in that participants are not randomized into treatment and control groups. Most quasi-experimental studies on healthcare demand can be more precisely characterized as natural experiments. Natural experiments use exogenous variations found in the economic environment to determine the treatment's effects. As an instance, Cherkin et al. utilized the Group Health Cooperative of Puget Sound's introduction of copayments to calculate the impact of price on the demand for healthcare services. The foundation of this methodology is a comparison of use prior to and following the policy change. The primary concern is that the researcher needs to account for any other variables that might have changed concurrently. If not, all other unobserved factors that changed during the analysis period will be included in the estimated effect of the policy change. As an illustration, let's say that a major flu pandemic struck the year following a change to the health insurance plan that included copayments. Assume further that after the plan is put into action, there is no discernible change in use. At first glance, it would seem that copayments have no impact on the demand for medical services. But this conclusion is not correct. The difference between the incidence of the flu in the pre-and post-time periods and the impact of the copayment adjustments are reflected in the change in use, or lack thereof. The researcher needs to be able to account for any additional variables that might have had an impact on use during the analysis period in order to get estimates of the actual impact of the policy change. To help answer the question of what would have happened if the policy had not been changed, a comparison group—which is comparable to the control group in the experimental design—that does not receive the policy change is frequently used. The degree to which the investigator managed to account for potential confounding variables needs to be taken into account when analyzing outcomes derived from natural experiments.

It is also discovered that the demand for health is income inelastic. The income elasticity of demand estimates between 0 and 0.2. The elasticity measure's positive sign signifies that the demand for healthcare services rises in tandem with income. On the other hand, the elasticity's magnitude indicates that the demand response is minimal. Research employing extended time series data typically presents greater income elasticities. Studies that use long time series data account for the effects of changes in medical technology, which explains the variation in estimates over different time periods.

2.3.1. Price Elasticity of Demand for Healthcare

Healthcare service pricing schedules can be very intricate. Coinsurance, deductibles, maximums for out-of-pocket expenses, premiums, and the cost of the good or service itself all affect how much a customer pays. Any modification to one of these variables will impact the patient's out-of-pocket medical expenses.

There are various methods to measure the amount of healthcare provided. In the studies we analyze, the primary quantity measures utilized are the total number of physician visits and total medical expenditures. In the evaluation of each study, as well as in the summary table, we will specify the specific healthcare quantity measure on which the reported price elasticity estimate is based. It is crucial to consider this when comparing elasticity estimates from different studies.

In 1971, Feldstein carried out one of the first investigations into the price elasticity of demand for healthcare. The findings, which were the first of their kind to be deemed statistically reliable, were based on microdata collected at the hospital level. The American Hospital Association Survey of Hospitals between 1958 and 1967 provided the study's data. Using differences in the cost of hospital stays, coinsurance rates, and the percentage of the population insured across states, a time series regression was used to determine the impact of price on the mean length of stay for hospitalized patients. Feldstein calculated that the demand for healthcare has a price elasticity of about –0.05. According to this elasticity estimate, the mean hospital stay will decrease by 0.5% for every 1% increase in the coinsurance rate, indicating that demand for healthcare services is relatively inelastic. Feldstein subsequently estimated a two-stage least squares model using state-level data, yielding a marginally larger price elasticity estimate of –0.67. A two-stage estimation procedure was employed to try to account for the possibility that the insurance price was endogenous.

Similarly, Fuchs & Kramer analyzed data at the state level to study the price elasticity of demand for healthcare services. They found that the estimates of elasticity based on net prices ranged from –0.15 to –0.20, which were notably lower than the estimates by Feldstein. These findings suggest that the demand for physician visits is not very responsive to changes in prices. However, there are several issues with using aggregate data to estimate the price elasticity of demand. The most significant problem is that combining data from multiple individuals and service types decreases the level of variation in the data and may result in biases in the analysis.

Rosett and Huang's study was one of the first to use individual-level data in an observational study on the demand for health. The impact of prices on demand for healthcare was examined using data from the 1960 Survey of Consumer Expenditure. Rosett and Huang estimated that when the out-of-pocket cost of healthcare is 20% of the market price, the price elasticity of demand was –0.35 using constructed measures of coinsurance. They discovered that medical costs were far more sensitive at higher out-of-pocket costs (elasticities up to –1.5). They may have built the coinsurance measures in a way that contributed to the comparatively large demand elasticities. The approach taken could cause price responsiveness to be overestimated.

Phelps and Newhouse estimated price elasticities of healthcare demand across coinsurance ranges using data on insurance plans in the US, Canada, and the UK. An estimate of the price elasticity for coinsurance rates ranging from 20 to 25% was –0.12. The elasticity dropped to –0.07 when coinsurance rates reached a range of 15 to 20%. Furthermore, price elasticity estimates of −0.04 were obtained for coinsurance rates between 10 and 15%. These findings suggest that the demand for healthcare will only be slightly affected by low cost-sharing.

Wedig approached the question in a slightly different way, looking at the relationship between the demand for doctor visits and price responsiveness. Data from the 1980 National Medical Care Utilization and Expenditure Survey were used to estimate elasticity. According to the findings, those who thought their health was fair or poor responded to prices less favorably (−0.16) than those who thought it was good or excellent (−0.35).

Eichner estimated the price elasticity of demand for healthcare using data from insurance claims from a single large employer. Eichner used variation in out-of-pocket costs within a plan with an annual deductible during a calendar year to isolate the behavioral response to price changes. As members of these plans reached their deductible, the cost of care decreased over the course of the year due to the plan's structure. According to him, the disparity in spending between people who have reached their deductible and those who haven't is a result of their behavior in response to fluctuations in the price of healthcare. The price elasticity of healthcare demand was estimated to be between −0.75 and −0.62.

Many researchers started utilizing the occurrence of natural experiments as an alternative estimation strategy in the early 1970s. Scitovsky and Snyder conducted research in 1972 on the impact of adding cost-sharing requirements to the health plan that Stanford University provided for its faculty, staff, and their dependents. In April 1967, a 25% coinsurance rate was instituted. The effects of coinsurance on demand were ascertained by analyzing changes in the utilization of healthcare services from 1966 to 1968. The findings demonstrated a high degree of inelasticity in the demand for healthcare, with the price elasticity of demand for doctor visits coming in at −0.14. Scitovsky and Snyder were able to examine some issues more thoroughly than had been possible in the earlier literature because they could use individual-level data. Their findings suggested that demand reacted to changes in healthcare costs does not significantly differ among socioeconomic and demographic groups. Scitovsky and McCall discovered in a related study that the institution of coinsurance does not result in a temporary decrease in service utilization. During the four-year follow-up period, at least, service use stayed at the lower level.

Beck researched the impact of copayments on healthcare utilization in Saskatchewan, Canada, during the same time frame. The province's health plan instituted a copayment program in 1968 that demanded $1.50 for each medical visit. Beck analyzed a random sample of 21,900 households, comprising over 40,000 individuals. The results showed that there was a −0.07 price elasticity of demand for healthcare services. The fact that this study's elasticity estimate was marginally lower than previous reports could indicate that Saskatchewan's physician practice patterns have changed. The effect would typically work in the opposite direction of the individual demand response if doctors responded to lower use by prescribing more intensive treatments for those who do use their services. As a result, Beck's estimate would underestimate the true impact of prices on the demand for healthcare services.

A more recent study examined the impact of copayments on the demand for healthcare services among people covered by Group Health Cooperative of Puget Sound (GHC) insurance, and it was based on a natural experiment.

Copayments of $5 for outpatient visits and $25 for ER visits were introduced by the plan in July 1985. Cherkin, along with others, enhanced the analysis from the 1970s by introducing a control group that was not subjected to the policy modification. Price elasticity of demand estimates of –0.04 for all visits were obtained from the comparison of use patterns before and after the policy change. Additionally, Cherkin et al. discovered that demand reactions to price changes were the same for all income levels. These studies' estimates cannot be directly compared to the estimates that were previously discussed. In Seattle, Washington, there is a large staff model HMO called The GHC. Prices will probably have a varied impact on the demand for healthcare services depending on the kind of health plan. Customers are subject to more restrictions as a result of the care management in HMOs, which influences their choice of services.

The government funded a social insurance experiment intended to address several significant questions regarding the demand for healthcare, in response to the relatively wide range of price elasticity estimates in the early health demand literature. Families in six locations were randomized into various insurance plans as part of the RAND Health Insurance Experiment (HIE), which took place between 1974 and 1982. The plans differed in terms of deductible size, out-of-pocket maximum, and degree of cost-sharing. The HIE was carried out about 20 years ago, but the associated studies' findings are still regarded as the "gold standard" for estimates of health demand elasticity. Researchers can avoid all of the selection and endogeneity issues that arise from observational studies thanks to the experimental design. The HIE analysis contrasts the utilization of healthcare services by individuals with varying insurance plans. Interestingly, the out-of-pocket maximums did not affect the use of healthcare services in the HIE. As a result, all insurance plans having the same coinsurance structure were regarded as identical for estimation purposes. It was discovered that the price elasticity of medical expenses was –0.17 for coinsurance rates ranging from 0% to 25%. The demand for healthcare was found to be somewhat more price-sensitive as the coinsurance rate increased, which is consistent with the trends observed in observational studies. Coinsurance rates ranging from 25% to 95% in the HIE produced elasticity estimates of –0.22. The HIE estimates of elasticities have magnitudes that are towards the lower end of the range of earlier estimates.

It was discovered that cost-sharing in the HIE greatly lowers per-person medical costs. Per capita spending was found to be 46% higher in the group receiving free care (0% coinsurance) than in the group receiving 95% coinsurance. Moreover, it has been discovered that higher deductibles, independent of coinsurance rates, lower healthcare utilization. Instead of lowering the intensity of treatment once a patient entered the healthcare system, the cost-sharing strategies reduced the number of treatment episodes. The decreases in episodes occurred in both scenarios where medical intervention would be very beneficial (an infection treatable with antibiotics) and where it would probably have the least impact (a virus-induced flu). This finding suggests that reducing less appropriate care through cost-sharing is an imprecise method.

While the experimental findings of the HIE are considered to be of high quality, there have been concerns raised about their external validity. The study was conducted in only six locations, which may not accurately reflect the healthcare utilization patterns of the entire population due to regional differences. Despite efforts to choose diverse sites for the study, the results are now outdated as the healthcare industry has evolved significantly since the experiment took place. With the rise of managed care and advancements in medical technology, it is uncertain if the HIE results can accurately predict consumer behavior in the current healthcare landscape. Additionally, the limited number of participants in each study site may not fully capture the effects of reduced demand on healthcare providers if cost-sharing plans were to be widely implemented. Thus, it is unclear how applicable the HIE results are to the broader healthcare market.

2.3.2. Income Elasticity of Demand for Healthcare

Despite the abundance of research on the income elasticity of demand, we have limited our discussion to the most important conclusions. Income is a crucial variable to take into account when making policy decisions, but it is difficult to manipulate. More research is necessary to determine how changes in factors that the policymaker can influence, like deductibles and coinsurance rates, will affect things.

Under full insurance, the effect of income on the demand for medical care should be negligible, if not zero. A customer's ability to receive medical services shouldn't be impacted by changes in income if they have access to free care. Theory and empirical estimates in the literature are in agreement. Phelps used the findings of an HIE study to compute income elasticities. He discovered that the demand for medical care was not very affected by changes in income. Calculations showed that the elasticities were 0.2 or less. This can be read to mean that the demand for healthcare will rise by 0.2% for every 1% increase in income. The conclusions drawn from data derived from the HIE are supported by the findings of several observational studies.

The level of medical technology available is held constant by income elasticities based on time series data covering a brief period or cross-sectional data. The overall demand for novel medical technologies and innovative treatment modalities rises along with the population's real income, and innovation quickens. The patterns of healthcare utilization will change as a result of technical change. The sensitivity of healthcare demand to changes in income is generally much greater when income elasticities are estimated from long-time series data. Feldstein estimated an income elasticity of 0.5 using data spanning from 1958 to 1967. Similarly, McLaughlin used data from 1972 to 1982 and discovered an income elasticity of 0.7. In a recent study, DiMatteo & DiMatteo discovered a similar income elasticity of 0.8 using data from 10 Canadian provinces between 1965 and 1991. The effects of technical change have been incorporated, as evidenced by the larger elasticities from the time series studies.

2.3.3. Time Price Elasticity of Demand for Healthcare

Although the demand for medical care is known to be significantly influenced by prices over time, there isn't much empirical data to support the claim that changes in time prices will have a minimal impact on the demand for healthcare. On the other hand, one study specifically addresses the time price elasticity of demand. Janssen estimated the demand for healthcare using information from the Netherlands Central Bureau of Statistics' National Health Interview Survey, giving special consideration to the impact of time prices on demand. The amount of time spent and the value of that time make up the time price of a doctor's appointment. Janssen defined the duration of time as comprising travel, waiting, and treatment duration. In certain situations, an individual's market wage determines the value of the time spent visiting the doctor; in other situations, their employment status does. Time price elasticities were discovered by the study to be between -0.09 and -0.14. According to these findings, the likelihood of seeing a general practitioner will drop by roughly 0.11% for every 1% increase in the time cost of medical care. The time price elasticity of demand is small and negative for all employment groups, indicating that people are not very sensitive to changes in time prices. Despite the estimates being grouped, full-time managers and directors were found to have one of the highest time price elasticities. This outcome makes sense because these individuals probably have large time opportunity costs.

Given that the majority of care is given at MTFs, where there is no out-of-pocket expense to the patient, time costs might be especially significant in the context of the MHS. In these situations, time costs play a crucial role in identifying usage patterns. Many individuals who are qualified for care at MTFs opt to use other providers who charge a copayment. This decision probably represents the impact of time pricing on the demand for healthcare services if waiting times are longer in the MTF setting.

2.4. Special Issues Regarding the Elasticity of Demand for Health

It is less simple to estimate the elasticity of demand for health because the demand for health is somewhat more complex than the demand for a typical product.

2.4.1. Measures of Healthcare Demand

Although they cannot directly buy health, consumers still have a demand for it. They have to pay for the medical services that are necessary to achieve health. Michael Grossman first addressed the notion that there is a derived demand for healthcare as opposed to a direct one in a 1972 article.

The number of inpatient days, outpatient visits, or prescriptions used can be used as a proxy for the amount of healthcare that is required. The majority of the time, the combination of services measured in various quantity units is possible because it is measured by the total cost of the services. Standard demand elasticities can be estimated using any of the measures.

Elasticities in terms of insurer costs are not typically expressed in studies. There may be differences in the elasticity between insurer and total costs, especially if the health plan has an out-of-pocket maximum and deductible.

2.4.2. Price of Healthcare

The healthcare services pricing schedule is quite intricate. A cost-sharing plan (coinsurance rates or copayments), a deductible, an upper limit on out-of-pocket expenses, and premiums all affect how much a consumer must pay for healthcare services. As a result, the quantity of services used can affect how much health services cost. Because of this, it can be challenging to estimate the price elasticity of demand for healthcare services. The effective price that the consumer would pay for an additional unit of health services must be identified by the researcher to calculate the true impact of price changes. For instance, it stands to reason that a person who has hit their annual out-of-pocket maximum and is therefore at zero cost will probably choose differently from a person who hasn't hit their deductible and must pay the entire cost of medical services.

2.4.3. Time Prices and Healthcare

The time required to buy a product is a component of its total cost. When it comes to medical care, time is often of the essence. The length of time patients must wait to see a doctor can have a big impact on how much people need to pay for medical services. Two common categories for waiting times are the amount of time spent in the doctor's office and the amount of time waiting to get an appointment. The majority of the research on how time prices affect the demand for healthcare generally concentrates on waiting times at work. This distinction is frequently made because the patient has to make a significant trade-off because they are unable to work or engage in other activities while they wait in the doctor's office.

Time prices can restrict access to medical services even in systems where the consumer's out-of-pocket expense is very low or nonexistent. People will only choose to see a doctor if the advantages of receiving medical care outweigh the time commitment. Therefore, we would anticipate that people who have lower opportunity costs of time would use medical services at higher rates than people who have higher opportunity costs of time. According to theory, cross-price time elasticities will be positive, and own-time price elasticities will be negative. The demand for medical services will decline as waiting times lengthen, according to the negative own-time price elasticity. Because of this, it's critical to take into account both the financial and time costs of medical care when analyzing the demand for healthcare.

2.4.4. Types of Healthcare

The range of healthcare services available makes it reasonable to assume that the elasticity of demand for any given service type would also differ. When prices change, the demand for inpatient services might react differently than the demand for outpatient services. In a similar vein, disparities in the responsiveness of acute and preventive care demand might be anticipated. Moreover, X-rays, medications, office visits, lab work, and a wide range of other products and services can be included in healthcare services. Because of this heterogeneity, it may be useful to estimate distinct demand elasticities for every category of health services.

2.4.5. Interrelationships Between the Demand for Health Insurance and Healthcare

It is a little more complicated to comprehend the demand for healthcare covered by a specific health plan than it is to comprehend the demand for healthcare in general. Any change in the out-of-pocket expenses for medical services has two significant effects when analyzing the demand faced by an individual plan. First, more customers will decide to enroll in a specific insurance plan if the out-of-pocket expenses for care in that plan decrease. Furthermore, people already enrolled in the plan will use more services than they did previously due to the cost reduction. As a result, changes in these variables combine to affect the amount of services rendered as a result of a price change. The combination of two distinct elasticities can be used to determine the overall impact of a price change on the demand for medical services covered by a specific insurance plan. The first illustrates how variations in the number of health insurance plan enrollees affect demand. The second illustrates how current enrollees' demand for medical services is impacted by the price change. If the health plan has a deductible and an out-of-pocket cap, additional information is needed to calculate the change in insurer costs related to a change in the demand for healthcare. For people who don't exceed the deductible, those who exceed the deductible but not the cap, and those who exceed the cap, the demand change should be assessed individually. For each of these three groups, the insurer's cost share will then vary. If the cost-sharing under the plan varies or the providers charge different prices for the same treatment, the analyst may also need to account for shifts in the demand for various providers.

2.4.6. Selection Effects

The presence of adverse selection is a significant factor to take into account when calculating demand elasticities in healthcare. Adverse selection happens when individuals in poor health opt for higher-benefit insurance plans, while those in good health may avoid these plans due to the high cost. If adverse selection is present, elasticity estimates will reflect the varying needs of individuals with different health and socioeconomic statuses, in addition to how quantity responds to price changes. Researchers have shown interest in measuring the extent of adverse selection in some cases, using advanced statistical methods to break down the overall impact on demand.

2.4.7. Moral Hazard

Moral hazard makes estimating the demand for healthcare even more difficult. When an individual's incentives to take action to help prevent a loss are undermined by the existence of insurance, this is known as ex-ante moral hazard. Ex-post moral hazard applies after the disease or injury has already manifested. The consumer is protected from having to cover the entire cost of medical services when they have insurance. Consequently, the patient uses more medical services than he would have in the absence of insurance. Therefore, researchers must comprehend how moral hazard contributes to the rise in the demand for medical services. The incentives that a person faces will alter in response to any price changes. For instance, an individual's share of the cost of any used healthcare service decreases as their out-of-pocket expenses rise. People consequently demand greater healthcare services (Morgan et al., 1999; Himsworth et al., 1999).

2.5. Empirical Estimation

Many studies have tried to measure medical demand empirically by taking into account different factors. Even though the research methods and analytical scope varied greatly among the studies, some general conclusions could be drawn. Regrettably, it is exceedingly challenging to measure the dependent variable that denotes the quantity of medical services used. The quantity demanded should ideally account for both the intensity and the use of medical services. Since these types of data are not available, the quantity of medical services demanded is typically determined by some utilization measure, such as the number of doctor visits or hospital patient days. To account for variations in quality, proxy variables are then included as independent variables. Results are skewed when quality control is not implemented correctly. This is because variations in the quality of care rendered may be the cause of shifts in demand, which may be mistakenly attributed to variations in other variables.

For economists, determining the out-of-pocket cost of medical care also poses a challenge. The growing importance of third-party payers has made this issue worse in recent years. In an ideal world, the consumer's out-of-pocket costs for medical services would match the amount they pay after taking insurance. Unfortunately, it is rare to find such data, so economists are frequently forced to make do with variables like the average cost of medical services provided.

The inclusion of a further variable in the equation is then done to account for health insurance. The demand for medical care should be negatively impacted by price, but the quantity demanded should be positively influenced by insurance.

Time cost variables account for the effects of waiting and travel expenses on demand, while an income variable measures the influence of purchasing power on demand. Demand is predicted to be positively impacted by the income variable and negatively impacted by the time cost variables. The regression equation should also take into account the costs of different complements and substitutes in terms of consumption. With the growing interconnectedness of the medical markets in recent years, this has taken on even greater significance.

For instance, we should account for the costs of physician services and hospital outpatient services (which could be complementary or substitute services) when estimating the amount of inpatient services that a hospital is expected to provide. The remaining variables, which are known as control variables and account for the potential influence of different noneconomic factors on the demand for healthcare services, are tastes and preferences, the rate at which health depreciates, the stock of health, and the quality of care.

2.5.1. Own-Price, Income, Cross-Price, and Time-Cost Elasticity Estimates

Globally, there is a wealth of empirical research on the elasticity of demand for primary healthcare. For example, according to studies where the dependent variable is medical expenditures, the own-price elasticity of demand varies from 20.04 to 20.7. Similar findings are found in other studies that examine the demand for physician and hospital services. All things considered, the estimates point to a 20.1–20.7 own-price elasticity of demand for primary healthcare, which implies that a 10% increase in the out-of-pocket cost of medical services causes a 1–7% drop in the quantity demanded. Ceteris paribus, the inelastic estimates also suggest that overall spending on medical services, including hospital and physician visits, rises as the out-of-pocket cost increases.

Overall, the study shows that the demand for specialty care is marginally more elastic to price than the demand for primary care. That is not surprising at all considering that hospital and physician services typically have the lowest percentage of out-of-pocket payments. As the percentage of the bill that is paid out of pocket rises, consumers should grow more price-sensitive, all other things being equal. For instance, Manning & Phelps discovered that patient age and sex, as well as the type of service rendered, all influenced the demand for dental services, which was found to be somewhat more elastic in terms of price. The demand for dental services by adult males and children appears to be slightly more price elastic, while the price elasticity of demand by adult females appears to vary between 20.5 and 20.7. Moreover, compared to primary medical services, the demand for nursing home services seems to be more elastic in terms of price. Chiswick discovered that nursing home services have an own price elasticity of 22.3, and Lamberton et al. estimated it to be 20.76. In conclusion, Headen discovered that the probability of entering a nursing home has an own price elasticity of 20.7.

There is a need for discussion regarding the wide range of empirical estimates for the income elasticity of demand. Healthcare is generally found to be a normal good with an income elasticity below 1.0 in studies that use household or individual data. These findings stand in stark contrast to research that examines the relationship between income and healthcare costs over time or between nations using data at the national level. Finding out how economic growth affects national healthcare spending is the aim of these studies. It's interesting and warrants an explanation why the macro- and micro-estimates differ from one another. According to Newhouse, the reason for this discrepancy is that, for instance, in the US, the average patient only ever pays a small percentage of the total cost of medical care, but eventually the entire nation is required to cover the entire cost of care. Because consumers are less price-conscious, income elasticity should decrease as the average consumer's out-of-pocket healthcare costs decline. If, for instance, the average person's out-of-pocket medical expenses are eliminated, they will likely receive treatment regardless of their financial situation. At its extreme, income elasticity is equal to zero. Nonetheless, the nation will be far more sensitive to changes in income and price because it must bear the full cost of healthcare.

If healthcare is a luxury good or not is one of the more intriguing questions this research raises. A luxury good is defined by economists as one with an income elasticity greater than 1.0. In this instance, a rise in income causes the amount of the goods consumed to increase even more. Assume that a good's income elasticity is equal to 0.5. In this instance, a 10% increase in income causes the good's consumption to rise by 15%. This implies, of course, that as income rises, so does the percentage of one's budget allotted to the good's consumption.

A demand-side explanation for the rise in healthcare costs in the United States relative to national income over the previous few decades may be found if the total income elasticity of healthcare is greater than 1.0. Since healthcare is a luxury good, the U.S. has dedicated a larger share of its income to it as its economy and per capita income have grown over the past few decades. Consequently, a bigger portion of the economic pie went to the healthcare industry.

The demand for medical services also seems to be significantly impacted by time costs. Studies show that the own-price elasticity of demand and the travel time elasticity of demand are roughly equal. Acton, Phelps, and Newhouse state that the travel time elasticity of demand falls between 20.14 and 20.51. Gravelle et al. used a data set produced in the United Kingdom and discovered that the elasticity of admissions to distance equaled 20.35. When combined, these studies indicate that the quantity demanded for medical services is reduced by approximately 3% for every 10% increase in travel time. Additionally, it seems that customers are willing to pay for the duration of their medical service waits. Martin and Smith discovered that the wait time elasticity was equal to 20.20, but McCarthy found that it varied from 20.36 to 21.14. Furthermore, Gravelle et al. calculated the admissions elasticity about waiting time to be 20.25. The decision to seek medical attention is also influenced by time costs; Frank et al. discovered that the probability of finishing childhood vaccinations on time is influenced by travel time costs in an elasticity of about 20.

It's unclear right now how much different medical service kinds complement or replace one another in terms of consumption. Regarding whether hospital services—outpatient and inpatient—complement or replace one another, for instance, there doesn't seem to be much agreement. According to Davis and Russell, there is a substitute relationship between the cost of inpatient services and the number of outpatient visits, with the cross-price elasticity ranging from 0.85 to 1.46. Gold subsequently provided qualitative confirmation of these findings. Customers therefore depend more on outpatient services to save money when the cost of inpatient hospital services rises. Conversely, Freiberg & Scutchfield discovered that there is no interchangeability between these two categories of medical care. Alternatively, Manning et al. indicated that their consumption complements one another.

2.5.2. The Impact of Insurance on the Demand for Medical Care

The demand for medical care has been significantly impacted by the expansion of both public and private health insurance. We will concentrate on a study carried out by the RAND

Corporation rather than going over the findings from the numerous studies that examined how insurance affected the demand for medical care. Without a doubt, the most thorough study to date is the RAND Health Insurance Study (HIS). In a controlled experiment, families were enrolled in various health insurance plans from six sites (Dayton, Ohio; Seattle, Washington; Fitchburg, Massachusetts; Charleston, South Carolina; Georgetown County, South Carolina; and Franklin County, Massachusetts). The purpose of the experiment was to determine how variations in insurance coverage affected the demand for medical care.

2.5.3. The Impact of Noneconomic Factors on the Demand for Medical Services

The empirical research also shows that the demand for medical care is influenced by a wide range of other factors, including tastes and preferences as well as the state of health. Most researchers concur that while an individual's overall health has an inverse relationship with their demand for medical care, age and the severity of their illness have a direct impact on that demand. However, there doesn't seem to be agreement on how education affects the desire for medical care. This may suggest that the inverse effect of education—a greater capacity to provide healthcare at home—offsets the direct impact of education on the demand for medical care, which is a greater willingness to seek care, or that more research is necessary in this area.

It's interesting to observe that some researchers have concentrated especially on how medical knowledge affects the demand for healthcare services. There seems to be a positive correlation between consumers' medical knowledge and their desire for medical care, in contrast to the findings regarding general education. This indicates that people who have had more medical training typically use more medical services. For instance, Hsieh & Lin discovered that older people with better health understanding were more likely to receive preventive medical care, while Kenkel discovered a positive correlation between consumers' medical knowledge and their likelihood of visiting a doctor for medical care. According to both studies, consumers who lack medical knowledge frequently overestimate the importance of receiving medical care and consequently don't take the recommended dosage. It's also possible that having more medical knowledge improves a person's capacity to use healthcare services efficiently, raising the marginal product of medical care. As a result, as consumer knowledge grows, so does the need for different kinds of medical care.

Lastly, Hsieh & Lin discovered that income, medical insurance, years of education, and employment in the medical field all had a positive impact on the amount of health knowledge a person learned. They also discovered that the amount of health data gathered was negatively impacted by an individual's age and whether or not they smoked or drank. It seems that while smokers and drinkers benefit less from any improved health that may come from additional medical knowledge, older people seem to absorb less new information because they have fewer years to live and enjoy the benefits of that knowledge.

2.6. Managing Demand in General Practice

General medical services are facing pressure from rising patient expectations. The population's use of primary care services has changed and continues to change in response to pressures from technology and demographics, even though empirical evidence of rising demand is hard to come by. Over the past 10 years, the number of consultations has slightly increased, but the number of out-of-hours calls has increased significantly.

The majority of chronic illnesses can be controlled without much help from specialists, but patients are becoming more aware of advancements in diagnosis and treatment. The information revolution has increased demand in the public sector for easily navigable services with continuous quality improvement. Users look for pertinent information that is expertly conveyed by the healthcare provider of their choice. People's desire to participate in management decision-making is growing. The perception of an expanding divide between the needs and desires of their patients and the resources available to the service creates a stressful undercurrent in general practitioners' professional lives.

The main utilitarian goals of demand management are to maximize the total amount of needs that are met for the largest number of people while utilizing the available resources. The process may involve increasing demand for underutilized services that are known to be cost-effective, in addition to merely reducing demand for ineffective services. Three target audiences exist for demand management initiatives: patients, healthcare providers, and the health system as a whole. Perceived need for care, treatment preferences, and non-health-related motivations impact both physicians and patients. Patients' and physicians' responses are influenced by broader environmental factors like financial incentives.

In some ways, the only thing involved in providing primary medical care is managing demand throughout the patient's journey through the system. Some of the tactics that can be used more methodically in everyday practice are depicted in the figure. All the initiatives are motivated by the desire to increase transparency in decision-making and information sharing. General practitioners and other team members are increasingly able to impact demand outside of the clinic by commissioning activities, taking on new clinical roles (like those in casualty departments), or doing educational work in schools or workplaces.

2.6.1. The Patient-Practice Interface

2.6.1.1. Health Education

We are aware that giving patients the right information can enable them to take care of minor ailments on their own without seeking medical assistance. There is uncertainty regarding the effects of health promotion programs that involve people in making decisions about their care, including whether healthier people who feel more in control of their health make less (expensive) use of health services. Before the advantages of a longer-term decrease in consultation fees become apparent, they might cause a brief spike in demand. Nonetheless, studies have demonstrated that self-care manuals can reduce medical visits and save two to three times the cost. In the US, a few health maintenance organizations are covering the cost of self-help videos for their members. Health promotion aims to do more than just control demand. Similarly, risk reduction—a traditional form of health promotion—offers only a single facet of all-encompassing demand management.

Better management of the shift from self-care to professional care requires a deeper comprehension of how individuals respond to their illnesses. The likelihood of seeking care depends on several factors, including prior experience contacting someone in a similar circumstance, how serious the symptoms are thought to be, and belief in the effectiveness of the treatment. Extra guidance given during a consultation for a minor ailment can motivate self-care in the future. For instance, the chance of a recurrent upper respiratory tract infection is decreased when antibiotic prescriptions are appropriately postponed.

2.6.1.2. "Contracts" with Patients

The Patient's Charter is seen by many medical professionals as overemphasizing entitlements and creating unwarranted demand. Creating clearer "contracts" between users and their providers could be one approach to better balance rights and obligations. Pietroni has detailed an effort of this kind to encourage patients to get in touch when it is necessary but discourage them in other situations.

2.6.1.3. Telephone Advice and Triage

Approximately 25% of primary medical care in the United States is provided over the phone. Compared to the conventional chain of referral, "patient risk assessment" employing iterative computer-generated algorithms and protocols may (more quickly) guarantee that the appropriate patient receives the right care from the appropriate health professional. There is growing evidence regarding the advantages of telephone triage. After getting advice from specially trained nurses, many people who called for urgent appointments were able to take care of themselves, according to an evaluation of telephone advice software conducted in south London. Numerous general practitioner cooperatives are currently using the system, which has proven effective at the national level in other nations.

The introduction of a nurse-led helpline (NHS Direct), for which pilots have already begun, and the white paper on the NHS in England reaffirmed the value of phone helplines. To determine whether telephone advice software at a distance is sensitive enough to diagnose conditions and whether certain patient categories are more vulnerable than others, more research is needed. In contrast to for-profit deputizing services, cooperatives seem to "convert" a higher percentage of house calls into phone conversations or consultations at an after-hours center. Once more, additional proof is needed to assess the caliber of the services they provide.

2.6.2. Other Means

Self-help resources are starting to become available online thanks to energizing practices. The UK has one of the highest rates of personal computer ownership among all countries. Will all practices utilize their website in the future to control the demand for their services? These developments will have a significant impact on the resources and education required of various primary healthcare team members.

Copayments are still favored by decision-makers looking for an easy way to balance their budget. However, evidence from both developed and developing nations indicates that the people most likely to be discouraged by charges are those who are least fortunate. Therefore, although this is still conjectural, the health service may be burdened more financially if illness manifests later. It's unclear how much professional support there is for these accusations.

2.6.3. Clinical Decision Making

Technological advancements in near-patient testing and electronic data interchange may reduce the need for urgent referrals by delivering test results more quickly. However, it is currently unknown how cost-effective a large portion of the available biochemical and hematological near-patient testing equipment is. Likewise, it's unclear what advantages come with the recent expansion of outreach clinics. By making specialists more accessible, referral activity may increase rather than decrease and referral thresholds may be lowered. The chance for educational exchange that outreach clinics offer is rarely taken advantage of by general practitioners.

2.6.3.1. Prescribing

Right now, the most advanced demand management is being done in the prescription space. In Britain, mechanisms include formulary development, feedback on precise prescribing data from the PACT (prescribing activity and cost) database, one-on-one "academic detailing" from medical or pharmaceutical advisers, and downward pressure on prescribing budgets.

There are numerous data points indicating that physicians tend to overestimate their patients' expectations. For instance, around 25% of patients leave general practice consultations with prescriptions they did not expect to receive. Conversely, patients who believe that antibiotics can solve all their current issues could significantly influence doctors' prescribing habits. Unhappy patients are more likely to seek a second opinion. Inappropriate prescribing and medication waste may result from discrepancies between patients' preferences and doctors' perceptions. Prescriptions are often used by doctors to conclude consultations, but it is time-consuming to thoroughly explore patients' beliefs, reasons for seeking advice, treatment preferences, attitudes toward medications, and past experiences. Ironically, this could lead to unreasonable demands by reinforcing patients' misconceptions.

Surprisingly, there has been little research on how guidelines impact professional practice. Reducing inappropriate care can be achieved through well-designed, effectively distributed, and implemented guidelines. These guidelines should be backed by reliable data, tailored to the community, and disseminated through engaging educational activities involving influential community members. Demand may increase when there are numerous unmet needs. It is also expected that the development of integrated care pathways will reduce resource wastage. Innovative software like Wax may enhance the effectiveness of local providers by providing desktop access to guidelines, evidence, and crucial information (such as wait times). Lastly, guidelines can form the basis for audits.

2.6.4. The Interface with Secondary Care

The rates of secondary care referrals by general practitioners are influenced by numerous factors. Scholars have endeavored in vain to elucidate the fluctuations in referral behavior. Only a small percentage of the variation can be explained by factors related to doctors, patients, and services. The "referral thresholds" of particular practitioners and their ability to handle uncertainty have drawn a lot of attention lately. A significant amount of the variation in health service use among general practitioners in small-area analyses is likely due to variations in this threshold both within and between general practitioners.

Three interrelated questions are relevant to attempts to change professional behavior at this interface:

- What is the purpose of seeking the specialist's opinion?
- What are the alternatives to referral to secondary care? and
- What incentives exist for general practitioners to change current practice?

Frequently, general practitioners fail to explain their referral decisions to patients. If one needs assurance or guidance on management, a quick phone call could offer the required assistance.

General practitioners rarely cross-refer to colleagues with specialized skills and interests before referring to a hospital, even though it may not always meet patients' expectations. In primary care groups, the incentives for doing so might get stronger. In the US, payment might be contingent upon a second medical opinion. In the future, teleconferencing consultations might offer a useful substitute for standard outpatient referrals.

Referral criteria may lower the number of inappropriate referrals, better prepare those who are being referred, and guarantee that patients in greater need receive hospital referrals as soon as possible. Sharing responsibility for these clear standards lessens the general practitioner's burden of rejection. An essential component of this process is the patients' and providers' informed, active participation.

Large fundholding practices and multi-funds have set the standard in the UK for tracking and disclosing information about the doctors they refer business to, as well as for allocating work among large teams to more effectively utilize pre-existing skills. There is, however, little data regarding how feeding back to practices affects their relative referral rates. Low referral rates do not always indicate that a practice is good. Data by itself won't have a meaningful or long-lasting impact on outliers due to the inherent difficulties in interpretation. It could be more beneficial to focus on recognized indicators of high-quality healthcare. Markers of cost-effective practice may be found in specific diagnostic tests (radiography for back pain, for example) or prescription patterns (the ratio of inhaled steroids to bronchodilators, for example). It also needs more investigation to see if outcome metrics like acute asthma admission rates accurately represent the caliber of care given.

Advocates of managed care in the US style have brought in a lot of rhetoric but not much else. This could alter: clinical governance in primary care groups may take on different forms depending on the utilization management strategies used by health maintenance organizations. With significant potential to alter the location of care, some of the more creative ideas in the personal medical services (PMS) pilot programs foreshadow the vertical integration of healthcare. However, a negative effect of unified budgets might be the rise in low-priority, revenue-generating activities. These misgivings arose from the surge in minor surgery that followed the 1990 contract modifications.

2.6.5. A Strategic Approach

Primary care groups will have an increased incentive to manage demand more methodically as they become independent entities accountable to their health authorities and take on responsibility for devolved budgets. Savings ought to be reinvested in patient care. But as a buyer and a provider, these agreements and the personal medical services pilots pose difficult ethical dilemmas for general practitioners. It makes sense that doctors are still reluctant to be held responsible for their cash-constrained budgets for on-demand services. Both individual and group patient participation will be required in the decision-making process.

It is risky to overemphasize individual approaches in isolation given the variety of approaches available for demand management. It will take a variety of approaches to alter patient and physician behavior at the practice level. These must be based on credible data, endorsed by other primary healthcare team members, and supported by them (Murphy et al., 1998; Perdersen et al., 1996) (Figure 2.4).

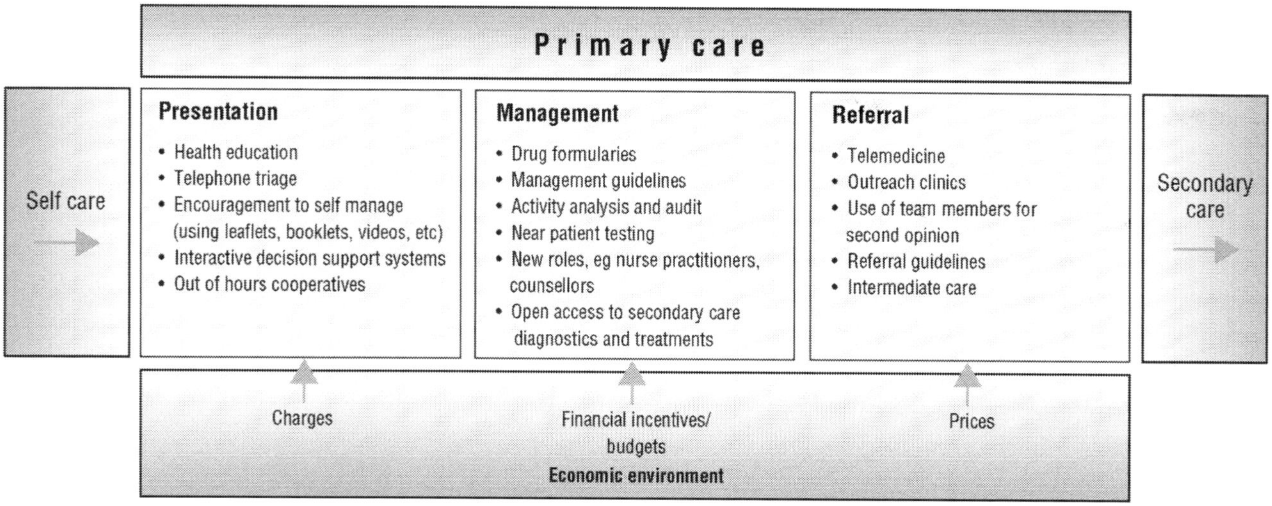

Figure 2.4. *Approaches to demand management in primary care.*

Source: https://www.ncbi.nlm.nih.gov/pmc/articles/PMC1113367/.

2.7. The Limits to Demand for Healthcare

There are numerous reasons why the National Health Service (NHS) has historically been underinvested, including historical, political, and economic factors. However, one significant deterrent to expansion is the belief that any increase in funding will only lead to more failures, despite higher costs. Additionally, the imbalance between the growing demand for healthcare services and the limited supply is expected to worsen as the population ages, new technologies emerge, and expectations increase. This belief has become so ingrained that questioning the connection between specific failures in healthcare delivery and the overall mismatch between supply and demand is often disregarded as an unrealistic denial.

The term "rationing" is most frequently used to discuss these issues. Restricting access to healthcare through measures that, in the opinion of the commentator, are most likely to increase effectiveness, be efficient, equitable, ethical, advantageous to the independent sector, or be politically feasible, is the concern with rationing. During a recession, the rationing debate gained prominence, meaning that decisions about healthcare "choices" involved deciding to provide less. The conventional, if implausible, insistence that the term "rationing" has a neutral meaning will be put to the test in the welcome new context of the United Kingdom's anticipated significant increase in healthcare spending.

2.7.1. Rationing the Evidence

The rationing controversy is incredibly non-scientific. The literature is dominated by assertion, political analysis, and ethical debate, and the problem it seeks to address is assumed rather than expressed in any form that can be refuted. In other fields of public health, claims need to be backed up by evidence. For instance, if the argument for a national health concern about the consequences of childhood obesity were based solely on accidental observations of obese children, it would not be accepted; instead, representative body mass index data from samples large enough to support reliable population estimates would be needed. In contrast, there isn't much relevant data in the rationing debate. Any specific failure is interpreted as proof of a worldwide deficiency in resources, which is the epidemiological equivalent of using the occasional obese person as proof positive enough to support an anti-obesity initiative.

The concepts of bias and representativeness are now widely acknowledged in the clinical setting to the point where certain observations are criticized for being anecdotal and therefore not suitable for generalization to a larger population. It is possible to demonstrate the epidemiological naivete that permeates discussions of health policy by examining current patterns of provision and utilization trends.

The persistent inability to meet the need for various efficient and high-volume medical procedures has long been seen as a sign of poor management of demand within the NHS. However, a closer examination suggests that this may not necessarily be due to an overall imbalance between supply and demand. For instance, in December 1999, approximately 1,10,000 individuals in England were waiting for day-case treatment in general surgery, with around 21,000 of them having waited over six months. While there are significant shortages in some regions, the majority of centers are able to meet demand effectively. The question then arises as to which group is truly representative: the 10% causing 35% of the issues, or the 10% with no issues at all? The common assumption that those failing to meet demand are indicative of a wider problem is akin to using a few overweight individuals to represent an entire population (Figure 2.5).

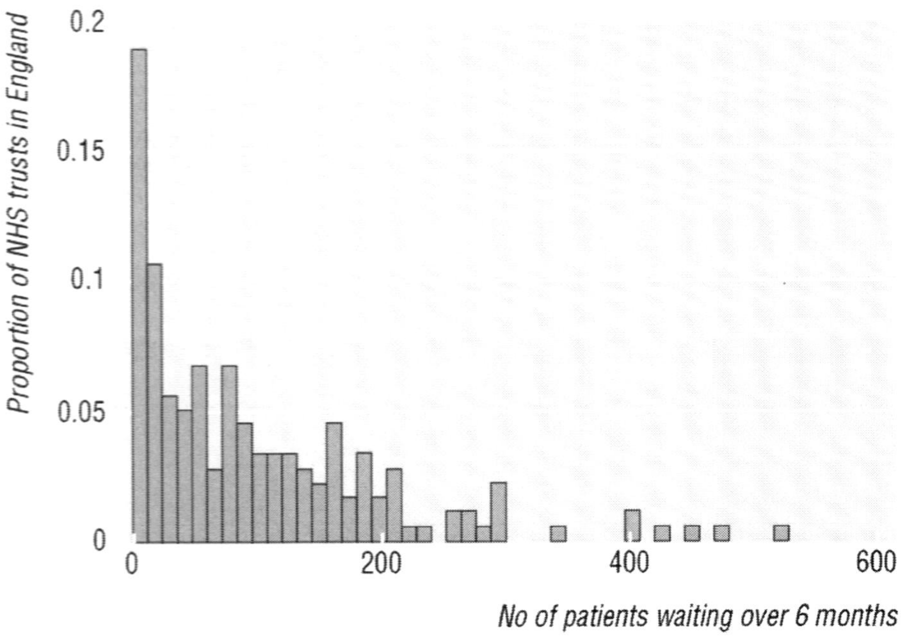

Figure 2.5. *Proportions of NHS trusts in England that had patients waiting more than six months for day-case general surgery.*

Source: https://www.ncbi.nlm.nih.gov/pmc/articles/PMC1127687/.

It is more common to voice concerns about a trend rather than raise doubts about it when it is believed that the demand for healthcare is rising. During times of increased demand, high rates of bed occupancy in the UK inevitably result in bed crises. These recurring issues are understood to be manifestations of the unstoppable rise in demand brought on by an aging population. In actuality, emergency admission rates are rising in certain regions while supposedly rising in others are mainly the result of counting patients transferred between hospital consultants. This is more of a situation that calls for further contextual investigation than it is an example of a worldwide, unsolvable problem. Fascinatingly, population-based utilization metrics in the UK, like the percentage of the population admitted to hospitals annually, have stayed remarkably stable over the last 15 years. Between 1988 and 1993, the Oxford area's total ordinary admissions "increased" by -0.3%. Throughout the decade from 1981–1982 to 1991–1992, the number of consultations in primary care increased by just 2–4%, from 33,961 to 34,785 per 10,000 person-years at risk. This is hardly an insurmountable challenge for the NHS.

2.7.2. The Epidemiology of Indications

It is challenging to explain the traditionally pessimistic forecasts regarding the relationship between demand and supply by looking at the overall epidemiological trends, which are generally positive. The rates of coronary heart disease and stroke, which contribute to healthcare demand, have been decreasing since the 1970s. Cancer rates vary between different age groups, with a decrease among younger men but an increase among older men, and a similar pattern occurring for women at age 50. Despite these varying trends, the overall outlook is positive as cohort effects gradually impact the population. However, this broad analysis may not be useful, as the true demand on the healthcare system is determined more by the need for beneficial forms of care rather than just the incidence of disease.

2.7.2.1. Examples of Failure

As an alternative to taking such a broad approach, breaking down the different areas of care can teach us a lot about evaluating the relationship between supply and demand. Demand is met in most areas of provision, meaning that everyone who is at risk is given care, such as in cases of major trauma, cancer, and childbirth. The NHS's reactions in other cases, like counseling and cosmetic surgery, are erratic. Although the boundaries between the mandatory and discretionary care poles of the continuum are clearly defined, they become more arbitrary in the vicinity of the marginal cases. Conditions for which there are waiting lists and conditions for which relief is ostensibly an obligatory NHS service, but the obligation is frequently not fulfilled, are examples of the failure to meet demand. Two of the most well-known instances of these are total hip replacement and cataract extraction, two elective surgical procedures that are relatively inexpensive and have a profoundly positive impact on patients' lives.

Conventional epidemiology is not able to estimate the potential demand for total hip replacement because the relationship between pathology and the likelihood of benefiting from treatment is not clear. A study was therefore carried out on a sample of 28,080 people to determine the prevalence of total hip replacement among the English population. Patients who indicated a preference and were deemed suitable for surgery needed 46,600 primary replacement procedures annually on average. This is in contrast to the approximately 43,500 primary total hip replacements currently provided in NHS and private hospitals in England. This minor discrepancy would be eliminated if every NHS orthopedic hospital performed slightly more hip replacements each month. Thus, the current state of affairs regarding access to this surgery cannot be explained by the magnitude of potential demand. Though they are not accompanied by under-provision, it is noteworthy that the levels of need for total hip replacement surgery in the United States and the United Kingdom are comparable.

Cataract surgery is a relatively inexpensive, safe, and effective treatment for one of the most common causes of irreversible vision loss in the elderly. Poorer nations are likely to lack access to cataract surgery, but it is unclear why older people in wealthy nations like the UK suffer from such easily reversible morbidity. To make treatment decisions, it is important to take into account factors other than the traditional pathology measurements, such as the pathology's effect on the patient's quality of life and surgical suitability. An estimated 3,25,000 people in England were estimated to require cataract extractions based on a study that used a random sample of 2,783 people. This population is served by about 600 ophthalmic surgical teams. The service could handle about 3,00,000 cataract extractions annually if each of them offered two surgical lists per week and removed five cataracts from each list (an acceptable level of activity). In Brighton, there was one instance of demand satisfaction. There don't appear to be many significant obstacles standing in the way of this being accomplished nationwide, where existing access uncertainties are to be replaced by booking systems based on established surgical criteria.

Such treatments have historically been rationed based on a patient's willingness to pay or wait, and previous inability to meet demand has frequently been invoked as an excuse for more stringent rationing. By breaking down the care areas where demand has not been satisfied, it is possible to move even these instances of failure from the NHS's discretionary to required areas with minimal impact on current treatment costs. The core mistake underpinning the health economists' hegemony in this discussion is the conviction that a sound macro-level assumption—that decisions must be made regarding the allocation of limited resources—can be blindly applied to the micro-level, where it may or may not be applicable. It is important to challenge accepted beliefs in other care domains if the notions of an inevitable mismatch between supply and demand in the sentinel conditions under consideration have minimal epidemiological support.

2.7.3. Changing Patterns of Demand and Supply

When we consider that the current adverse balance is negatively impacted by the three frequently mentioned adverse pressures of rising life expectancy, new technologies, and increased public expectations, the question of whether we can keep up with today's problems may become moot. Why is this trio being portrayed in such a negative light when each could alternatively be viewed as a symbol of desirable advancement?

2.7.3.1. Age

Policymakers are fond of doomsday scenarios and demographic time bombs; they do not appear to be deterred by the fact that earlier crisis forecasts have not come to pass. It is crucial to understand that the relationship between aging and healthcare costs is, for the most part, one of association rather than causation. The number of older people is growing and will continue to grow if life expectancy rises. The process of dying has a strong correlation with healthcare costs. Although the amount of time spent in the hospital tends to increase with age, even for the elderly, this increase is typically limited to the period just before death. Healthcare expenses will decrease as people live longer, but this is the price of dying, not growing older. Given that people are more likely to be in their final years as they age when healthcare costs will be concentrated, cross-sectional data are especially misleading in this regard. There is no proof that older patients in the US require more acute care, and long-term data indicate that, once the remaining lifetime is taken into account, healthcare spending does not appear to be influenced by age. In addition, a rising standard of living may shorten the time between the onset of illness and death, leading to a compression of morbidity; in fact, the percentage of people in the UK who needed assistance with everyday tasks was cut in half between 1976 and 1991. According to recent projections, accounting for the increasing fitness of successive cohorts of older adults in the UK lowers the population burden of disability by approximately three times, from 3.5 million to 1 million by 2051.

It would be inaccurate to characterize longevity as merely a burden on society since it is one of the benefits of prosperity. An aging population will have an impact on healthcare, but the full impact won't become apparent until further research is conducted. It is not acceptable to accept the conventional wisdom that a wealthy nation like the United Kingdom must inevitably struggle to care for its citizens when it is required.

2.7.3.2. The Cost of Innovation

Innovation is embraced in most domains, but in the medical field, new technologies are frequently viewed as a threat to stability. The presumption that new technology must result in significant cost increases that are most likely unachievable is not sufficiently challenged or backed by empirical data. It is unclear whether increased spending during the 1970s was caused by or a result of new technology, and an analysis of new medical technology introduced during that time would not support the assumption that new technologies increase costs.

One issue with pricey new technologies is that their modest clinical effectiveness often belies the high expectations placed on them. Only specific innovations and specific problems can be used to judge this issue; some innovations will cost more while others will save money. According to a study on the evolving trends in peptic ulcer diagnosis and treatment, new technology has reduced costs. For other conditions, this may or may not be the case. For instance, the expenses of the 1950s practice of delayed mobilization following myocardial infarction, at today's prices, may very well turn out to be similar to those of contemporary intensive interventions and brief hospital stays. Drugs like statins, which are too costly for general use, lower the number of coronary revascularizations, which saves money but in a different area of the healthcare system.

The introduction of several expensive drugs, such as sildenafil (Viagra) or the influenza drug zanamivir (Relenza), which were either marginally beneficial or marginal to conventional clinical practice, led to the recent political acknowledgement that an open-ended commitment was unsustainable for the NHS. The growing expense of medications is frequently brought up in these talks as an unavoidable limitation. This is untrue: complex commercial judgmental factors and broader political interest in a crucial industry determine prices. For example, the fact that statins cost roughly one-seventh of what the NHS pays in India disproves the notion that they should be rationed and restricted to treating people who have an abnormally high risk of coronary heart disease to lower mortality from the condition. The cost-effectiveness of these medications would be on par with other secondary preventive measures in the UK if they had equivalent pricing. There is obviously some discretion in the costs of these kinds of innovations, at the very least.

2.7.3.3. Public Expectations

The third argument in favor of pessimism is the claim that the needs of a better-informed public must grow faster than the ability of the health system to meet them. The empirical foundation for such future projections must be very thin when there is so little information available about current expectations. The patient should be the real expert and the main decision-maker when the illness is not life-threatening or when there are only questionable benefits to the treatment. The treatments that people prefer and what is offered sometimes diverge dramatically. Treatment non-compliance is a persistent problem, but how this is understood is changing. Increasingly, the 30–50% of people who refuse to take prescribed medications are not viewed as non-compliant; rather, their actions are understood as logical choices made by people who may have a better understanding of their issues than the doctor. Robust evidence suggests that an informed public is equally apt to refuse treatments as they are to call for increased availability of them.

Ultimately, the majority of people prefer to pass away at home, but passing away in an institution is becoming more common. Evidence that other public expectations can rise as well, most notably the expectation of protection from treatments for which the risks are likely to outweigh the benefits from the individual's point of view, must temper the oversimplified assumption that "increased public expectations" equates with overwhelming demand. It is impossible to forecast how these contradicting implications will balance out, but it might be influenced if the public is led toward safety rather than misinformation.

2.7.4. The Social Construction of Pessimism

Thus, these various factors will gradually moderate the extent of reasonable demand. One explanation for the prevalence of the pessimistic interpretation is the ongoing informal examination of healthcare experiences, their constant media coverage, and their role as a seasoning for much political discourse, all of which contribute to the difficulty of making an informed prediction of the outcome's balance.

Modern health systems may reassure the well-affected and solve or lessen many issues related to diseases that were previously incurable, but their main focus is on a wave of suffering, fear, humiliation, and death. Thus, a happy health service is a bit of a contradiction. Rather than being the result of an insufficient health system, many of the issues that spark discussions about rationing have more to do with an unwillingness to accept that certain disease processes are unavoidable. Sensitivity to the feelings of sick individuals and their families or the bereaved often prevents informed comment in cases like the child case, in which a health authority denied additional treatment to a child with non-Hodgkin's lymphoma. Prosperity accentuates this kind of denial of mortality and the irreversibility of much morbidity, which could explain the otherwise strange correlation between a nation's wealth and its obsession with rationing.

The widespread emphasis on failure also contains a thread of professional self-interest. One of the biggest employers in the UK is the National Health Service (NHS). Disinterested evidence does not always imply unfulfilled demand. Ordered coping is rarely rewarded in the competitive process of bidding for additional resources. The potential for abuse that comes with a system that provides financial incentives for deliberately low productivity is still present with surgical waiting lists. The National Health Service (NHS) continues to rely on a remarkable reservoir of compassion; however, it would be naive to claim that staff interests and public interests always align. It is less probable to arrive at a fair evaluation of the system's ability to satisfy demand when there are undercurrents in the information flow. With the pool so shallow, it can be hard to see why the NHS should be viewed as drowning (Coast et al., 1995; Cropper et al., 1977).

A Closer Look

Economic Development and Health

It is commonly known that good health can lead to better opportunities for growth and development, or that poor health can have the opposite effect and lead to slower rates of economic growth and development. It is hypothesized to relate to: (i) labor productivity and growth regarding nutrition; (ii) population dynamics and fertility concerning growth; and (iii) child and youth health concerning growth. This is not a one-way relationship, though, as wealth growth (through economic development and the ensuing spending on health services) is thought to be beneficial to health.

The development of the modern economy since the early 19th century has resulted in improvements in life expectancy and a decrease in infant mortality. These metrics have improved as a result of technological advancements (such as vaccinations and antibiotics) as well as a better knowledge of the factors that contribute to illness, such as inadequate sanitation. Many illnesses are incapacitating rather than deadly. For those afflicted, the financial burden of these illnesses consists of lost wages and out-of-pocket medical expenses. Low productivity and the upfront expenses of medical care are the nation's two biggest financial burdens. New medications and better hygienic conditions became more widely available in low-income nations during the second half of the 20th century as a result of the dissemination of knowledge and technology in these areas. The improved services would not have been affordable without the wealth increase that made this possible. Even at low-income levels, significant improvements in health can be achieved. Because of the intricate relationships between income levels and the costs of infrastructure, health services, education, clean water, better housing, sanitation systems, etc., individuals worldwide live nearly 25 years longer now than they did in 1900 at comparable income levels. It's crucial to remember, though, that there is a nonlinear relationship between wealth and health.

Once a critical threshold is reached, improvements in health can be achieved even with low-income levels. At this stage, even small advancements in economic growth can lead to significant enhancements in health outcomes. The significance of collaboration between various sectors is emphasized, as it often increases the efficiency of health programs, particularly in low-income settings. For instance, infrastructure investments such as roads can help pregnant women reach delivery services promptly and ensure vaccines reach health facilities without compromising their quality. Additionally, basic education has been shown to empower mothers to make informed decisions when dealing with health issues.

Better health has a demographic connection that can also support economic growth. Even though they are less evident, changes in a population's demographic makeup can arise from more children living to adulthood, which raises the ratio of people who are employed to those who are not. It is argued that this "demographic dividend" has the potential to be a major force behind economic expansion if the more liberal policy framework permits these workers to find gainful employment. Given the synergistic achievement of intra-sectoral linkages, it is anticipated that the population's per capita income will rise quickly in response to the changing age structure of the population. For instance, in East Asia, the population of working age increased several times quickly between 1965 and 1990 than the population of dependents. This change has been ascribed by a number of studies to the decrease in infant mortality brought about by the development of new medical technologies like antibiotics and anti-malarial medications as well as broad advancements in clean water and sanitation.

Good health is essential for economic growth, while poor health can hinder it significantly. This is especially evident in poorer countries, where disease burdens are often higher. Poor health can impact economic development by reducing both the quantity and quality of the workforce available. As a result, the number of hours worked decreases, negatively affecting national income. If unhealthy trends persist, the rate of economic growth will be greatly impacted. This leads to a decrease in resources available for investment in areas such as education, healthcare, and living conditions. Ultimately, this creates a cycle of poor health and poverty that becomes increasingly difficult to break.

Summary

- The amount of goods or services that consumers plan to buy depends on the prices of other goods and services.
- Medical care consists of countless goods and services that maintain, improve, or restore a person's health.
- Demand requires people to seek a service they can afford and are willing to pay for it. The need for healthcare is the care that doctors believe is essential for a person to stay healthy or healthy.
- Demand for healthcare depends on the level of consumption of an individual in case of illness; the amount of consumption can differ according to the factors affecting the demand, such as income, service price, education, norms, social traditions, and quality.
- Developing countries are focused on promoting healthcare as an essential policy to improve health outcomes and fulfill international obligations and universal coverage of health services.
- Grossman used human capital theory to explain the demand for healthcare. According to human capital theory, people invest in themselves through education and health to increase their income.
- The Grossman model of health demand is a model for studying the demand for health and medical care outlined by Michael Grossman in a monograph in 1972 entitled: "The demand for health: A theoretical and empirical investigation."
- The demand for health is somewhat more complicated than the demand for a typical product and estimating the elasticity of demand for health is less straightforward.
- The types of healthcare services offered vary widely and we might expect that the elasticity of demand for specific service types would vary.
- Understanding the demand for healthcare paid for by a particular health plan is somewhat more complex than understanding the demand for healthcare in general.
- Adverse selection is an important consideration in the estimation of demand elasticities for healthcare. Adverse selection occurs when persons with poor health tend to choose insurance with high benefits and persons with good health tend to avoid such insurance because of its high cost.
- The growth of health insurance, both public and private, has had a profound impact on the demand for medical care.
- The objectives of demand management are essentially utilitarian: the maximization of total met need for the greatest number within available resources.
- As primary care groups take responsibility for devolved budgets and become freestanding bodies accountable to their health authorities, the incentive to manage demand more systematically will grow.
- It is difficult to justify the conventionally unfavorable forecasts of the relation between demand and supply of overall epidemiological trends, as these are broadly favorable.

- Modern health systems resolve or ameliorate many problems with illnesses that until recently were insoluble and they may provide reassurance to those who are well, but their predominant concern is with a tide of pain, fear, indignity, and death.

References

1. Acton, J. P. (1975). Nonmonetary factors in the demand for medical services: Some empirical evidence. *Journal of Political Economy, 83*(3), 595–614.
2. Bagust, A., Place, M., & Posnett, J. (1999). Dynamics of bed use in accommodating emergency admissions: Stochastic simulation model. *BMJ, 319*(7203), 155–158.
3. Coast, J., Inglis, A., Morgan, K., Gray, S., Kammerling, M., & Frankel, S. (1995). The hospital admissions study: Are there alternatives to emergency hospital admission? *Journal of Epidemiology & Community Health, 49*(2), 194–199.
4. Cropper, M. L. (1977). Health, investment in health, and occupational choice. *Journal of Political Economy, 85*(6), 1273–1294.
5. Finkelstein, A., Taubman, S., Wright, B., Bernstein, M., Gruber, J., Newhouse, J. P., Allen, H., Baicker, K., & Oregon Health Study Group. (2012). The Oregon health insurance experiment: Evidence from the first year. *The Quarterly Journal of Economics, 127*(3), 1057–1106.
6. Frankel, S. (1989). The natural history of waiting lists: Some wider explanations for an unnecessary problem. *Health Trends, 21*(2), 54–56.
7. Frankel, S., Eachus, J., Pearson, N., Greenwood, R., Chan, P., Peters, T. J., et al. (1999). Population requirements for primary hip-replacement surgery: A cross-sectional study. *Lancet, 353*(9161), 1304–1309.
8. Grundy, E. (1997). The health and health care of older adults in England and Wales, 1841-1994. In J. Charlton & M. Murphy (Eds.), *The health of adult Britain 1841–1994* (pp. 182–203). London: Stationery Office.
9. Himsworth, R., & Goldacre, M. (1999). Does time spent in hospital in the final 15 years of life increase with age at death? A population-based study. *BMJ, 319*(7221), 1338–1339.
10. Morgan, K., Prothero, D., & Frankel, S. (1999). The rise in emergency admissions—Crisis or artifact? Temporal analysis of health service data. *BMJ, 319*(7203), 158–159.
11. Murphy, S. (1998). Does new technology increase or decrease health care costs? The treatment of peptic ulcer. *Journal of Health Services Research & Policy, 3*(4), 215–218.
12. Perdersen, T. R., Kjekshus, J., Berg, K., Olsson, A. G., Wilhelmsen, L., & Wedel, H. (1996). Cholesterol lowering and the use of health care resources: Results from the Scandinavian Simvastatin Survival Survey. *Circulation, 93*(10), 1796–1802.

Chapter

SUPPLY IN HEALTHCARE

3

Contents

Introduction

Supply in healthcare refers to the intricate network of resources essential for the provision of medical services and the maintenance of patient well-being. This multifaceted system encompasses a wide array of components, ranging from pharmaceuticals and medical equipment to human resources and infrastructure. Understanding the dynamics of healthcare supply is paramount, as it directly influences the accessibility, quality, and efficiency of healthcare delivery.

Healthcare supply management involves the strategic coordination of resources to ensure timely access to essential goods and services while optimizing cost-effectiveness. This encompasses the procurement, distribution, utilization, and disposal of various supplies within healthcare facilities. Effective supply management not only addresses the immediate needs of patients but also plays a crucial role in safeguarding public health, particularly during emergencies and pandemics.

Orientation and Directional Terms:

Term	Definition	Illustration
Healthcare delivery	A healthcare delivery system includes all the people, institutions, and services that assist in care coordination, patient flows, diagnosis, disease management, and promotion of health maintenance programs.	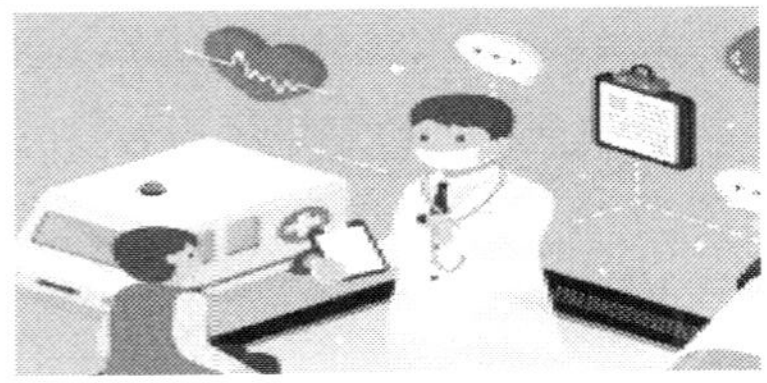
Supply curve	The supply curve is a graph that shows the quantity supplied at each price. Sometimes the supply curve is called a supply schedule because it is a graphical representation of the supply schedule.	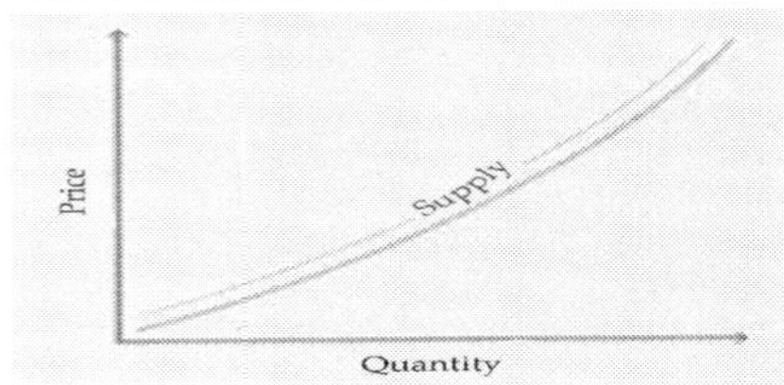
Product curves	Product curves are upside-down. Bowl-shaped curves that show the relationship between additional inputs, such as labor or capital, and how much of a good is actually produced.	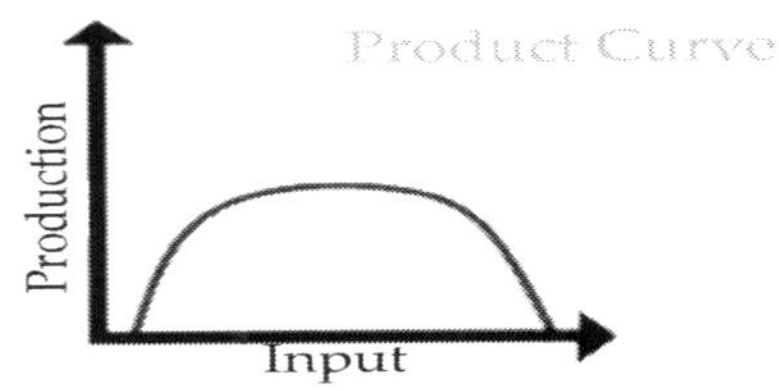
Average product curve	The average product curve is U-shaped, with the peak of the curve representing the point of diminishing returns. The point of diminishing returns refers to the point at which the marginal return (the output from one additional unit of input) begins to decline.	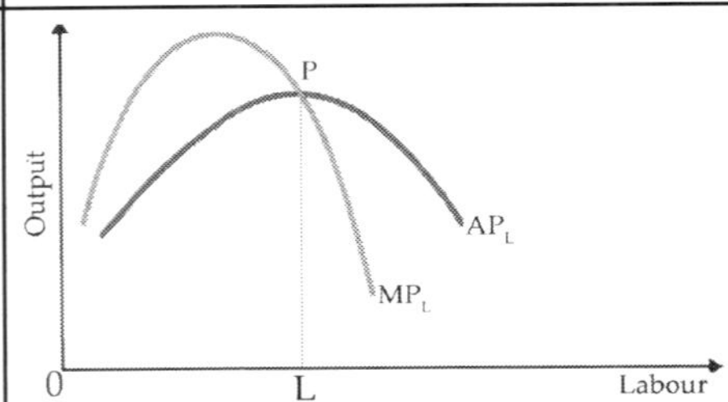
General practitioner	A general practitioner or family physician is a physician who treats acute and chronic illnesses and provides preventive care and health education to patients of all ages.	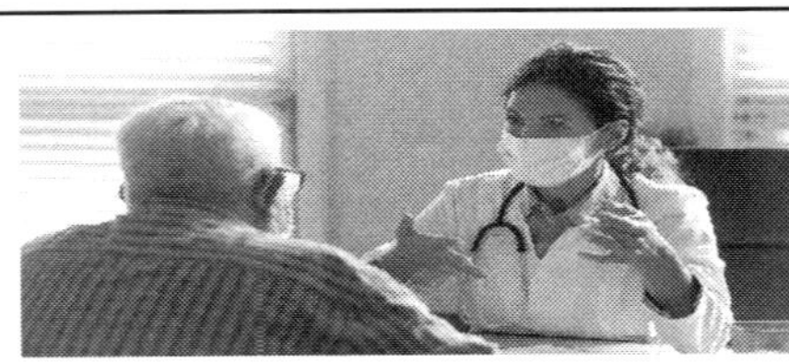

3.1. The Nature of Supply

The approach to the supply of healthcare is comparable to that of the demand for it. Hospitals, which offer healthcare services directly, as well as manufacturers of pharmaceuticals and medical equipment, which supply raw materials for the healthcare industry, are examples of suppliers. Theories of firm behavior—often referred to as the theory of the firm—have a significant impact on the supply side of the market.

In economics, theories of the firm that are predicated on the idea that their primary goal is to maximize profits frequently dominate analyses of supply. There are two ways to look at this. Firstly, these theories can be useful in positive economics to produce predictions about how markets and firms function since they are plausible explanations of the objectives of certain firms. That being said, a common feature of healthcare operations is that companies don't even try to maximize profits—rather, they don't even try to make any extra money at all. To stay in business over the long term, all firms need to generate a normal rate of return or profit. Most insurance and pharmaceutical companies want to make money, so maximizing profits might be a reasonable objective for them. In contrast, maximizing profit is not the goal of the majority of hospitals, nursing homes, and certain insurance companies. Though they offer a helpful set of performance benchmarks against which firms' actual performance can be compared, theories based on profit maximization have another use. Therefore, we will emphasize that while profit maximization models are important, other theories will be more appropriate for a large portion of the healthcare industry.

A supply curve with an upward slope for office visits is depicted in Figure 3.1. It shows, for instance, that if the cost was $90 per office visit, doctors would be willing to provide ten. Perhaps at a $100 fee, more visits would be available.

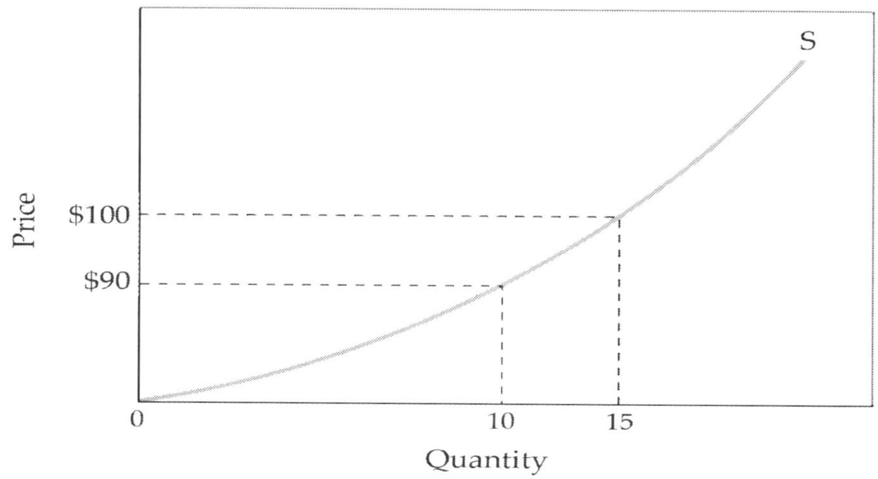

Figure 3.1. *Supply of office visits.*

Source: Data from – Johnson-Lans, (2004). A Health Economics Primer. Boston: Pearson Addison Wesley.

3.1.1. Factors That Affect Supply

We might come up with a list of supply shifters. The following are the variables that underlie the supply curve and are considered exogenous determinants of supply. The relationship between the output's price and the quantity supplied at the given prices is represented by the supply curve. One theory of an endogenous supply determinant is output price:

1. **Changes in Technology:** Healthcare products become more affordable to produce as technology advances. Undoubtedly, technological advancements that raise the price of goods without enhancing their quality are disregarded. As production costs decrease, suppliers are more inclined to offer a higher quantity of the product for sale at a given price. The supply curve moves to the right and increases.
2. **Input Prices:** If the wages of physicians were to rise, this increase in input cost would result in suppliers' willingness to offer as much for sale at the original price. The supply would decrease, shifting the curve to the left.
3. **Prices of Production-Related Goods:** The price of a good related to production, such as a rise in the price of radiology services, would also be relevant. Because physicians can use radiology for diagnosis as well as treatment, this will cause the supply to decrease, thus shifting the supply curve to the left.
4. **Size of the Industry:** As more firms enter the market, the supply of the product will be greater. Therefore, the entry of firms will cause the supply curve to shift to the right.
5. **Weather:** For several products, acts of God such as weather will tend to affect production. The direction of the effect is obvious: good weather increases supply.

3.2. Short-Run Production Function of the Representative Medical Firm

The Representative Medical Firm's Short-Run Production Function: Producing and selling medical output generates income for all medical organizations, including hospitals, doctor's offices, assisted living facilities, and pharmaceutical companies. Production and retailing activities take place under any ownership structure (public, not-for-profit, or for-profit). Microeconomics may provide important insights into the management and planning procedures of medical businesses since these activities take place in an environment where resources are limited.

To simplify our discussion of short-run production, we make five assumptions. First, we assume the medical firm produces a single output of medical services, q. Second, we initially assume only two medical inputs exist: nurse hours and a composite capital good, k. We can think of the composite capital good as an amalgamation of all types of capital, including any medical equipment and the physical space in the medical establishment. Third, since the short run is defined as a period over which the level of at least one input cannot be changed, we assume the quantity of capital is fixed at some amount. This assumption makes intuitive sense because it is usually more difficult to change the stock of capital than the number of nurse-hours in the short run. Fourth, we assume for now that the medical firm faces an incentive to produce as efficiently as possible. Finally, we assume the medical firm possesses perfect information regarding the demands for its product.

A production function shows the possible combinations and transformations of different inputs to get a final output. In this case, the production function shows the various combinations of capital and nurse hours that can be used to generate different levels of medical services. Every level of output can potentially be produced by multiple combinations of the nurse and capital inputs, according to the production function. Since each combination produces the highest output possible given the state of technology, it is assumed that each combination is technically efficient. It will become clearer later on that a unique least-cost, or economically efficient, method of production is determined by both technical and economic factors.

In the present example, the short-run production function for medical services can be mathematically generalized as:

$$q = f(n, \bar{k}). \quad (1)$$

Eqn. (1)'s short-run production function for medical services shows that the level of medical services is dependent on a fixed (by a bar) capital input and a variable nurse input. Assuming that the capital input $\bar{k}$, is fixed, we start our analysis by looking at the relationship between a higher quantity of the variable nurse input, *n*, and the level of medical services, *q*. The precise relationship between the amount of total output and the employment of the variable input is ascertained through the application of several production theories and microeconomic principles. The law of diminishing marginal productivity is a key microeconomic concept from production theory. This statement, which is more of a generalization about production behavior than a true law, indicates that, while all other inputs remain constant, total output initially increases at an increasing rate but eventually decreases in response to an increase in a variable input.

Figure 3.2 illustrates how the law of declining productivity works. It displays a graphical relationship between the number of nurse hours on the horizontal axis and the quantity of medical services on the vertical axis. Because it shows the total output produced by various levels of the variable input while holding all other inputs constant, the curve is also known as the total product curve, or TP. Take note of the fact that the number of services first rises steadily over the nurse-hour range of 0 to n_1. The slope of the curve at each point indicates the rate of increase. Through this range of nurse hours, the tangent lines get steeper, increasing the value of the slope of the total product curve.

Beyond point n_1, however, further increases in nurse hours cause medical services to increase, but at a decreasing rate. That is the point at which diminishing productivity sets in. Notice that the slope of the total product curve gets smaller as output increases in the range from n_1 to n_2 (as indicated by the flatter tangent lines). At n_2, the slope of the total product curve is zero, as reflected in the horizontal tangent line. Finally, beyond n_2, we allow for the possibility that too many nurse hours will lead to a reduction in the number of medical services. The slope of the total product curve is negative beyond n_2.

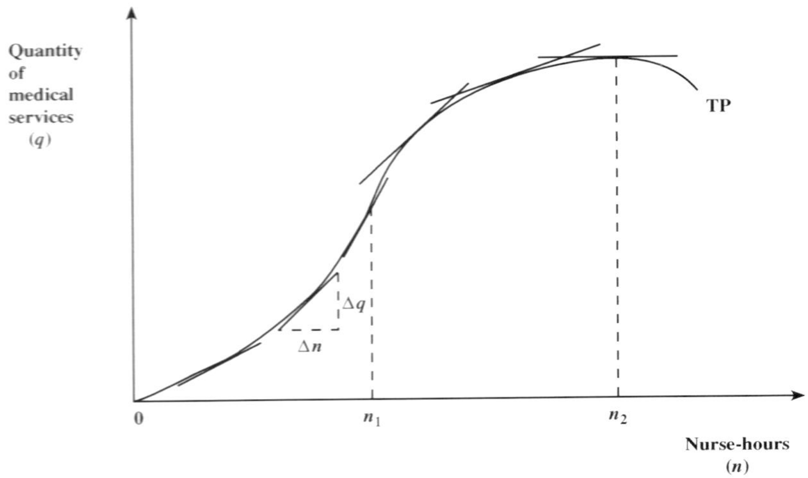

Figure 3.2. *The total product curve.*

Source: Rexford, E. S., & Stephen, P. N., (n.d.). Health Economics, ISBN-13: 978-0-324-78908-9.

The specific logic behind the law of diminishing marginal productivity has not yet been taken into consideration with regard to the production decision made at the firm level. The fixed short-run inputs are cited by economists as the cause of declining productivity. For instance, there is initially a significant amount of capital, the fixed input, available to produce medical services when nurse hours are increased. The availability of capital makes it possible to hire more nurses and provide ever-higher volumes of medical services. Furthermore, a synergy effect might take center stage at first. Because of labor specialization, for example, nurses who collaborate as a team can produce more output than they could individually. This is known as the synergy effect.

Eventually, the fixed capital is constrained about the variable input (such as insufficient medical space or equipment), and more nurse hours produce fewer and fewer incremental units of medical services. In the worst-case scenario, when more nurses are jammed into a medical facility that can only accommodate a certain number of staff members, congestion may start to reduce the number of services provided as unintended production issues arise.

3.2.1. Marginal and Average Products

Instead of using the total product curve to show the essential traits connected to the production process, we can also use the marginal and average product curves. The change in overall output resulting from a one-unit change in the variable input is commonly referred to as the marginal product. In terms of our example, the marginal product or quantity of medical services associated with an additional nurse-hour, MP_n, can be stated as follows:

$$MP_n = \Delta q/\Delta n. \quad (2)$$

The extra amount of medical services generated by each additional nurse-hour is indicated by the size of the marginal product of a nurse-hour. It is a measurement of the nurse-hour's marginal contribution to the output of medical services. Since the total product curve in Figure 3.2 measures the rise (vertical distance) over the run (horizontal distance), or $\Delta q/\Delta n$, it indicates the marginal product of a nurse-hour at each point. Therefore, by analyzing the slope of the total product curve at each level of nurse hours, we can ascertain the marginal product of an extra nurse hour. Figure 3.3 provides a graphic representation of a nurse-hour's marginal product. Marital productivity increases cause MP_n to increase from its initial positive value throughout the range of 0 to n_1. Because diminishing marginal productivity has set in, the marginal product is positive but decreasing in the range of n_1 to n_2. The marginal product of a nurse-hour is zero at n_2, and then it turns negative. According to the marginal product curve, it is not possible to anticipate that a nurse-hour will contribute the same marginal amount to overall output as the one before it. Because some other inputs are fixed, the law of diminishing marginal productivity states that, over time, a level of output will eventually be reached where an incremental increase in the number of nurse-hours results in progressively fewer additions to the total output.

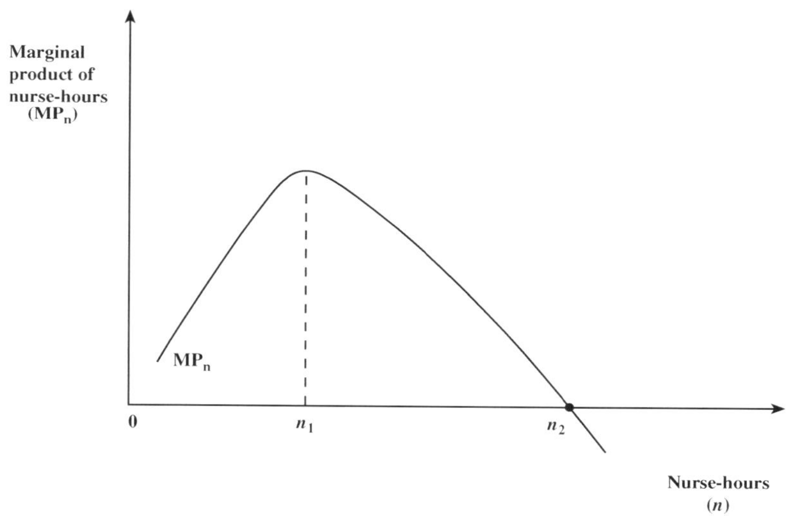

Figure 3.3. *The marginal product curve.*

Source: Rexford, E. S., & Stephen, P. N., (n.d.). Health Economics. ISBN-13: 978-0-324-78908-9.

Apart from MP_n, the mean value of a nurse hour can also offer valuable information about the manufacturing procedure. Generally speaking, the average product is calculated by dividing the total output by the variable input level. For this example, the total number of medical services divided by the total number of nurse hours yields the average product of a nurse hour, or AP_n:

$$AP_n = q/n. \tag{3}$$

The average amount of medical services provided in an hour is measured by the average product of a nurse-hour. For instance, let's say that the number of daily patient hours at a medical facility is how we (roughly) calculate the total amount of medical services. Furthermore, let's say that 200 nurse hours are needed to attend to 300 patient hours per day. In this case, 300/200, or 1½ patients per hour, is the average product of a nurse-hour.

We can also derive the average product of a nurse-hour from the total product curve, as shown in Figure 3.4(a). To derive AP_n, a ray from the origin is extended to each point on the total product curve. The slope of the ray measures AP_n for any given level of nurse hours since it equals the rise over the run, or q/n. In Figure 3.4(a), three rays labeled 0A, 0B, and 0C emanate from the origin to the total product curve. The slope of ray 0A is flatter than that of 0B and therefore is of a lower magnitude. As it is drawn, ray 0B has a greater slope than any other ray emanating from the origin. At this level of nurse hours, the average product is maximized. The slope of ray 0C is flatter and of a lower magnitude than that of 0B. The implication is that the average product initially increases over the range from 0 to n_3, reaches a maximum at n_3, and then decreases, as shown in Figure 3.4(b). It is the law of diminishing marginal productivity that accounts for the shape of AP_n.

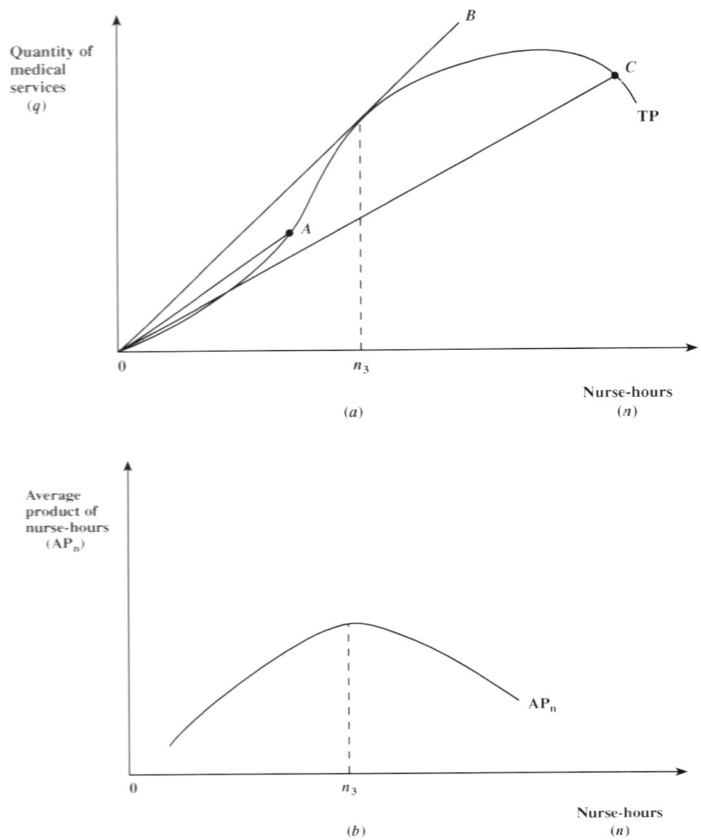

Figure 3.4. *Deriving the average product curve from the total product curve.*

Source: Rexford, E. S., & Stephen, P. N., (n.d.). Health Economics. ISBN-13: 978-0-324-78908-9.

The marginal and average product curves are superimposed in Figure 3.5 to show their relationship. A few noteworthy aspects of the relationship between these two curves are as follows. The average product curve is first cut at its maximum point by the marginal product curve. When the average reaches its extreme value, the marginal equals the average according to a widely accepted mathematical principle. Secondly, when AP_n is rising, MP_n is always higher than AP_n. This also illustrates a widely accepted mathematical concept, so the reader shouldn't be too surprised. For instance, if you receive an A on the final exam and your average grade in the course is B+ up until then, the incremental improvement in grade will raise your final average. Third, when AP_n is decreasing, MP_n is below AP_n. It should also come as no surprise that the marginal and average values relate to one another.

Putting the grades aside (because learning is more important than grades—right?), we can discuss the relation between the marginal and average product curves in terms of our example concerning nurse hours and the production of medical services. For this discussion, it helps to think of the marginal product curve as the amount of medical services generated hourly by the next nurse hired. Also, we can think of the average product curve as the average quantity of medical services generated by the existing team of nurses within an hour—that is, the "team" average.

Recalling Figure 3.5, you will see that, up to point n_3, the newly hired nurse consistently produces more services per hour than the team average. As a result, each extra nurse helps the team reach its average production level up to this point. However, after n_3, the team average declines because the newly hired incremental nurse produces fewer services per hour than the team average. It is crucial to understand that the unique skills of each additional nurse hired have no bearing on any increase or decrease in the marginal product. Instead, it has to do with the law of declining marginal productivity. The fixed input constraint causes the incremental nurse to become less productive at a certain point in the production process. The average productivity of the nursing team is influenced by the marginal productivity.

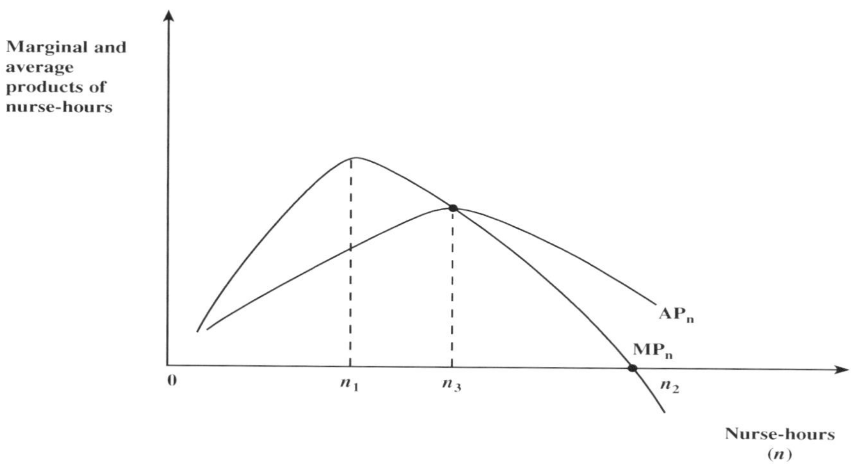

Figure 3.5. *Relation between the marginal and average product curves.*

Source: Rexford, E. S., & Stephen, P. N., (n.d.). Health Economics. ISBN-13: 978-0-324-78908-9.

It would seem reasonable to assume that a medical company would like to produce at a point similar to n_1 or n_3 in Figure 3.5. They are, after all, the locations where the average or marginal product is maximized. Generally speaking, though, a medical practice would prefer to hit a certain financial benchmark, like a break-even or maximum profit level. Therefore, before we can determine the ideal level of production, we need more details regarding the revenue and cost structures the medical firm must contend with.

3.2.2. Elasticity of Input Substitution

We have only considered one variable input up to this point. In practice, though, the medical company uses multiple variable inputs in the near term. As a result, any two variable inputs may be substituted in certain situations. For instance, in the provision of inpatient services, licensed practical nurses frequently take the place of registered nurses, and in the provision of ambulatory services, physician assistants occasionally take the place of physicians. Technical and legal considerations determine the true extent of substitutability between any two inputs. For instance, in the majority of states, it is illegal for physician assistants to write prescriptions. Furthermore, licensed practical nurses typically lack the technical expertise required to carry out all registered nurse responsibilities.

In general terms, the elasticity of substitution between any two inputs equals the percentage change in the input ratio divided by the percentage change in the ratio of the inputs' marginal productivities, holding constant the level of output, or

$$\sigma = \frac{\Delta(I_1/I_2)}{I_1/I_2} \div \frac{\Delta(\mathrm{MP}_2/\mathrm{MP}_1)}{\mathrm{MP}_2/\mathrm{MP}_1} \quad (4)$$

I_i(I = 1, 2) stands for the quantity employed of each input. The ratio of marginal productivities, MP_2/MP_1, referred to as the marginal rate of technical substitution, illustrates the rate at which one input substitutes for the other in the production process, at the margin. For example, suppose the marginal product of a registered nurse-hour is four patients and the marginal product of a licensed practical nurse-hour is two patients. It follows that two licensed practical nurse hours are needed to substitute completely for one registered nurse hour.

Theoretically, σ (Greek letter sigma) takes on values between 0 and $+\infty$ and identifies the percentage change in the input ratio that results from a 1% change in the marginal rate of technical substitution. The magnitude of s identifies the degree of substitution between the two inputs. For example, if $\sigma = 0$, the variable inputs cannot be substituted in production. In contrast, when $\sigma = \infty$, the two variable inputs are perfect substitutes in production. In practice, it is more common for σ to take on values between these two extremes, implying that limited substitution possibilities exist.

3.2.3. A Production Function for Hospital Admissions

Jensen & Morrisey (1986) provide one of the more interesting empirical studies on the production characteristics of hospital services. In keeping with Eqn. (1), Jensen & Morrisey estimated a production function for admissions at 3,540 non-teaching hospitals in the United States as of 1983 in the following general form:

Case-mix-adjusted hospital admissions = f(Physicians, nurses, other non-physician staff, hospital beds, X) (5)

Observe that the output is measured in terms of hospital admissions. However, because hospital services vary widely, this output measure was multiplied by the Medicare patient index to account for variations in case-mix among hospitals. This index is the weighted total of the Medicare patient proportions at the hospital across various diagnostic categories, with the weights representing the average case costs for each diagnostic category. The labor inputs were represented by the number of beds; the capital input was represented by the number of physicians, nurses (full-time equivalent [FTE] units), and other non-physician staff (FTE); X stood for several other production factors that were not relevant to the discussion.

Jensen and Morrisey specified a translog production function to transform Eqn. (5) into a format that can be estimated using a multiple regression technique. It is sufficient to mention that the translog is a flexible functional form that places very few constraints on the estimated parameters because the form and properties of this specific mathematical function are too complicated to briefly describe.

Jensen and Morrisey were able to calculate estimates of the marginal product of each input from the empirical estimation. The marginal products were all positive, as would be expected. As the law of diminishing marginal product suggests, Jensen & Morrisey observed that the marginal product of each input decreased in magnitude with increased usage. According to the estimated marginal product of a doctor, 6.05 more case-mix-adjusted annual admissions were produced by an extra doctor. The most fruitful input was by far that of the nurse. Specifically, the marginal nurse was accountable for approximately 20.3 more annual admissions adjusted for case-mix. It was discovered that the marginal products of beds and other non-physician staff were, respectively, 6.97 and 3.04 case-mix-adjusted annual admissions.

Additionally, the estimating process produced enough data for Jensen and Morrisey to quantify the input substitution options that hospitals have. Every input was discovered to serve as a stand-in for the others during production. Specifically, it was reported that the substitution elasticities between nurses and beds, physicians and nurses, and physicians and beds were, respectively, 0.547, 0.175, and 0.124. The average hospital can more easily switch between these two inputs, as indicated by the relatively large elasticity of 0.547 between physicians and nurses. According to this specific input elasticity estimate, ceteris paribus, a 10% increase in a doctor's marginal productivity results in a 5.47% increase in the nurse-to-doctor ratio. These positive substitution elasticities imply that by substituting with other inputs, hospital policymakers may be able to mitigate part of the price (wage) increase in any one input. For instance, a pay increase for nurses might be partially offset by adding more hospital beds to maintain a certain level of admissions (American Medical Association, Center for Health Policy Research (1998; Association of American Medical Colleges, 2002).

3.3. Short-Run Cost Theory of the Representative Medical Firm

We must address the distinction between the terminology used to describe costs by accountants and economists before moving on to our examination of the medical firm's cost curves. Specifically, when calculating the accounting profits of a medical firm, accountants only take into account the explicit costs of doing business. A recent market transaction can be used to calculate an exact cost; explicit costs are simple to quantify. Medical firms bear explicit costs in the form of electric utility bills, medical supply expenses, and wage payments to hourly medical staff because the amounts of these expenditures can be ascertained by consulting disbursement records.

Economists, unlike accountants, consider both the explicit and implicit costs of production. Implicit costs reflect the opportunity costs of using any resources the medical firm owns.

For instance, the physical assets (clinic, medical equipment) needed to provide physician services could belong to a general practitioner (GP). It is not possible to ascertain the cost of using these assets in this instance based on a recent market transaction. Nevertheless, there is an opportunity cost associated with using them since the physical assets could have been rented out for a different purpose. One possible course of action would be to remodel the clinic and lease it out as a beauty salon, while another doctor could lease the medical equipment. The opportunity cost of using the GP's physical assets is thus reflected in the rental payments that were forfeited.

Consequently, economists take into account the entire cost of doing business, including both explicit and implicit costs, when calculating the economic (as opposed to accounting) profits of a company. Economists think it's critical to ascertain whether enough revenues are coming in to pay for using all inputs—owned and rented alike. For instance, the GP may benefit more from renting out the physical assets than from keeping them for personal use if the rental return on those assets is higher than the return on use.

3.3.1. The Short-Run Cost Curves of the Representative Medical Firm

Cost theory is based on the production theory of the medical firm previously outlined and relates the quantity of output to the cost of production. As such, it identifies how (total and marginal) costs respond to changes in output. If we continue to assume the two inputs of nurse-hours, n, and capital, $\bar{k}$, the short-run total cost, STC, of producing a given level of medical output, q, can be written as:

$$STC(q) = w \times n + r \times \bar{k}, \quad (6)$$

where; *w* and *r* represent the hourly wage for a nurse and the rental or opportunity cost of capital, respectively. Input prices are assumed to be fixed, which means the single medical firm can purchase these inputs without affecting their market prices. This is a valid assumption as long as the firm is a small buyer of inputs relative to the total number of buyers in the marketplace.

Eqn. (6) suggests that the quantities and prices of the inputs used will determine the short-term total costs of production. The total wage bill, which reflects all variable costs of production, is equal to the wage rate multiplied by the number of nurse hours. Variable costs adjust in response to variations in the output level. The total fixed costs of production are calculated as the product of the capital quantity and the rental price. Given that the amount of capital is fixed in the short term, it follows that this cost component is not affected by variations in output.

The total product curve not only identifies the quantity of medical output produced by a particular number of nurse hours but also shows, reciprocally, the number of nurse hours necessary to produce a given level of medical output. With this information, we can determine the short-run total cost of producing different levels of medical output by following a three-step procedure. First, we identify, through the production function, the necessary number of nurse hours, n, for each level of medical output. Second, we multiply the quantity of nurse hours by the hourly wage, w, to determine the short-run total variable costs, STVC, of production, or w × n. Third, we add the short-run total fixed costs, STFC, or r × $\bar{k}$, to STVC to derive the short-run total costs, STC, of production. If we conduct this three-step procedure for each level of medical output, we can derive a short-run total cost curve like the one in Figure 3.6.

Take note of the reciprocal relationship between Figure 3.2 short-run total product curve and Figure 3.6 short-run total cost function. In Figure 3.6, for instance, short-run total costs increase at a decreasing rate up to point q_1, while total product increases at an increasing rate up to point n_1. This is because the overall costs of production rise more slowly as productivity increases in this range. The slope of the total product curve indicates that output increases at a decreasing rate beyond point n_1 in Figure 3.2 and that this causes the short-run total costs to increase at an increasing rate beyond q_1 in Figure 3.6. Observe that the only reason the overall costs rise with an increase in output is because more nurses are hired. Additionally, Figure 3.6 illustrates how the short-run total cost for the level of output q_2 can be broken down into its variable and fixed components.

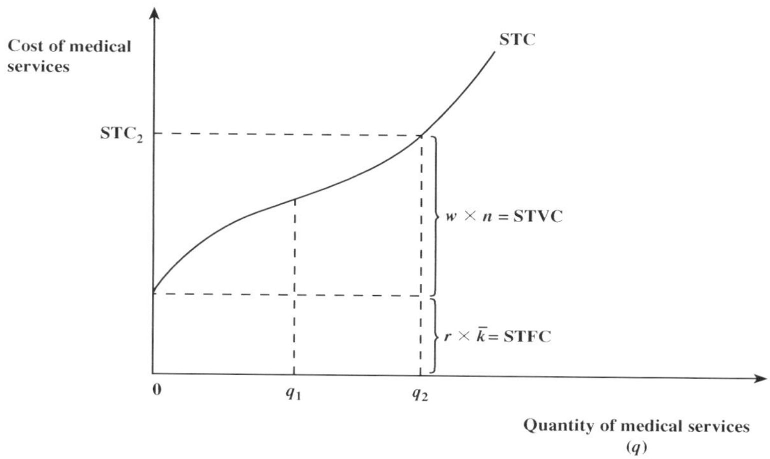

Figure 3.6. *The short-run total cost curve.*

Source: Rexford, E. S., & Stephen, P. N., (n.d.). Health Economics. ISBN-13: 978-0-324-78908-9.

Differentiating between fixed and variable costs can be especially difficult in practice. Keep in mind that fixed costs remain constant regardless of changes in the actual amount of output produced, while variable costs fluctuate proportionately. In the short term, during what is known as the "operating period," fixed costs arise because certain input levels are fixed. During the long-term planning phase, on the other hand, when future budgets are being created, for example, all inputs are variable. Because it takes a long time to build a new facility or move to a larger location, the physical size of a production facility is frequently regarded as a fixed input. Hourly employees can be quickly hired or fired based on the desired change in output, so they are usually viewed as a variable input. You can see that the fixity of costs and inputs is greatly influenced by time. Consequently, extended contracts add more fixed expenses to a company's budget even though they might have compensating advantages.

3.3.2. Short-Run Per-Unit Costs of Production

Another way to look at the reciprocal relation between production and costs is to focus on the short-run marginal and average variable costs of production. The short-run marginal costs, SMC, of production, are equal to the change in total costs associated with a one-unit change in output, or

$$SMC = \Delta STC/\Delta q. \qquad (7)$$

In terms of Eqns. (6) and (7), the short-run marginal costs of production look like the following:

$$\text{SMC} = \Delta(w \times n + r \times \bar{k})/\Delta q. \quad (8)$$

Because the wage rate and short-run fixed costs are constant concerning output, Eqn. (8) can be rewritten in the following manner:

$$\text{SMC} = w \times (\Delta n/\Delta q) = w \times (1/\text{MP}_n) = w/\text{MP}_n. \quad (9)$$

Notice on the right-hand side of Eqn. (9) that short-run marginal costs equal the wage rate divided by the marginal product of nurse hours. The short-run average variable costs, SAVC, of production, equal the short-run total variable costs, STVC, divided by the quantity of medical output. Because STVC is the total wage bill (that is, w × n):

$$\text{SAVC} = \text{STVC}/q = (w \times n)/q = w \times (1/\text{AP}_n) = w/\text{AP}_n \quad (10)$$

Such that, SAVC equals the wage rate divided by the average product of a nurse-hour. Notice that the short-run marginal and average variable costs are inversely related to the marginal and average products of labor, respectively. Thus, marginal and average variable costs increase as the marginal and average products fall, and vice versa. Figure 3.7 shows the graphical relation between the per-unit product and cost curves.

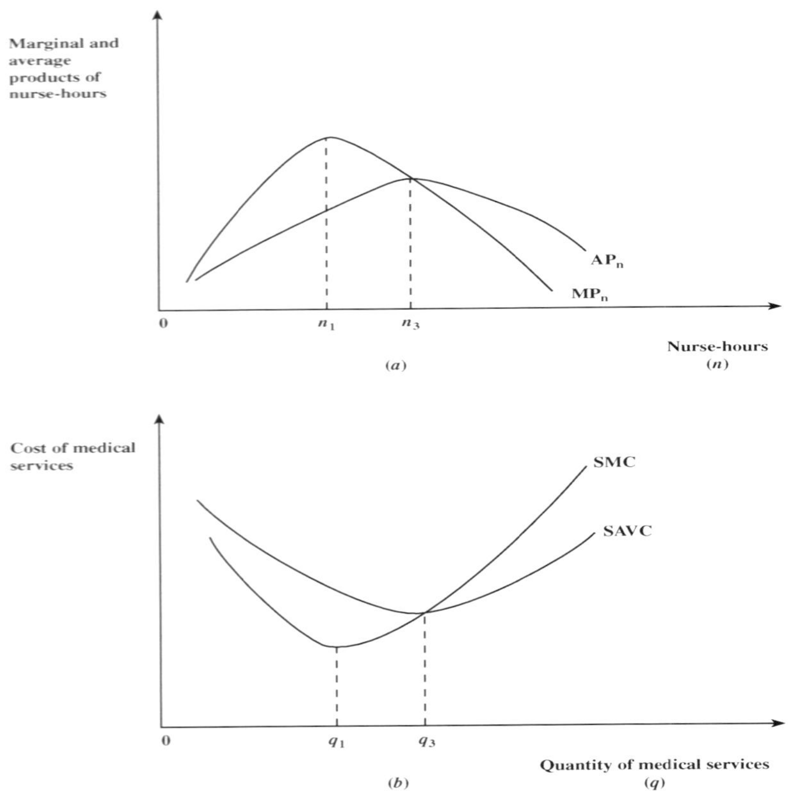

Figure 3.7. *Relation between the per-unit product and cost curves.*

Source: Rexford, E. S., & Stephen, P. N., (n.d.). Health Economics. ISBN-13: 978-0-324-78908-9.

The two graphs in Figure 3.7 make the reciprocal relationship between costs and production evident. For instance, diminishing productivity kicks in and the marginal product starts to drop after point n_1 in Figure 3.7(a). Because of this, given a fixed wage, the short-run marginal costs ($=w/MP_n$) rise above output level q_1. Similar to how the average product of a nurse-hour decreases after n_3, so do the average production variable costs after q_3. The law of diminishing marginal productivity is reflected in the shapes of the average variable cost and marginal cost curves. Production and costs are two different ways to observe aspects of the production process because of this reciprocal relationship.

Eqns. (9) and (10) make it clear that the minimum points on the marginal and average variable cost curves coincide exactly with the maximum points on the marginal and average product curves. It can be observed in Figure 3.7(b) that the short-run average variable cost curve's minimum point is crossed by the short-run marginal cost curve. Furthermore, when the SAVC curve is rising, the SMC curve is above it, and when it is falling, it is below it.

To put it simply, Figure 3.7(b) shows how costs change in response to short-term output changes made by the medical firm. First, the average and marginal variable costs of production decrease as the medical firm hires more nurses and increases output. The fixed inputs eventually cause diminishing productivity, which raises average and marginal variable cost. Thus, the amount of output a medical company produces in the short term affects both the marginal and average variable costs of production.

Besides the marginal and average variable costs of production, decision-makers are interested in the short-run average total costs of operating the medical firm. Following Eqn. (6), we can find the short-run average total costs of production by summing the average variable costs and average fixed costs. Short-run average fixed costs (SAFC) are simply total fixed costs (STFC) divided by the level of output.

$$\text{SAFC} = \text{STFC}/q. \quad (11)$$

The SAVC decreases as the value of the denominator, medical services, rises because the numerator in Eqn. (11) is by definition fixed in the short run. Therefore, as output increases, the average fixed costs of production decrease because total fixed costs, also known as overhead costs, are dispersed over an increasing number of units.

SMC, SAVC, and short-run average total cost (SATC) are graphically related, as Figure 3.8 illustrates. Keep in mind that the average total cost curve is cut at its minimum point by the marginal cost curve. It should be noted that the average fixed costs of production are represented by the vertical distance between the average total and variable cost curves at each level of output. Given that total costs comprise both variable and fixed costs, this shouldn't come as a surprise. Because the SAVC gets closer to zero as output rises, the vertical distance between the two curves decreases. The model's conclusion is that average total costs rise at a certain output level because, in the end, declining productivity's cost-enhancing effect triumphs over average fixed costs' tendency to decrease costs.

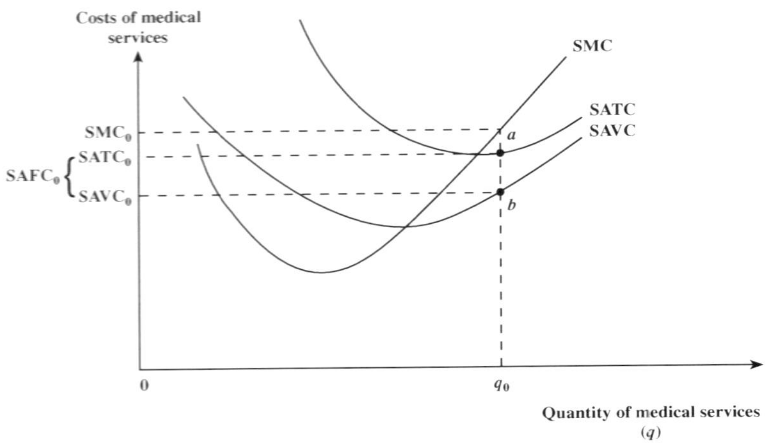

Figure 3.8. *Relation among short-run marginal, average variable, and average total costs.*

Source: Rexford, E. S., & Stephen, P. N., (n.d.). Health Economics. ISBN-13: 978-0-324-78908-9.

Because average costs are minimized, the uninformed reader might conclude that the medical firm should decide to produce at the minimum point on the SATC curve. However, as was already mentioned, the medical firm's output level decision is based on its goals (such as reaching a break-even or maximum profit level). Thus, in addition to the cost structure, a proper analysis also needs to have an understanding of the revenue structure. We discuss some other goals that might spur medical companies' production practices. Let's assume that the company has decided to produce the level of medical output, q_0, shown in Figure 3.8 for educational purposes. Let us ascertain the different expenses linked to the production of q_0 units of medical output.

The identification of the per-unit cost of producing a given level of output is a fairly easy matter. We can determine the per-unit cost by extending a vertical line from the appropriate level of output until it crosses the cost curves. For example, the average total cost of producing q_0 units of output is $SATC_0$, while the average variable cost is $SAVC_0$. The average fixed cost of producing q_0 units of output is represented by the vertical distance between $SATC_0$ and $SATC_0$, or distance ab. In addition, SMC_0 identifies the marginal cost of producing one more unit assuming the medical firm is already producing q_0 units of medical services. Now suppose that instead of the per-unit costs, we want to identify the various total costs (STC, STVC, and STFC) associated with producing q_0 units of output. We can do this by multiplying the level of output by the per-unit costs of production.

3.3.3. Factors Affecting the Position of the Short-Run Cost Curves

The locations of the per-unit and total cost curves are impacted by a range of short-term conditions. These include the patient case mix, the prices of the variable inputs, the level of care, and the quantities of the fixed inputs. The cost curves shift upward or downward in response to changes in any one of these variables, depending on whether costs are rising or falling. For instance, the cost curves will move upward to reflect the higher production costs if input prices rise in the near term (particularly since $SAVC = w/AP_n$ and $SMC = w/MP_n$). In the event of a short-term decline in input prices, the cost curves will shift downward to show reduced production costs.

Additionally, the cost curves respond by moving upward if the medical practice adopts a more severe patient case-mix or raises the standard of care. This is because a unit of labor can produce less in a given amount of time when the patient case mix is more severe or the quality of care is higher. According to our formal analysis, a more severe patient case mix or higher quality of care lowers the labor input's average and marginal productivity, which increases production costs. For instance, when patients are not as sick and care quality is not as important, a nurse can tend to many more patients in an hour. On the other hand, lower cost curves are linked to lower quality of care or a less severe patient case-mix.

Finally, a change in the amount of fixed inputs can alter the costs of production. For example, it can be shown that excessive amounts of fixed inputs lead to higher short run costs.

In sum, a properly specified short-run total variable cost function for medical services should include the following variables:

STVC = f(output level, input prices, quality of care, patient case-mix, quantity of the fixed inputs) (12)

We believe that these variables may account for variations in costs between medical practices within the same sector. In particular, output affects short-run variable costs by dictating the medical firm's location along the cost curve, while other factors influence the curve's location. High-cost medical practices are probably linked to higher output, better pay, higher-quality patient cases, more severe patient case mixes, and/or an overabundance of fixed inputs.

3.3.4. Estimating a Short-Run Cost Function for Hospital Services

Cowing & Holtmann (1983) empirically estimated a short-run total variable cost function for a sample of 138 short-term general care hospitals in New York using 1975 data. Along the lines of Eqn. (12), they specified the short-run total variable cost, STVC, function in the following general form:

$$\text{STVC} = f(q_1, q_2, q_3, q_4, q_5, w_1, w_2, w_3, w_4, w_5, w_6, K, A). \quad (13)$$

Each q_i (i = 1, 5) represents the quantity of one of five different patient services—emergency room care, medical-surgical care, pediatric care, maternity care, and other inpatient care— measured in total patient days; each w_j (j = 1,6) stands for one of six different variable input prices for nursing labor, auxiliary labor, professional labor, administrative labor, general labor, and material and supplies; K is a single measure of the capital stock (measured by the market value of a hospital); and A is the fixed number of admitting physicians in the hospital.

Cowing and Holtmann's specification of the cost function is more intricate and adds more realism to the empirical analysis than Eqn. (12) does. First, the hospital is viewed as a multiproduct company that can actually produce and market five distinct patient service categories at the same time. Second, six distinct variable input prices are specified as opposed to our single variable input price, which is the hourly nurse wage. Lastly, due to their significant influence on the process of producing hospital services, Cowing & Holtmann have included the number of admitting physicians in the model.

For Eqn. (13), the authors used a multiproduct translog cost function. It is sufficient to say that this flexible form allows us to evaluate a wide range of real-world characteristics related to the production process; we do not go into detail about the properties associated with this particular functional form.

First, the different outputs can interact with one another thanks to this functional form, allowing economies of scope to be investigated. The cooperative sharing of related resource outputs, such as nurses, auxiliary workers, and administrative labor, leads to economies of scope. If the combined cost of producing two outputs is less than the total cost of the two outputs separately, scope economies are present. For instance, because of alleged cost savings from economies of scope, many colleges and universities jointly offer graduate and undergraduate degrees. The same academic staff, library staff, and physical spaces can be utilized to concurrently produce both learning outcomes.

Cowing and Holtmann discovered some extremely fascinating findings. First, their research shows evidence of short-run economies of scale, which denotes that short-run total variable costs rise less than proportionately to an increase in output. The representative hospital is operating to the left of the minimum point on the short-run average variable cost curve, which suggests that larger hospitals are producing in the short run at a lower cost than smaller ones. This is evidence of short-run economies. They note that this finding supports the theory that closing a few small hospitals and combining the services of the remaining ones could lower overall hospital costs.

Secondly, Cowing & Holtmann found little evidence for economies of scope concerning pediatric care and other services, in contrast to economies of scale. Additionally, they discovered scant evidence in favor of diseconomies of scope in relation to emergency and other services. Indeed, they contended that considering the importance of the scale effects and the general absence of any significant economies of scope, the results for both scope and scale economies suggest that larger but more specialized hospitals might be more efficient.

Third, Cowing & Holtmann also noted that the short-run marginal cost of each output, $\Delta STVC/\Delta q_i$, declined and then became constant over the levels of output observed in their study. For example, the marginal cost of an emergency room visit was approximately \$32 for 54,000 visits per year and about \$20 for 1,00,000 visits per year. For medical surgical care, marginal cost was found to fall from \$255 per patient day for 6,000 annual patient days to around \$100 for 3,00,000 annual total patient days. For maternity care, the evidence suggests that the marginal costs of \$540 per patient day for hospitals with 1,500 total annual patient days declined to \$75 for hospitals with 20,000 total annual patient days. Eventually, each of the marginal costs leveled off.

Finally, Cowing & Holtmann estimated the short-run elasticities of input substitution between all pairs of variable inputs. They reported that the results indicate a substantial degree of substitutability between nursing and professional workers, nursing and general workers, nursing and administrative workers, and professional and administrative labor.

3.4. Long-Run Costs of Production

The concept of "long-run economies of scale" describes how labor and capital specialization lead to a decrease in average costs as a medical practice grows physically larger. Bigger medical companies can use more and bigger specialties for the different labor tasks that are part of the production process. For instance, when someone does a task repeatedly, they usually become very skilled at it. Larger companies can therefore produce more at a lower cost thanks to specialization. The long-run average total cost curve (LATC) in Figure 3.9 exhibits a downward-sloping portion that represents economies of scale.

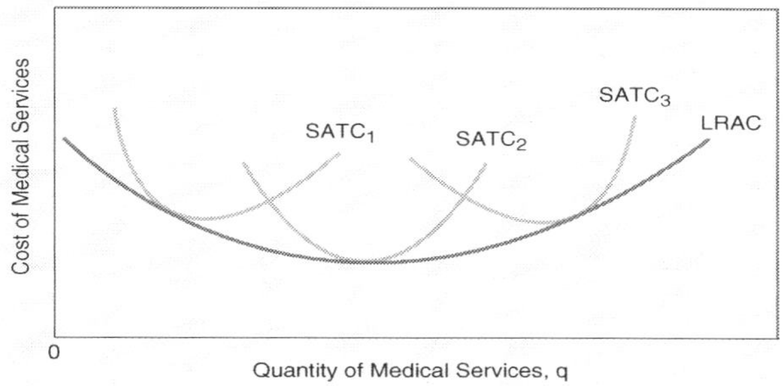

Figure 3.9. *Long run average cost curve.*

Source: Data from - Johnson-Lans, (2004). A Health Economics Primer. Boston: Pearson Addison Wesley.

An alternative approach to understanding long-term economies of scale is to consider the relationship directly between inputs and output, or returns to scale, as opposed to output and costs. Growing returns to scale are in line with long-term economies of scale. When an increase in all inputs yields an output increase greater than proportionate, this is known as increasing returns to scale. Increased returns to scale, for instance, can be seen when all inputs are doubled and the output is tripled. Likewise, a production process demonstrates economies of scale, or long-term increasing returns, if a doubling of output is possible without doubling all inputs.

The majority of economists think that diseconomies of scale eventually take over when economies of scale are depleted. When a medical company grows too big, diseconomies of scale occur. Top-to-bottom communication channels collapse, and bureaucratic red tape spreads widely. Poor decisions are occasionally made as a result. Long-term average costs therefore rise as the company grows too big. The upward-sloping portion of the LATC curve in Figure 3.9 is indicative of diseconomies of scale.

Diseconomies of scale can also be understood as decreasing returns to scale, where an increase in all inputs leads to an output increase that is less than proportionate. For instance, if a dentist's office experiences a doubling of painter hours and the decision-maker is required to increase each input by three times (staff, office space, etc.). Diseconomies of scale, or declining returns, are a feature of the dental office's production process that allows for a slight increase in services.

An additional possibility depicted in Figure 3.9 is that there are continuous returns to scale in the production process. When inputs and outputs are doubled, for instance, there is a constant return to scale. Constant returns suggest a horizontal LATC curve in terms of long-term costs, which suggests that average long-term costs are independent of output.

3.4.1. Shifts in the Long Run Average Cost Curve

A collection of long-term factors, such as patient case mix, quality, and the cost of all inputs, influence the long-term average cost curve's location. The long-run average cost curve moves upward or downward when these conditions change over time, depending on whether the change results in higher or lower long-run production costs. A technology that reduces costs, for instance, usually causes the long-term average cost curve to move downward (Becker et al., 1965; Bellemore et al., 1998).

3.5. The Healthcare Workforce Market

3.5.1. The Market for Physicians and Nurses

American attitudes toward medical professionals have been characterized by two opposing points of view. One concludes that there are not too many financial benefits to practicing medicine after focusing on the significant financial and psychological costs of the extensive training program, long workdays, and heavy responsibilities that come with the job. The opposing argument contends that by charging fees above what would be typical in a market with some degree of competition, doctors and other healthcare providers have been able to collect economic rents.

3.5.2. The Physician's Market

Public policy and individual career decisions work together to determine the supply of physicians. Medical associations and state and federal governments have engaged in interactions to regulate the practice of medicine since the mid-1800s. Decisions affecting training opportunities are also made by hospitals and medical schools that offer residency programs. The ability of people to enter the profession and the financial rewards for doing so are therefore not dependent on the invisible hand of supply and demand in the private market.

The professionalization of medical training and the practice of medicine date from the mid-19th century, when at the urging of the American Medical Association (AMA), state licensing boards were established to set examinations for doctors of medicine (MDs). Licensing limited the scope of activity of other medical practitioners: homeopaths, osteopaths, chiropractors, midwives, etc. In the 20th century, the AMA also began to oversee the quality of medical education. In 1910, a commissioned study that came to be known as the Flexner Report. This highly critical review of medical education led to the closure of many United States medical schools and the addition of a second requirement for becoming a licensed physician graduating from an accredited medical school. The MD degree requires four years of medical school, plus a year-long internship of practical training in hospitals. Physicians must pass examinations in a particular state to be licensed to practice there. Most physicians in the United States also undertake additional postgraduate training in the form of hospital residency in some specialty. This is now often combined with the internship. In addition, many become board-certified specialists. A board-certified specialist must complete one or more residencies and pass an examination in one of two specialist fields chosen. A physician can practice in a specialist field, such as cardiology, without being board certified, but the certification carries with it prestige and the likelihood of higher earnings. Some specialists, such as neurosurgeons, require very long residencies. A physician's training often requires a commitment of more than a decade. In 2001, approximately 67% of the total actively practicing physicians in the United States were board-certified specialists.

3.5.3. Physician Shortage

3.5.3.1. Health Planners' Evaluation of the Physician Supply

Health planners assess the physician supply by calculating the theoretical number of doctors needed to provide the medical care that a community requires. They estimate this need by consulting data on the prevalence of disease in a given population. With the uneven geographic distribution of practicing physicians, it was concluded using this definition that there was a physician shortage in the early 1960s, especially in some regions.

3.5.3.2. Economic Analysis of Physician Supply

When the amount supplied at a given market price is less than the quantity demanded, this is referred to by economists as a shortage. In a field where a large percentage of practitioners are independent contractors, shortages are difficult to quantify. There is a paucity of information regarding vacancy rates, except for hospital-employed junior physicians in training. Therefore, relative earnings or relative returns to training are studied by researchers looking at professional markets.

A medical degree can be thought of as a stock of human capital that yields a stream of returns over time. A convenient way to evaluate the return on any form of investment is to find its discounted present value (DPV), where:

$$DPV = \Sigma[R_{t=} + R_{t+}/(1 + r) + \ldots + R_{t+n/}(1+ r)^{t+n-1})]$$

The discount rate that will bring the discounted present value of the return streams and the discounted present value of the training costs into line is the internal rate of return. In competitive markets with free entry, it would be expected that internal rates of return in various professions would eventually converge. Increased rates of return could be a sign of what are known as dynamic shortages. These happen when supply and demand don't adjust at the same time. Because supply and demand conditions may change during the training period, there may be long delays and miscalculations about the economic return on the part of those entering the field in a career where training can take more than 10 years. On the other hand, persistent differences in internal rates of return offer circumstantial evidence of market imperfections because people are drawn to fields with higher returns.

Compared to other professions, physicians were found to have higher internal rates of return on their training in the 1950s and 1960s. As a result, health planners and economists agreed that there was a physician shortage.

3.5.3.3. Barriers to Entry

Barriers to entry into the medical field contribute to the higher returns on investment associated with medical education. The higher-than-equilibrium returns to medical training may be explained by the tight restrictions on foreign-trained physicians' admission due to immigration policy, medical school capacity constraints, and licensing requirements in the United States. Some economists connected the AMA's profit-maximizing actions to the high returns. The AMA was perceived as a guild that restricted admission to the profession and enforced stringent apprenticeship standards. Even if the limitation is for quality control, limiting the number of doctors will result in higher costs for their services if demand stays the same. Furthermore, even in situations where multiple providers of the same service exist, monopoly-level prices may arise if regulations that forbid price competition are combined with entry restrictions. It was reasonable to assume that there was no price competition because county medical associations had the authority to penalize doctors for not cooperating. Among other things, the penalties might be expulsion from the medical association and loss of hospital privileges.

In a competitive market with freedom of entry, the equilibrium price for a service would be PC and the equilibrium quantity would be qC. Restrictions on supply are shown in Figure 3.10 as a movement from SS to S_{1S1}, with a resulting competitive price of P*. If physicians' associations set prices collusively within local areas, the profit-maximizing price will approach P_m in Figure 3.10.

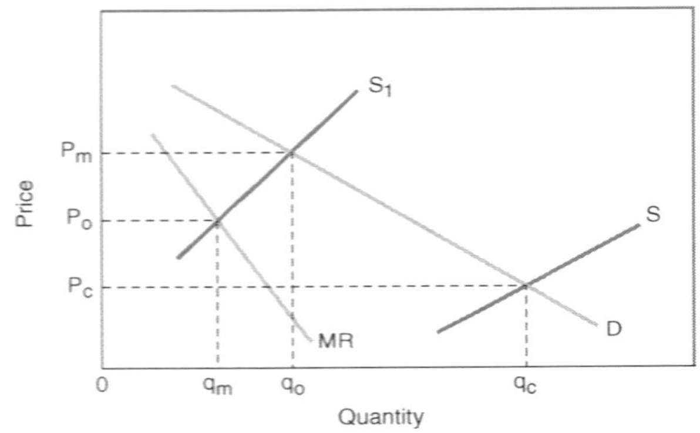

Figure 3.10. *Pricing of physician services.*

Source: Data from - Johnson-Lans, (2004). A Health Economics Primer. Boston: Pearson Addison Wesley.

3.5.3.4. Policy Responses to a Shortage

The goal of 1960s public policy was to alleviate the scarcity of doctors. Internationally trained doctors now have an easier time practicing medicine in the US thanks to the Immigration Act of 1965. The Health Professions Education Act of 1965 gave medical schools more federal funding, but to be eligible, they had to enroll more students. Between 1965 and 1980, the number of physicians increased significantly due to these measures, roughly doubling the size of physician training programs.

Returns on medical education, after accounting for hours worked, were still greater than those of other graduate-degree-requiring professions by 1970, but were now roughly comparable to those of attorneys and dentists. Internal rates of return for physicians by 1991 were lower than those for business or law training, though they were still comparable for primary care physicians.

3.5.3.5. Choice of Specialization

There is diversity among physicians. Nowadays, very few doctors in the U.S. only hold a basic MD degree. Typically, residents in internal medicine or geriatrics finish their training before becoming primary care doctors. Between 1986 and 1994, the percentage of U.S. medical school graduates pursuing internal medicine residencies fell by more than 30%. This indicates that a growing number of primary care physicians received their training outside of the U.S. In urban areas, the number of office-based primary care physicians decreased by 45% during the same period. Medical professionals were drawn to other specializations by better pay, more prestige, and more consistent work schedules. However, the percentage of doctors practicing primary care stabilized and stayed relatively constant between 1996 and 2001.

3.5.3.6. Economic Incentives to Alter the Distribution of Physicians

The private costs of training are significantly lower than the total costs to society (or social costs) as a result of subsidies for medical education provided to teaching hospitals, medical schools, and students in the form of below-market and deferred interest-bearing loans. People base their decisions about how much training to invest in on their costs and benefits. People will keep going to further training until the private marginal return on each extra training unit is exactly equal to the private marginal costs. From the perspective of society, this could lead to a less-than-ideal distribution of specialists.

From a societal perspective, the last unit of an item or service produced has reached optimality when the marginal social benefit and marginal social cost are equal. If society's objectives and the incentives offered by the private sector differ, it is unlikely that society will achieve its goals unless the incentive system is altered.

3.5.3.7. Public Policy to Change Incentives

Under the National Health Service Corps, the U.S. government offers physicians the opportunity to have a portion of their student loans forgiven if they commit to practicing in underserved areas. It is also possible to see Medicare fee schedule modifications that benefit primary care physicians as a kind of public policy intended to modify the availability of doctors in other specializations.

3.5.3.8. Private Insurance Market Incentives

Primary care physicians have more opportunities as a result of managed care organizations' increased use of them. The earnings gap between primary care physicians and specialists like radiologists, anesthesiologists, and pathologists was found to have shrunk between 1985 and 1993 as managed care insurers gained more market share. Between 1987 and 1997, the number of specialists and physicians overall grew at slower rates in metropolitan areas with higher penetration of managed care organizations, while the growth rate of general practitioners remained constant.

3.5.4. The Result of Changing Incentives

3.5.4.1. Fields Chosen by Younger Physicians

Taking age into consideration changes the pattern of the physician distribution by specialty. In 2001, internal medicine, family practice, and pediatrics employed more than half of female physicians and more than 40% of male physicians under 35. Since roughly 1991, when Medicare payment reforms were already in place and managed care was beginning to make significant inroads into national markets, physicians under the age of 35 who received their training in the United States would have been making decisions about specialty fields. Aside from these considerations, other factors that impacted the specialty choices were shorter residency training periods, more rigid work schedules, and guaranteed vacations.

3.5.5. Projections About the Supply and Demand of Physicians: Economic and Health Planning Viewpoints

It was commonly accepted by the late 1970s that there had been an overshoot in policy and that there would soon be an overabundance of doctors. Congress created the Council on Graduate Medical Education out of concern that Medicare would stop funding residency programs with several billion dollars annually. This indicated that the general physician-to-population ratio would be high by 2000. Additionally, it was projected that there would be 60% more specialists than were required. It suggested that hospital residency program subsidies be cut and more medical students be assigned to primary care positions. The quantity of positions in American medical schools steadied and stayed largely unchanged.

The number of doctors in the future is predicted to vary. Some believe there will soon be a shortage, but not everyone shares this opinion. A roundtable discussion in 2001 offered a representative sample of opinions on this matter. This representative sample of expert views highlights the differences between the perspectives of economists and health planners.

3.5.6. The Market for Nurses

In this chapter, the term "nurses" will refer to registered nurses (RNs). To become a registered nurse, one can take one of three routes. Four-year colleges offer BA programs alongside two-year associate programs in community colleges and three-year diploma programs in hospitals. There are also graduate nursing programs that lead to an MA or PhD. Similar to doctors, registered nurses can pursue further education in specialized fields. The need for nurses is impacted by shifts in the healthcare production function.

Although the percentage of registered nurses working in hospitals had dropped to roughly 60% by the end of the 1990s, hospitals have historically been the primary employers of registered nurses. The need for hospital nurses rises with the intensity of care provided in acute care hospitals, but employment in hospitals tends to decline with decreased use of inpatient hospital services. The need for nurses in nonhospital settings tends to rise to the degree that managed care organizations and other integrated healthcare delivery systems can replace doctors in ambulatory settings with nurses.

The decisions made by individuals to enroll in training programs and pursue employment in the nursing field upon completion of their education determine the availability of nurses. The training opportunities available to nurses are determined by public policy in the same way that they are for physicians. The supply is certainly influenced by the occupation's relative rate of return when compared to other jobs requiring similar training. Undoubtedly, opportunities for women to pursue careers as doctors offer an alternative to those who might otherwise choose to become nurses. We cannot assume that the increase in other professional opportunities for women will be significantly offset by the replacement of male nurses with female nurses since the percentage of male registered nurses has remained below 5%.

3.5.7. Is There a Nursing Shortage?

Using the definitions of shortages provided by economists and healthcare planners, there have been numerous claims of a nursing shortage. To bolster its allegations of a nursing shortage in the 1950s and 60s, the American Hospital Association pointed to the high percentage of open positions for registered nurses and the replacement of RNs with less experienced licensed practical nurses. At the going rate of pay, there was a greater demand for nurses than there were available. Hospital nurse vacancy rates never dropped below 13% between the 1940s and the early 1960s, peaking at 23% in 1962.

Congress responded by passing the Nurse Training Act (NTA) in 1964, which began a tradition of government subsidization of nurses' training. Using vacancy rates in hospitals as an indicator, the legislation that supported nurses' training appears to have mitigated the shortages. Vacancy rates fell to below 10% by 1971.

Between 1971 and the present, there appear to have been several periods of adjustment in which high vacancy rates were followed by policies to expand nurses' training, followed by reductions in shortages. Wages have responded, for the most part, to shortages. Because the training period is much shorter, responses to imbalances in supply and demand are more rapid than in the case of physician training.

3.5.7.1. Cyclical Shortages and Responses

The choices made by nurses regarding whether to join the workforce and how many hours to work are highly cyclical. This is because a large number of nurses are married and come from two-earner households. They enter and exit the labor force in response to changes in real wages and employment opportunities, as well as changes in their spouses' employment circumstances. During recessions, there are usually a lot fewer nursing vacancies.

Early in the 1980s, there was a recession that led to a record low of less than 5% for the vacancy rate and an increase in the labor force participation of trained nurses. But by the end of the 1980s, it was higher than 12%. The resurgence of the shortage was caused by a decrease in nurses' participation rates when the economy improved, an increase in the need for hospital nurses, and a decrease in the number of people enrolling in nursing programs in the early 1980s. As a result, the Nurse Shortage Reduction Act of 1988 and the Nurse Relief Act of 1989 were passed, easing restrictions on the immigration of nurses with foreign training and providing additional funding for nursing education. Consequently, the number of nurses available increased quickly. By the middle of the 1990s, there had been another decline in vacancy rates, partly because of the 1992 recession and higher nursing participation rates. However, since then, there has been a resurgence of rising vacancy rates across much of the country.

3.5.7.2. Wages

Despite high vacancy rates, nurses' wages decreased from the 1940s to the early 1960s when compared to other female professionals. In the same time frame, nurses working outside of hospitals saw a rise in pay relative to their counterparts in the hospital industry.

The establishment of Medicare in 1965 brought about a change in the situation. In comparison to their non-hospital counterparts, hospital nurses' salaries rose, and they eventually caught up to the earnings of other occupations with a high female employment rate that required an equivalent degree of education. Nurses' pay increased after price controls were lifted in 1974, but they had been restricted in the 1970s. Wage levels remained constant in the 1980s. Real wages for nurses rose from 1983 to 1993, then experienced a brief decrease from 1993 to 1997. Because vacancy rates decreased during the same period, the Nurse Shortage Reduction Act of 1988 likely contributed to the increase in the supply of nurses. Demand-side forces, though, might have also played a role. Hospitals have often been accused of cutting corners on nursing care as a result of managed care insurers' cost-containment strategies. On the other hand, it seems that the 1990s short-term real wage decline for nurses was only partially explained by the entry of managed care organizations into the market. Hospital nurses' pay has grown since 1998, both in absolute terms and concerning other women with similar levels of education.

3.5.8. The Monopsonistic Market for Nurses

There has been a widespread perception that there is a chronic shortage of registered nurses and that nurses are underpaid in the nursing market. It seems illogical to associate shortages with low wages. A shortage should be filled in a healthy competitive market by raising wages until equilibrium is restored, as shortages arise when the quantity supplied at a given wage is less than the quantity demanded. A common explanation for this phenomenon is the monopsony model. A monopoly employer or buyer of nurses is known as a monopsonist. One common textbook example of monopsony is the market for registered nurses. If the area is home to just one hospital, it may have monopoly power over the nursing staff. The outcome would be the same if multiple hospitals banded together to fix the pay scale for nurses.

The supply curve for labor must be upward-sloping for monopsony to have an impact on market outcomes; this implies that the employer must raise wages to draw in more workers. If we assume that everyone performing the same work is paid the same wage, the supply curve represents an average factor cost curve from the employer's perspective. A company is considered a wage setter if it is the only one hiring a particular type of worker. It must therefore consider the marginal costs of adding more employees. As Figure 3.11 illustrates, the marginal factor cost curve rises more sharply when the supply curve is upward-sloping. If the company needs to pay more to attract new employees, it also needs to pay more to the people it already has on staff.

The demand schedule for any input into production is its marginal revenue product curve. The demand curve shows the maximum amount that an employer will pay for any given quantity of workers hired. A hospital will not pay more for an extra nurse than the marginal contributions to revenue. A firm will hire workers up to the quantity where the marginal factor cost (MFC) of the last worker just equals the marginal revenue product (MRP) of the last worker. This satisfies the profit-maximizing criterion MR = MC. In Figure 3.11, (Wg, ND) shows the quantity of nursing help that will be employed and the wage that will be paid by the monopsonist. At (Wg_1, ND_1), the quantity demanded exceeds the quantity supplied by ND_1–NS_1. This difference measures the amount of the vacancy. The monopsony model can explain the coexistence of high vacancy rates and lower-than-competitive wages of nurses.

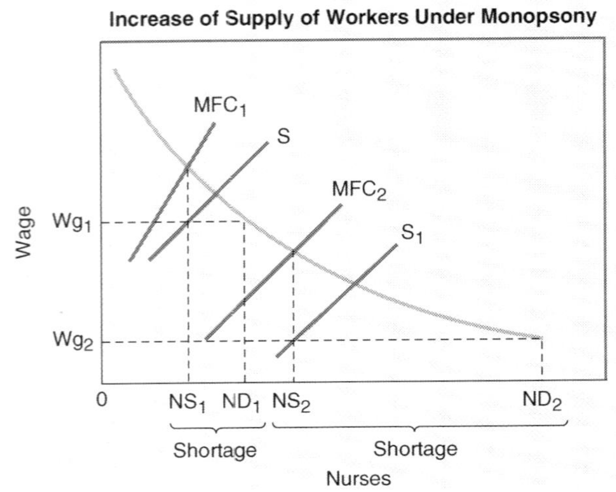

Figure 3.11. *Increase of supply of workers under monopsony.*

Source: Data from – Johnson-Lans, (2004). A Health Economics Primer. Boston: Pearson Addison Wesley.

From the 1940s until the mid-1960s, the monopsony model seems to fit the data fairly well. That being said, this model does a poor job of explaining the patterns in employment and pay for registered nurses during the Medicare era. Real nursing wages rose in tandem with demand after 1965. Without mentioning monopsony, the drop in nurses' pay between 1993 and 1997 can be attributed to both a sharp rise in supply and some downward pressure on the demand for hospital nurses.

Economists have, nevertheless, reexamined the problem of nursing market monopsony. It has been discovered that hospitals set wages, and there is a strong wage inelasticity in the short term for the supply of nurses. When employers have more market power, nurses are forced to work harder. A review of the nursing markets in Australia provides compelling evidence of monopsony in those markets. In a time of high job vacancy rates, Australian nurses receive pay that is around 20% less than that of other workers in a similar position. Policies intended to eliminate shortages by increasing the labor supply may, in cases where monopsony occurs, actually make shortages worse. The adverse effects of the nursing shortage, which result in excessive work hours and rotations to services for which training and experience are insufficient, have been highlighted by the American Nurses Association.

According to a government estimate from the United States, by 2010 there will be more demand than supply for registered nurses. This presumes that the real wages of nurses remain constant, that is, that they are modified by anticipated increases in the price index.

Using contract labor is a creative solution to the hospital nurse shortage. Short-term nurse supplies are provided by agencies. When nurses work for these agencies, they give up job security and benefits in exchange for greater pay and more flexible schedules. In a field where married women predominate, this trade-off might be better for the employer and the worker. Hospitals with wildly fluctuating demand for nurses may find it effective to use temporary registered nurses. Additionally, in areas where hospitals have monopsony power, employment of nurses may increase more than would otherwise be predicted because salaried nurses' pay is unaffected by the pay paid to temporary workers.

3.6. Technology in Healthcare

The role of technological change in healthcare is of particular interest to health economists and policy analysts because of the need to evaluate its effects on healthcare costs as well as its benefits. Cost containment may slow down the pace of technological advancement and its spread, which is a related worry. The demand for technologically advanced healthcare increased as a result of healthcare advancements in the second half of the 20th century, which raised expectations about achievable levels of health. Because there were no cost controls imposed by the U.S. health insurance system during the 1940s and 1950s, the demand for healthcare increased. The demand for health insurance was further increased by improvements in healthcare efficacy and the ensuing rise in healthcare costs. Using the best technology available was further motivated by worries about possible medical malpractice lawsuits. These elements worked together to virtually ensure that any innovation would be demanded and that it would be demonstrated to offer even a slight improvement in treatment outcomes for the majority of the second half of the 20th century.

Technology has been the main driver of the rising trend in healthcare costs, according to the consensus of those who have worked to identify the factors contributing to the rising cost of healthcare. A combination of factors such as rising real income, supplier-induced demand, monopoly profits to suppliers, shifting population demographics, and the labor-intensive nature of healthcare can account for considerably less than half of the increase in healthcare costs over time.

3.6.1. Technological Change

3.6.1.1. Promotion of Innovation

Innovation is the process by which technologies advance. Creating and advertising new products is a component of innovation, which can be combined with the process of invention or discovery. According to Schumpeter, innovation is what propels a market economy. He dubbed the process "creative destruction," in which an inferior product or method is substituted with an improved one.

He underlined the importance of profits in fostering innovation and pointed out that businesses with significant market power—such as oligopolies or monopolistically competitive businesses—will be the ones to lead the charge in innovation. Along with government funding for basic research, other factors that may serve as important stimulants in the process of innovation include professional prestige and the sense of accomplishment that comes from curing diseases.

In the United States, health research takes place within the government-funded National Institutes of Health (NIH); in universities, where much research is also funded by NIH; the National Science Foundation (NSF); and private industry in general and within firms themselves. Studies show that the rate of product development is greater in firms that have more contact with academic institutions, which is particularly true with products that are radically new, rather than incrementally changed products.

Innovation cannot happen unless there is a market for products and an expectation of profits. Government funding for research is crucial for fostering innovation, but it might not always result in a direct pipeline for finished goods. For example, a significant amount of biotechnology research from Oxford and Cambridge Universities has led to the development of commercially valuable products in businesses outside of the United Kingdom. This might have been influenced by the National Health Service's price caps on prescription drugs. In the U.S., there's a persistent worry that cost-cutting measures slow down the pace of advancement in health technology. The Clinton healthcare reform plan's 1990s collapse may have been influenced by the inclusion of price controls on pharmaceutical products.

3.6.1.2. Intellectual Property Rights

Patent protection for intellectual property rights is another element that is thought to encourage innovation. Patents are licenses that provide the sole right of ownership over inventions or processes for a predetermined period. Drug and medical device patents in the US are currently granted for 20 years, including the testing phase. The effective patent life is frequently lowered to 10 years or less due to the protracted testing phase. For novel discoveries about specific genes, patent protection is also an option. If the Food and Drug Administration (FDA) has postponed releasing a new medication for that long, patents on biomedical and pharmaceutical innovations may be renewed for a maximum of five years. For an effective patent life of longer than 14 years, the extension may not be granted.

Without patent protection, innovation would be severely hindered unless governments provided funding for both fundamental research procedures and product development. Because duplication lowers the profitability of research and development (R&D) activities, there would be less of an incentive to innovate. Since development costs are much higher than production costs in the pharmaceutical industry, imitation is a serious problem. The substantial testing required to obtain government approval to market and sell the drugs is far more expensive than the cost of producing them.

The degree of patent protection and the rate of innovation have a complex relationship. Examining variations among nations serves as an illustration of this. Only in 1977 did Switzerland, home to three prosperous pharmaceutical companies, institute patent protection for pharmaceuticals. Up until 1987, Canada's patent laws were extremely lax. However, since tightening up on patent protection, the country has seen a notable rise in research and development (R&D) activity as a result of the research efforts of foreign multinational corporations.

3.6.1.3. U.S. Firms' Successful Innovation

The United States has been the world leader in the commercialization of biotechnical knowledge, although Germany, the United Kingdom, and Canada appear to be beginning to close the gap. The main reasons for the United States' success appear to be:

- The existence of a large stock of human capital and research institutions;
- Government support for basic research;
- Well-enforced patent protection;
- Historically generous insurance (third party) payers;
- Extensively subsidized employer-based private insurance for the majority of its citizens;
- Physicians and hospitals that are motivated to use the highest technology available.

3.6.2. Technological Diffusion

When it comes to the spread of the majority of medical technologies, the U.S. ranks highly. This is demonstrated by a study that contrasts this nation with Canada and Germany, two other nations renowned for having top-notch healthcare systems. In terms of the diffusion of all technologies examined, the United States came in first. Radiation therapy and magnetic resonance imaging (MRI) offered especially significant benefits. These two technologies demand extremely large investments in terms of both human and physical capital. These instances highlight the necessity for complementary support in the form of treatment facilities that are well-equipped and medical professionals who have received the necessary training to carry out the procedures when using advanced technologies.

3.6.2.1. Factors That Promote Technological Diffusion

It has been discovered that financial incentives have an impact on how quickly new, high-tech treatments spread. Studies conducted across multiple countries have revealed that countries with fee-for-service reimbursement systems—Japan, Korea, Australia, and France are among the examples—have higher rates of diffusion when it comes to the adoption of advanced technology treatments for heart attacks. The use of high-tech treatments is growing at an immediate rate in the United States, which combines prospective and fee-for-service payment systems. Despite this, the country still has more medical technology per person than any other country.

3.6.3. Measuring the Contribution of Technological Change

Technological change has been treated as a residual in empirical studies of healthcare costs, meaning that it is the unexplained variance that remains after all known factors have been taken into account. We refer to this as the Solow residual. Once the effects of other factors were considered, technological change came to be recognized as the primary cause of the rise in healthcare costs in the United States. More recently, a method that more precisely measures technological change has been developed by Newhouse, Cutler, McClellan, and others. Their methodology is limited to investigating the correlation between expenses and technological advancements in the management of particular illnesses, like heart care.

3.6.3.1. Cost Increasing versus Cost-Saving Innovations

A cost-increasing innovation in medicine is an innovation that increases the cost of treatment for a particular disease. Where there is no incentive to contain costs, it may be more profitable for firms to develop more expensive or cost-increasing technologies. A number of economists argued that at least until the mid-1980s, both Medicare and the prevalent indemnity form of private insurance encouraged a bias toward cost-increasing (as well as quality-increasing) innovation.

It may be useful to distinguish between process and product innovations. Process innovations are often cost-saving. For example, the introduction of more expensive and more effective new drugs has been shown to provide significant cost savings on non-drug expenditures that greatly outweigh the increase in expenditure on drugs for the treatment of similar diseases. Using data from 1986 to 1998, the reduction in non-drug expenditures associated with the use of newer drugs was found to be on average 7.2 times the increase in drug expenditures. For the Medicare population, the reduction in total expenditure on non-drug aspects of treatments, including both individual out-of-pocket expenditures and Medicare's contribution, was 8.3 times the increase in expenditure on drugs. These are examples of clear cost-saving improvements in technology.

An example of a cost-increasing innovation is laparoscopic cholecystectomy surgery to remove the gallbladder using a small inserted camera to direct the surgeon's instruments. It is particularly notable because of the rapid diffusion of this technique after it became available in the United States in the 1980s. By 1992, 80% of the cholecystectomies performed in this country were laparoscopic. The technique is more frequently used in the early stages of the disease among younger, non-Medicaid patients. Still, it has also come to be widely used among the elderly, including the very elderly for whom it is also appropriate and effective. The new technique has been shown to cut mortality rates in half for all age groups. Among the elderly, it has also greatly reduced the need for stays in skilled nursing homes. It has shortened the average recovery time. Patients can also return to work in an average of 15 days instead of 31 days, and hospital stays have been reduced from 4.3 to 1.6 days.

Even if the increase in the need for gallbladder surgery had not accompanied the development of the laparoscopic technique, the innovation defined narrowly is more expensive. Even though hospital stays are shorter, total surgeon and hospital charges are higher for laparoscopic surgery than for open surgery, and they outbalance savings in hospitalization costs.

Certain stages in the development of medical treatments may tend to involve initially higher costs followed by lower costs. Therefore, it depends on what point in the life cycle of the innovation the costs are measured. Scientific discoveries often have life cycles that lead to first- and second-generation technological improvements. The two stages have been called halfway technologies and high technology by Weisbrod (1991). Halfway technologies are usually more expensive than cures and are certainly cost-increasing when compared to no treatment or watching and waiting during certain disease stages. Compare the early treatments for polio mellitus, a disease that was life-threatening well into the 1950s in high-income countries. The iron lung was an expensive machine that kept paralyzed individuals alive but required intensive care. Contrast this with the second-generation innovation, the Salk and Sabin vaccines, which prevented the disease and were inexpensive and noninvasive. Here, the development of vaccines replaces expensive combinations of machinery and drugs.

3.6.3.2. Productive Efficiency

Studies of alternative technologies used for the treatment of specific diseases often compare treatment methods in terms of their productive efficiency. Productive efficiency compares the quantities of inputs used to produce a given output. Comparing production functions without reference to the prices of inputs is a fairly standard way of making intercountry comparisons of the use of various medical technologies. For example, Bailey & Garber (1997) compared the United States, Germany, and the United Kingdom in the treatments for diabetes, gallstones, breast cancer, and lung cancer. The United States was found to be more productively efficient than Germany in the treatment of each of the diseases except for diabetes, which requires long-term therapies and little high technology.

The lack of capacity of capital equipment imposed by the British National Health Service budget limited the use of laparoscopic surgery. In Germany as well, these techniques were less prevalent than in the United States. This resulted in more time and resources to achieve better or worse outcomes. Productive efficiency is therefore not independent of previous decisions made in several countries about how much to allocate to developing capital capacity and technology.

In the treatment of breast cancer, the United States and United Kingdom were both unambiguously more productive than Germany. The United States achieved a 9% better outcome using 38% fewer inputs, and the United Kingdom achieved a 6% better outcome using 53% fewer resources. Compared to the United Kingdom, the United States used 15% more inputs to achieve a 3% better outcome (Bindman et al., 1994; Cullen et al., 1994).

A Closer Look

Supply of Healthcare Services

Healthcare services encompass a broad spectrum of medical interventions, ranging from preventive care and diagnostics to treatment and rehabilitation, each crucial for promoting and maintaining individual and population health.

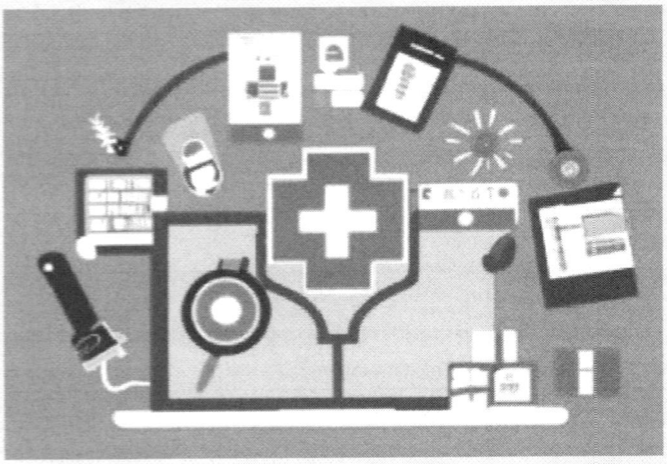

One fundamental aspect of healthcare service supply is its geographic distribution and accessibility. Disparities in healthcare access exist across regions, influenced by factors such as population density, infrastructure, and socioeconomic status. Rural areas often face challenges in accessing essential healthcare services due to limited healthcare facilities, healthcare workforce shortages, and transportation barriers. Addressing these disparities requires strategic planning and investment in healthcare infrastructure, telemedicine solutions, and healthcare workforce recruitment and retention initiatives to ensure equitable access to healthcare services for all individuals, regardless of their geographical location.

Furthermore, the availability and allocation of healthcare resources play a pivotal role in determining the capacity and efficiency of healthcare service delivery. Healthcare resources encompass a wide range of inputs, including medical personnel, medical equipment, pharmaceuticals, and financial resources. The adequacy of these resources directly impacts the ability of healthcare systems to meet the healthcare needs of their populations effectively. Shortages or mismatches in healthcare resources can lead to bottlenecks, delays in care, and compromised patient outcomes. Thus, healthcare organizations must engage in comprehensive resource planning and management to optimize resource allocation and utilization, ensuring that resources are allocated based on population health needs, evidence-based practices, and cost-effectiveness considerations.

Moreover, the quality and safety of healthcare services are paramount considerations in healthcare supply. Quality healthcare services are safe, effective, patient-centered, timely, efficient, and equitable. Achieving high-quality healthcare requires a multifaceted approach, encompassing clinical excellence, evidence-based practices, patient engagement, and continuous quality improvement initiatives. Healthcare organizations must implement robust quality assurance mechanisms, such as clinical guidelines, performance metrics, and accreditation standards, to monitor and improve the quality of care delivered. Additionally, ensuring patient safety involves identifying and mitigating risks, errors, and adverse events through proactive measures such as error reporting systems, medication safety protocols, and infection control practices.

Summary

- The supply of healthcare can be approached in a similar way as the demand for healthcare. Suppliers include hospitals, which provide healthcare directly, and medical equipment and pharmaceutical companies, which provide inputs to the healthcare production process. The supply side of the market is heavily dependent on theories of how firms behave—this concept is often called the theory of the firm.
- The Short-Run Production Function of the Representative Medical Firm: All medical firms, including hospitals, physician clinics, nursing homes, and pharmaceutical companies, earn revenues from producing and selling some type of medical output. Production and retailing activities occur regardless of the form of ownership (that is, for-profit, public, or not-for-profit). Because these activities take place in a world of scarce resources, microeconomics can provide valuable insights into the operation and planning processes of medical firms.
- A variety of short-run circumstances affect the positions of the per-unit and total cost curves. Among them are the prices of the variable inputs, the quality of care, the patient case mix, and the amounts of the fixed inputs. Whenever any one of these variables changes, the positions of the cost curves change through either an upward or a downward shift depending on whether costs increase or decrease.
- Long-run economies of scale refer to the notion that average costs fall as a medical firm gets physically larger due to the specialization of labor and capital. Larger medical firms can utilize larger and more specialties in the various labor tasks involved in the production process.
- The supply of physicians depends upon a combination of individual career decisions and public policy. Since the middle of the 19th century, medical associations have interacted with state and federal governments to regulate the practice of medicine. Medical schools and hospitals with residency programs also make decisions that affect the opportunities for training. As a result, one's ability to enter the profession and the financial returns of doing so are not left to the invisible hand of the supply and demand in the private market.
- Economists define a shortage as a situation in which the quantity supplied is less than the quantity demanded at a given market price. Shortages are not easy to measure in a profession where a high proportion of the members are self-employed. Except for young physicians in training employed by hospitals, there are few data on vacancy rates. Researchers studying markets for professionals therefore study relative earnings or relative returns to training.
- Health economists and policy analysts are particularly interested in the role of technological change in healthcare because of the need to assess both its benefits and its impact on the rising costs of healthcare.

References

1. American Medical Association, Center for Health Policy Research. (1998). *Physician Marketplace Characteristics, 1997–1998*. Chicago: AMA.

2. Association of American Medical Colleges. (2002). *AAMC Data Book 2002*. Washington, DC: AAMC.
3. Barzanski, B., et al. (1991). Education programs in U.S. medical schools. *Journal of the American Medical Association, 266*(7), 916.
4. Becker, G. (1965). A theory of the allocation of time. *Economic Journal, 75*(299), 493–517.
5. Bellemore, F. A. (1998). Temporary employment decisions of registered nurses. *Eastern Economic Journal, 24*(3), 265–279.
6. Bindman, A. B. (1994). Primary and managed care: Ingredients for health care reform. *Western Journal of Medicine, 161*(1), 78–82.
7. Cullen, T. J., et al. (1994). *The National Health Service Corps: Rural Physician Service and Retention*. Seattle, WA: WAMI Rural Health Research Center.
8. Currie, J., et al. (2003). Cut to the bone? Hospital takeovers and nurse employment (NBER Working Paper No. 9428). Cambridge, MA: National Bureau of Economic Research.
9. Escarce, J. E., et al. (2000). HMO growth and geographical redistribution of generalist and specialist physicians. *Health Services Research, 35*(4), 825-848.
10. Feldstein, P. J. (1999). *Health Care Economics* (5th ed.). Albany, NY: Delmar Publishers.
11. Friedman, M., & Kuznets, S. (1945). *Income from Professional Practice*. New York: National Bureau of Economic Research.
12. Hirsch, B. T., & Schumacher, E. J. (2004). Classic monopsony or new monopsony? Searching for evidence in nursing labor markets (IZA Discussion Paper No. 1154). Chicago: Institute for the Study of Labor.
13. Howak, M. J., & Preston, A. C. (2001). Can human capital theory explain why nurses are so poorly paid? *Australian Economic Papers, 40*(2), 232–245.
14. Johnson-Lans, S. (2006). *A Health Economics Primer*. Boston: Pearson Addison Wesley.
15. Kessel, R. A. (1958). Price discrimination in medicine. *Journal of Law and Economics, 1*(1), 20–53.
16. Lane, J., & Gohmann, S. (1995). Surplus or shortage: Economic approaches to the analysis of nursing labor markets. *Southern Economic Journal, 61*(3), 644–653.
17. Lee, B., et al. (1968). Migration, location, and remuneration of medical personnel: Physicians and dentists. *Review of Economics and Statistics, 50*(3), 332–347.
18. McKay, N. L. (1990). The economic determinants of specialty choice by medical residents. *Journal of Health Care Economics, 9*(4), 335–357.
19. Mennemeyer, S. T. (1978). Great returns to medical education? *Journal of Human Resources, 13*(1), 75–90.
20. Pasko, T., & Smart, D. R. (2003). *Physician Characteristics and Distribution in the U.S., 2003–2004 Edition*. Chicago: American Medical Association.
21. Rimlinger, G. V., & Steele, H. B. (1968). An economic interpretation of the spatial distribution of physicians in the U.S. *Southern Economic Journal, 30*(1), 1–12.
22. Scanlon, W. (2001). *Nursing Workforce: Recruitment and Retention of Nurses and Nurse Aides is a growing concern*. Washington, DC: U.S. Government Accounting Office.

23. Schumacher, E. J. (2001). The earnings and employment of nurses in an era of cost containment. *Industrial and Labor Relations Review, 55*(1), 116–132.

24. Simon, C. J., et al. (1998). The effect of managed care on the incomes of primary care and specialty physicians. *Health Services Research, 33*(3), 549–569.

Chapter 4

EQUITY AND HEALTH

Contents

Introduction

The ethical concept of justice and fairness in the allocation of healthcare resources, opportunities, and results among populations is embodied in equity in health. Regardless of socioeconomic status, race, gender, ethnicity, or other social determinants of health, it represents the idea that everyone should have the chance to reach their utmost level of health. In addition to being an issue of social justice, achieving health equity is also a vital part of public health and healthcare systems across the globe.

Disparities in health outcomes caused by systemic and unfair social, economic, and environmental factors are addressed by health equity. These discrepancies can take many different forms, such as variations in the quality of care, health-related behaviors, and health outcomes, as well as in access to healthcare services. For example, poverty, discrimination, inadequate insurance coverage, language barriers, and geographic isolation are some of the reasons why marginalized communities frequently encounter difficulties in accessing healthcare. As such, in comparison to more privileged groups, they suffer from higher rates of chronic conditions, preventable diseases, and early mortality.

A comprehensive strategy that tackles the underlying causes of health disparities, as well as their aftereffects on people and communities, is necessary to achieve health equity. This entails addressing the underlying social determinants of health, such as education, income, housing, employment, and environmental conditions, in addition to expanding access to healthcare services. Reducing structural barriers, empowering marginalized communities to participate in health-related decision-making, and promoting equitable resource distribution are all necessary.

Sustainable development, social justice, and human rights are strongly related to health equity. Achieving universal health coverage, lowering health disparities within and between nations, and advancing everyone's health and well-being are among the global health goals that depend on it. Societies can build more resilient, inclusive, and prosperous communities where everyone has the chance to live a long and healthy life by placing a high priority on health equity.

Orientation and Directional Terms:

Term	Definition	Illustration
Wealth gaps	The wealth gap, also known as income inequality, wealth disparity, or wealth and income differences, is the difference in assets and net worth across races and ethnicities.	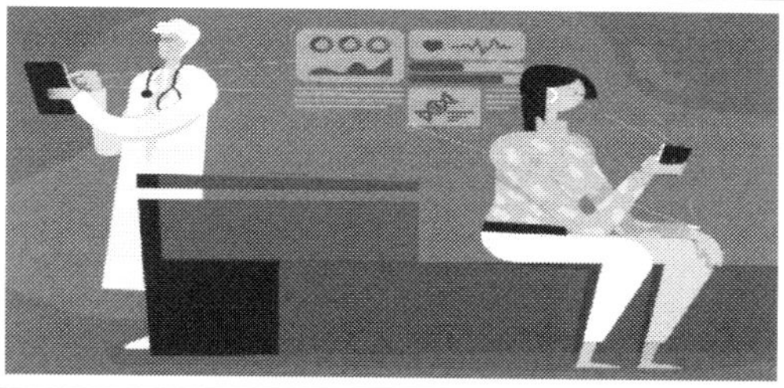
Health disparities	Health disparities are preventable differences in the experience of disease, injury, violence, or opportunities to achieve optimal health experienced by socially disadvantaged racial, ethnic, and other population groups, and communities.	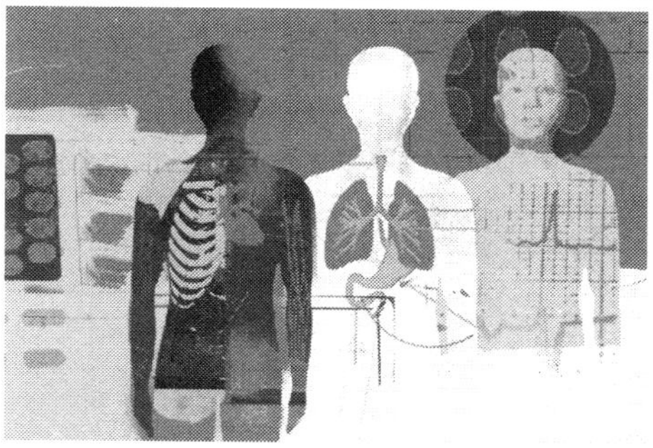
Health equality	Health equality is equal treatment and availability of healthcare services.	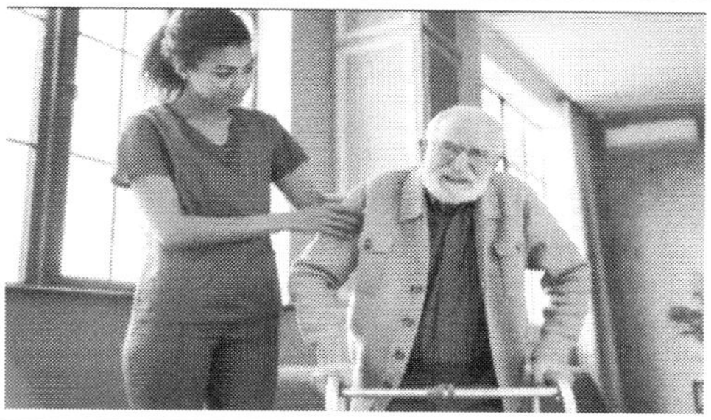
Healthcare	Healthcare, or healthcare, is the improvement of health via the prevention, diagnosis, treatment, amelioration or cure of disease, illness, injury, and other physical and mental impairments in people.	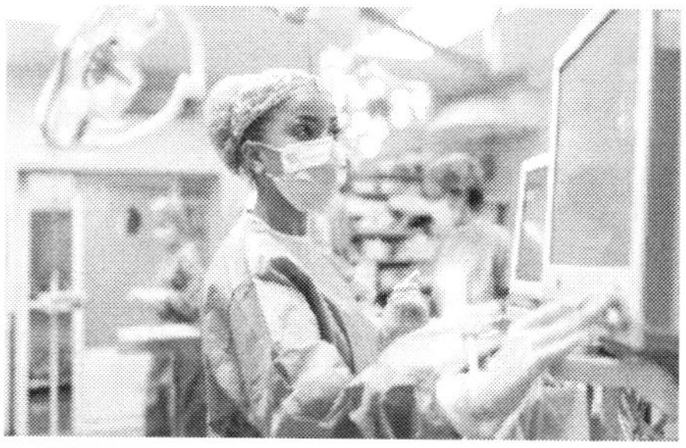
Endometriosis	Endometriosis is a chronic female reproductive system disease that causes tissue similar to the lining of the uterus to grow outside of the uterus.	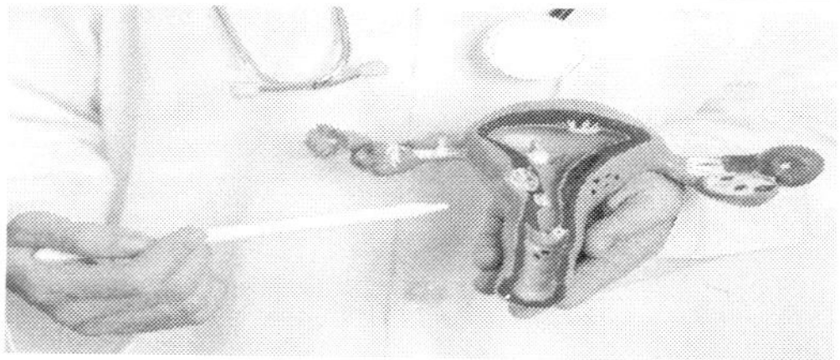

4.1. Equity in Healthcare

Ensuring that everyone has the opportunity to be as healthy as possible is known as health equity. However, an individual may be unable to reach their optimal level of health due to circumstances beyond their control. A couple of these factors are resource scarcity and discrimination.

To ensure health equity, all individuals must be given the chance to reach their optimal state of health. Unfortunately, there are a lot of social and environmental factors that can make it harder for someone to continue using healthcare and good health practices. These health disparities exist.

Examples of these obstacles include:

- Racial and ethnic discrimination;
- Lack of access to quality education;
- Income and wealth gaps;
- Inadequate housing or lack of housing;
- Unsafe environments.

Through minimizing, confronting, or conquering these barriers, individuals can attain health parity. But someone can rarely take care of this on their own. Governments, healthcare providers, and community organizations must instead make adjustments.

4.1.1. Health Disparity, Equality, and Equity

When it comes to getting healthcare, people use terms, such as health disparity, health equality, and health equity.

4.1.1.1. Health Disparity

A difference that impacts an individual's capacity to attain optimal health is known as a health disparity. Race, gender, education, income, disability, location, and sexual orientation are a few examples of health disparities. Health inequities are caused by health disparities.

Some people don't always have access to the same opportunities as others to improve their health because of their circumstances or differences. A health disparity is frequently uncontrollable by an individual. Health equality and health equity are two ideas that deal with how to address these disparities.

4.1.1.2. Health Equality vs. Health Equity

All people have equal opportunities when it comes to health. One example might be a community center that provides everyone with free or inexpensive health examinations. When people have opportunities based on their needs, it is said to promote health equity. One illustration might be the same health facility charging individuals according to their financial situation. While someone else may have to pay for the same care, someone who cannot afford it may get it for free.

To put it briefly, health equity refers to the provision of tailored care to each individual to raise their level of health. Health equality refers to the application of the same standard to all. Parity in health is not always desirable. For instance, a person who has to work in the morning cannot take advantage of a clinic that provides free morning examinations. Even though everyone is eligible for checkups at the clinic, some people are still unable to use the service. To ensure health equity, alternate afternoon and evening checkup times should be provided, allowing individuals to utilize the service whenever it is most convenient for them.

4.1.2. Examples of Health Equity

Examples of services that promote health equity include:

- Providing health seminars and courses that are specific to the needs of certain ethnic communities and racial groups.
- Providing low-cost services to those living in low-income households.
- Using mobile health screenings to help those who may not have access to transportation.
- Offering evening or late-night health appointments to those who work long hours or are unable to access care.
- Providing better education, testing, and treatment access to communities particularly impacted by certain conditions or diseases.

Government agencies and neighborhood associations must recognize and work to eliminate care-related obstacles to advance health equity. Groups that have historically been denied rights and subjected to discrimination without cause are those who lack health equity.

Examples include:

- Racial and ethnic minorities;
- People living in a low-income household;
- Members of the LGBTQ+ community.

People who live in these communities are more likely to encounter obstacles to care and health, such as homelessness, low income, and violent crime. It takes community, political, and individual efforts to achieve health equity. Most of the time, a person cannot address every element influencing their health equity. Programs and professionals who help them can be beneficial to them.

4.1.3. Promote Health Equity

Individuals and organizations can take steps to help individuals achieve health equity.

The following are some steps to take:

- Identify how health disparities in a community affect specific groups.
- Recognize that each person has their own racial and ethnic biases and learn how to recognize when a policy or environment may exclude (sometimes unintentionally) a person or group.
- Show respect to people of all groups and make efforts to involve all groups in enacting change.
- This means that if someone is going to start a policy or program that addresses health disparities, they should ask the people they are trying to reach if the particular program will help them.
- Frequently evaluate how well policies aimed at health equity are working. Make changes when necessary to ensure these policies are most effective.
- Encourage people to contribute, using their talents, time, and gifts. An example could include tutoring students to help them obtain their high school diploma or a healthcare professional volunteering their time to help at a clinic.
- To promote health equity, a person must work with others to lift healthcare barriers whenever possible.

4.1.4. Differences Between Health Equity and Health Equality

Both health equality and health equity seek to enhance access to care and improve outcomes, particularly for underprivileged and marginalized communities. In healthcare, equity and equality are two different concepts and ways of thinking that can produce quite different results.

Providing everyone with the same opportunities, treatment, and services is known as health equality. A physician may give the same information to every patient or administer the same test to every patient at the same interval, regardless of risk factors. The physician may also think that they are acting impartially if they treat everyone the same.

Removing the institutional and discriminatory barriers that cause inequality and health inequities is the goal of health equity. This encompasses elements found both inside and outside the healthcare system, such as poverty and unequal resource distribution, as well as elements found within the system, such as racism and sexism.

In policy, health equity places a higher priority on justice whereas health equality provides equal support for everyone to receive healthcare. Everybody would receive equal access to healthcare funding and services under an equality-based approach. Under an equity-based approach, a person's ability to access services and receive funding would be determined by their needs.

4.1.5. Health Equity

The foundation of health equity is justice. Ensuring equitable access to high-quality healthcare and overall well-being is the aim, even if this means providing additional resources and support to some individuals. Health equity considers socioeconomic status, access to resources, and diversity of culture. For instance, living in unsafe communities, having less access to nutrient-dense food, and experiencing more stress and trauma can all be consequences of poverty on one's health.

Health practitioners take into account the effects of social determinants of health and methods for resolving them within a framework for health equity. For instance, a physician who is aware that a patient has trouble getting nutritious food may collaborate with the patient to develop plans for overcoming this obstacle and lowering the likelihood of health problems. The physician may also advocate for laws that deal with this problem.

4.1.6. Health Equality

Ensuring equal access to healthcare and treating everyone equally are the main goals of health equality. Health equality may be able to reduce disparities in certain situations, particularly if those disparities are the result of unfair treatment.

For instance, a 2016 study discovered that racist myths about Black people, such as the idea that they experience less pain, are frequently believed by medical students and residents. Removing these racist assumptions and promoting equitable assessments by medical professionals could increase awareness of Black people's suffering and help mitigate certain health inequalities. Transgender people also commonly report experiencing discrimination and receiving subpar medical care. According to half of trans respondents in a National LGBTQ Task Force survey, they had to educate their doctors about trans healthcare. Furthermore, 28% of respondents said they had experienced harassment in a medical setting, and almost 5% said they had been denied care.

While eliminating harassment and discrimination against transgender people would be the main goal of a health equality lens, the issue would not be entirely resolved. An equity-based strategy would guarantee that medical professionals are qualified to treat transgender patients.

4.1.7. Health Disparity

A health difference and a health disparity are not the same. A difference merely indicates that the experiences of various groups differ. For instance, uterine individuals frequently become pregnant. This is not a discrepancy, but a biological difference. Individuals over 50 who have uteri have a lower chance of becoming pregnant than those under 30. Once more, there is a distinction but not a discrepancy.

A difference that is unfair and avoidable is called a disparity. Inequalities are impacted by society. Different groups experience different but avoidable outcomes from disease and health disparities. For instance, prostate cancer is a greater cause of death for Black men than for White men. A 2019 study indicated that there was no discernible difference in the death rates of Black and White men with prostate cancer after controlling for social and environmental factors, such as access to high-quality care.

This suggests that rather than any real predetermined differences, the high death rates of Black men with prostate cancer are due to preventable issues. These concerns include social inequality that compromises health, the type of care a person receives, and access to high-quality care. Health disparities can be addressed by both health equality and health equity, but the best strategy varies depending on the particular health issue.

4.1.7.1. Disparities Based on Racism

Melanoma is a very aggressive form of skin cancer that affects black people less frequently than white people. Nevertheless, because doctors frequently identify their cancer at a later stage, they have a higher chance of passing away from it. Equal access to skin cancer screenings for Black and White people would be the main goal of a health equality lens. This method would inform medical professionals about the reality that Black individuals can and do pass away from melanoma and urge them to exercise the same caution when observing suspicious growths on both Black and White skin.

Within this framework, scientists could try to address scientific disparities, like the exclusion of Black subjects from skin cancer studies.

While more Black people may receive cancer screenings as a result of this, other problems might not be addressed. A more thorough approach is taken when using an equity lens. Equal access to screenings would be emphasized in this framework. But healthcare professionals would also look at other factors, such as:

- Lobbying for funding for programs that ensure that Black people can access skin cancer screenings.
- Reaching out to black communities to overcome barriers to skin cancer screenings, such as lack of transportation or health insurance.
- Identifying any cultural barriers to seeking or getting treatment.
- Educating people about the risks of skin cancer.

4.1.7.2. Disparities Based on Sexism

According to the data, people who are assigned female at birth frequently have difficulty receiving a proper diagnosis for reproductive and gender-specific health issues. For instance, a 2020 study proposes that the time between the onset of endometriosis symptoms and diagnosis and treatment is typically more than 6 years. Certain approaches to health equality would not even partially address this issue. For instance, endometriosis and other female health issues would not be included if men and women had equal access to screenings.

Equal training in medical school and ongoing education on health issues specific to men and women could be another equality-based strategy. This might guarantee that physicians receive the necessary training, but it might not be the answer.

From the standpoint of health equity, one could examine the particular difficulties faced by women when visiting the doctor. Numerous studies indicate that people do not take their pain seriously, even medical professionals. For instance, a 2021 study discovered that observers believed men when it came to the pain of women, but they attributed female pain to mental health problems. Observers frequently misjudged the degree of pain experienced by women.

Interventions such as implicit bias training and education about the tendency of doctors to discount the pain experiences of women could be beneficial. Public health advocates could create campaigns that target conditions that physicians frequently underdiagnose and make sure the messaging is visible in locations that are convenient for people to access.

4.1.8. Health Inequity

The term "health inequality" describes preventable variations in health among various populations. Lower life expectancy, high rates of mental illness, and trouble accessing healthcare are a few instances of health inequity. Systems that have a detrimental impact on people's living situations, access to healthcare, and general health status are the cause of these pervasive disparities.

People from underprivileged or historically marginalized groups are most severely affected by health inequity. On the other hand, it is detrimental to everyone. Additionally, it will outline what health equity might entail and offer concrete instances of how health disparities impact individuals.

Health inequity is defined by the World Health Organization (WHO) as "systematic differences in the health status of different population groups." This indicates that because of the systems that affect their lives, some groups have poorer health and more difficulty getting access to healthcare. For instance, poverty may be influenced by political and economic structures. High rates of poverty may limit a person's access to things like secure housing, hygienic food, clean water, education, and healthcare, all of which have an impact on health. This leads to an unfair and preventable division between various groups. To address this, changes in governmental policy are required.

Health disparities transpire at the local, national, and international levels, impacting every nation. The effects of health disparities on individuals will be examined in more detail in the ensuing sections.

4.1.8.1. Lower Life Expectancy

A person's average life expectancy can differ significantly based on the area in which they were born. Socioeconomic status has a significant impact on this. For instance, children born in Japan can expect to live for 84 years, whereas children born in Sierra Leone, West Africa, can expect to live for 50 years. Significant variations in living circumstances, financial status, and access to healthcare services have led to this. This issue is not unique to nations with lower incomes. Men's life expectancy in Glasgow, United Kingdom, varies by up to 15 points and 5 years based on the neighborhood they live in.

4.1.8.2. Higher Rates of Mental Ill-Health

Chronic stress, which impacts one's physical and mental well-being, can also result from inequality. For instance, the Youth Risk Behavior Study (2009–2019) discovered that bullying and sexual violence against gay, lesbian, and bisexual youth in the US are more common than among heterosexual youth. Suicide and mental illness rates have gone up as a result of this. It may be more challenging for some people to seek treatment for their symptoms and go to work or school if they have mental health issues or feel unsafe.

4.1.8.3. Difficulty Getting Healthcare

Treatment and diagnosis delays may result from bias, discrimination, and prejudice. Doctors may also find it difficult to believe or take certain groups seriously. According to certain research, when women visit the emergency room, they typically have to wait longer than men to receive medical attention. Significant delays are also seen in the treatment of many conditions, such as lupus and bleeding disorders, in women. This has no medical explanation. Misdiagnosis rates are higher when people are unaware of the gender-specific variations in heart attack symptoms, and these misdiagnoses can be fatal.

4.1.8.4. Preventable Death

Preventable deaths are caused by health disparities. While there are numerous instances of this, the disparity in infant mortality and health between Black and White babies born in the United States is among the most glaring. Low birth weight babies are more common in Black people than White people. They also have a higher chance of losing a child. This is true regardless of socioeconomic status and is unrelated to biological variations between races. This indicates that there is no inherent or unavoidable reason for the increased infant mortality rate.

4.1.9. Root Causes of Health Inequity

Systems and structures created by humans that favor some groups while undermining or actively oppressing others are the cause of health disparities. The unequal distribution of resources and power is the cause of this.

For example, these structures include:

- Racism, which distributes more power and resources to one race over another, typically means that historically marginalized racial or ethnic groups — such as Black, Indigenous, Latinx, Asian, and Pacific Islander people — receive fewer resources.
- Sexism, which privileges one gender over another, meaning that in most cases, men have more privileges than women and other gender identities.
- Classism, which gives unfair advantages to those with wealth and social status and disadvantages to those with less.
- Xenophobia, which gives nonimmigrants more power and rights than immigrants.
- Heterosexism, which privileges heterosexuality over other sexual orientations.
- Ableism, which values able-bodied people and devalues people with mental or physical disabilities.

Because of their complexity and interdependence, these systems have an impact on one another. Numerous individuals are impacted by multiple of these systems.

People perpetuate these systems at every level, including at an:

- Institutional level, which includes how organizations and governments set their laws, policies, and practices.
- Interpersonal level, which includes how people behave toward each other.
- Internal level, which includes how people view themselves.

The result of this is environmental, social, and economic differences that impact people's health, leading to health inequity.

4.1.9.1. Impact

Everyone is negatively impacted by health inequity. It results in worse outcomes for those with more power and resources and for those who are directly impacted.

For example, health inequity:

- Makes it more difficult to contain and treat infectious diseases;
- Increases levels of crime and violence across communities;
- Fuels alcohol and substance misuse;
- Increases stress and anxiety by damaging social cohesion;
- Decreases productivity and employment, and, therefore, tax revenue;
- Pushes 100 million people into poverty each year and prevents at least half of the world's population from getting the healthcare they need.

Costs billions of U.S. dollars per year and raises the cost of healthcare for everyone. For people who health inequity directly affects, the impact is not just limited to their lifetime. Health inequity can affect their children and grandchildren, both psychologically and physically.

4.1.9.2. What Could Health Equity Look Like?

The antithesis of health inequity is health equity. It outlines a system that guarantees everyone receives excellent healthcare and standards of health. To do this, it would be necessary to eradicate the causes of health disparities and give each patient specialized care that is tailored to their needs. This means that instead of treating everyone equally, some groups will receive more resources and power than others.

In the healthcare system, this could involve:

- Financial risk protection for people who need to pay for healthcare.
- Affordable prices for medications and vaccines.
- Flexible appointment times for people who work long or unusual hours.
- Mobile health services for those in remote areas and people who cannot travel.
- Easy access to translators, care workers, and others who can help people understand and access medical care.
- Education for healthcare professionals on how inequity affects the care they provide to their patients.
- Financial and social support for trainee medical staff who come from diverse backgrounds.

Achieving health equity also involves societal change. This could involve:

- Provide financial investment to areas and groups that need it most.

- Cleaning up environmental pollution and instating laws to protect against it.
- Addressing problems with accessing healthy food, such as food deserts.
- Addressing barriers that prevent people from attending school, such as period poverty.
- Ensuring that all houses and workplaces are safe and accessible, as well as prohibiting exclusionary housing practices.
- Ensuring that everyone can access green spaces, parks, and trails for exercise.

4.2. Factors Affecting Health Equity (Social Determinants of Health)

The surroundings in which people live, learn, work, play, and worship have an impact on a variety of health risks and consequences. These environments are known as social determinants of health. Extended disparities in six fundamental domains of social determinants of health are interconnected and impact an extensive array of health and quality-of-life consequences and hazards. We can better understand how to promote health equity and enhance health outcomes by looking at these multilayered health and social inequities.

4.2.1. Social and Community Context (Including Discrimination and Racism)

A person's relationships with family, friends, coworkers, the community, and institutions, as well as their interactions with the places they live, work, learn, play, and worship, all form part of their social and community context. Interventions play a vital role in safeguarding the health and welfare of individuals who do not receive the necessary support to flourish within their social and community settings. For instance, children of detained or jailed parents may benefit from their parents' involvement in reentry programs that help with job placement or provide parenting support, and school-based initiatives to prevent bullying and reduce violence would be beneficial for high school students who identify as lesbian, gay, or bisexual and who are bullied.

Discrimination, or the unfair treatment of individuals or groups based on attributes like race, gender, age, or sexual orientation, is another aspect of the social and community context. There is discrimination in many societal systems, including those that are designed to safeguard health or well-being, like the criminal justice, housing, healthcare, and financial systems. Discrimination frequently has a detrimental impact on the individuals and groups that experience it, as well as some members of groups that have historically faced discrimination, such as those who are homeless, incarcerated, or have disabilities. Consequently, individuals subjected to discrimination may be impacted by complex health and social disparities.

An increasing amount of evidence demonstrates that racism has existed in American society for centuries at various levels and has harmed communities of color. Racism is a system that is upheld and sustained by governmental regulations, institutional frameworks, societal norms and values, and individual actions. For more than 400 years, racism in its many forms has defined and produced the majority of the unequal structures that still exist in our society today and contribute to health disparities. The three types of racism include:

1. **Structural, Institutional, or Systemic Racism:** Differential access to the goods, services,

and opportunities of society by race.

2. **Personally-Mediated or Interpersonal Racism:** Prejudice (differential assumptions) and discrimination (differential actions) by individuals towards others.
3. **Internalized Racism:** Acceptance by members of the stigmatized races of negative messages about their abilities and intrinsic worth.

Racism bases opportunities on a person's skin color or physical appearance. Additionally, it influences social and economic variables that raise the risk of poor mental health outcomes, health-related behaviors, chronic and toxic stress, or inflammation in certain members of racial and ethnic minority groups. Racism impedes millions of individuals from achieving optimal health, which in turn impacts the well-being of our country.

4.2.2. Healthcare Access and Use

Multiple barriers are more likely to be encountered by individuals with disabilities, members of certain racial and ethnic minorities, those living in rural areas, and White populations with lower incomes when trying to access healthcare. For instance, it may be difficult to visit the doctor due to structural obstacles relating to socioeconomic status, such as a lack of childcare, insurance, transportation, or time off from work. Language hurdles and cultural differences between patients and providers have an impact on the quality of healthcare as well as patient-provider interactions.

4.2.3. Neighborhood and Physical Environment

Finding decent, affordable housing disproportionately affects members of racial and ethnic minority groups. Segregation in American cities has been exacerbated by the practice of redlining, or rejecting mortgages to people of color. This has prevented these individuals from accessing public transportation, supermarkets, and healthcare. Since the 1970s, the federal government has passed laws to lessen urban segregation. This historical form of discrimination has restricted housing options for members of racial and ethnic minorities to areas and homes with underfunded school districts, higher-than-average rates of crime, and inadequate infrastructure. These circumstances may increase the frequency and severity of illnesses, diseases, and injuries in these populations. Furthermore, these populations might have less access to reasonably priced, nutrient-dense food options, and they might also see higher levels of environmental pollution in their communities.

4.2.4. Workplace Condition

Even among workers with identical jobs, there are differences in the risk of work-related health issues. Occupational health disparities are preventable variations in the incidence of work-related diseases, mental illnesses, or morbidity and mortality that are strongly associated with disadvantages related to social, economic, and/or environmental factors, such as contract work arrangements, sociodemographic traits (e.g., gender identity, sex, age, or class), as well as organizational elements (e.g., inadequate worker safety precautions, little or nonexistent health insurance benefits).

4.2.5. Education

Inequities in access to high-quality education disproportionately affect those who have historically been marginalized, such as members of racial and ethnic minorities, people with disabilities, and those with lower disposable incomes. The resources available in schools located in lower-income neighborhoods are restricted by laws that tie public school funding to a neighborhood's tax base. Residents of lower-income neighborhoods receive lower-quality education as a result, which can have negative effects on literacy and numeracy levels, high school graduation rates, and college admission barriers. Apart from educational obstacles, restricted availability of high-quality job training or programs catered to the language requirements of specific racial and ethnic minority groups may limit prospects for employment in the future and result in jobs that are less stable or pay less.

4.2.6. Income and Wealth Gap

Some racial and ethnic minorities, as well as other historically marginalized groups, also have a harder time obtaining better-paying jobs with benefits because they have less access to high-quality education, discrimination, language barriers, geographic location, and transportation issues. Individuals with few career options frequently earn less money, face obstacles to building wealth, and have higher debt loads. Due to the inability to pass down property and accumulate wealth, the historical practice of redlining and refusing mortgages to people of color has also created a lack of opportunity for homeownership. It could be challenging to manage spending, pay medical bills, and get access to affordable, high-quality housing, childcare, education, and food due to financial difficulties (Aghighi et al., 2008; Ameryoun et al., 2010).

4.3. Measurement of Equity in Health

According to the Pan American Health Organization's Plan of Action (1), efficiency and effectiveness are the other two fundamental characteristics of a health services system, and equity is one of them. While it is the case for many more specific goals like high life expectancy or low infant mortality, it is not surprising that no indicators of progress towards any of these concepts—which are all difficult to define or measure—have been adopted. Though there isn't a single way to measure equity, there are a number of straightforward indicators that can be used to infer some information about it.

4.3.1. Equity as Equality of Treatment

Treating every member of the population equally is the core concept of equity. Ensuring everyone has good health and, to the greatest extent possible, equal health is the goal, and this will be attained through curative or preventive care. Due to differences in needs, equity cannot simply be defined as equality in general; rather, equity can be evaluated by taking specific forms of equality into account. Though "to provide 100% of the population with access to health services" may be the stated goal, what matters most is that everyone should have the same level of access, regardless of their circumstances.

Whatever the causes, disparities in access to healthcare that keep some people from receiving medical care while allowing others to do so lead to inequality. It is not reasonable to expect that everyone will visit a doctor at the same frequency or that the cost of healthcare will be the same for all demographic groups because illness and accidents occur randomly and in non-uniform ways. Resources and treatment ought to be directed where they are most required. However, it is expected that for a given set of health problems, there will be certain probabilities that are the same for all population groups in an equitable healthcare system.

4.3.1.1. Probabilities of Illness, Treatment, and Recovery

Figure 4.1 depicts this concept schematically. A person may or may not become ill or injured within a certain amount of time; they may or may not receive treatment; and if treatment is provided, there may or may not be a cure or a recovery. There are just four probabilities that can fully characterize the transition from an initial state to a final state (health, illness, disability, or death), as shown by the bold arrows in Figure 4.1.

These are:

- P(S) the unconditional probability of needing medical care.
- P(T/S) the conditional probability of receiving treatment, given the need for it.
- P(C/T) the conditional probability of being cured by treatment.
- P(R/T*) the conditional probability of recovering without treatment.

If the chance of being treated when there is no need for it—shown by the dashed arrow—is excluded from consideration, then every other probability, including those of final good health and ill health, P(H) and P(H*), is just some combination of these four basic probabilities.

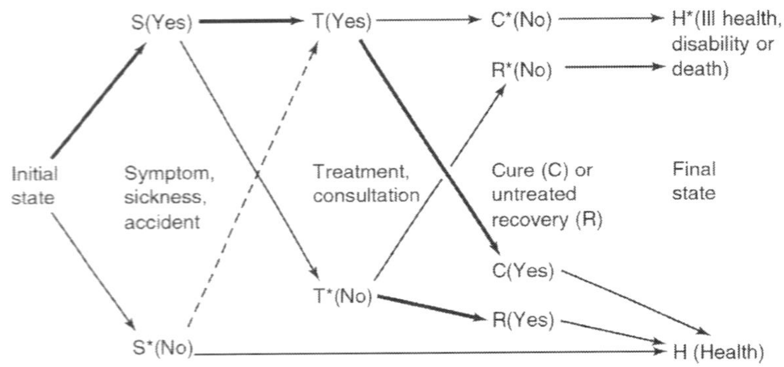

Figure 4.1. *Schematic stages of illness or accident, treatment, and outcome.*

Source: https://documents1.worldbank.org/curated/en/840211468779068549/pdf/279270PAPER0Health0economics.pdf.

4.3.2. Different Dimensions of Equity

This plan greatly simplifies matters, but it highlights various points to evaluate the fairness of a healthcare system. Key considerations include the subsections.

4.3.2.1. Which Stage of the Sequence Is Analyzed?

For instance, the system may give all patients receiving treatment about the same chance of recovery, but it may unfairly target some individuals for treatment far more easily than others.

4.3.2.2. The Difference Between Prevention, Which Acts on P(S), and Curative Treatment

It includes P(C/T) and P(T/S). Certain variations in the probability of becoming ill or injured shouldn't be regarded as unfair since they are linked to age or other risk factors that are primarily outside the purview of the healthcare system. Other P(S) disparities, such as the likelihood of contracting poliomyelitis or diphtheria, are unfair since prevention is within the system's purview and can be applied equitably to almost the whole population.

4.3.2.3. The Particular Condition, Illness, or Need, Studied

While everyone may have equal access to emergency care in the event of a car accident, there may still be significant disparities in the way that cancer and tuberculosis are treated in a healthcare system.

4.3.2.4. The Level of Quality of Treatment

The question of whether treating everyone for a given condition requires the same kind of care, or whether the system is considered equitable if all patients receive at least a minimally adequate level of care—even if some receive more complex, lengthy, or expensive treatment—also comes up when analyzing the distribution of income: is equality of incomes necessary for equity, or is a decent minimum income for everyone important? This question becomes especially relevant when analyzing expenditure on medical care.

4.3.2.5. The Interaction of Supply (Physical Availability of Services) and Demand (Individual Perception of Need) in Determining Who Does and Who Does Not Get Treatment

To what extent is it the government's responsibility to alter such cultural patterns so that medical needs and individual demands are related in the same way for the entire population? For instance, if the system offers relatively little care to a cultural group that is more stoic than average, or more likely to rely on home remedies or traditional healers.

The answers to all of these questions make it abundantly evident that there is no one way to quantify the equity of a healthcare system; one system may be blatantly unfair by some standards and fairly fair by others. Just as it is impossible to condense the health status of the populace into a single indicator, neither can the equity of a nation's health services be assessed by a single figure.

Lastly, there is a crucial matter that Figure 4.1 does not make clear. Some methods of grouping the population are necessary to estimate and compare probabilities. How this is carried out could have a big impact on the perceived inequality. The healthcare system may appear far more equitable in one area than another, much as income is usually distributed more unevenly among educational classes than among geographic regions. It is likely that more than one method of population division—for instance, based on socioeconomic factors and/or geography—will be necessary for a sufficient assessment.

Recent data from Peru can be used to illustrate a number of the above-discussed issues. These comprise household-level data from the 1984 National Health and Nutrition Survey, typical administrative data gathered by the Ministry of Health and examined by the Central Reserve Bank of the nation, and analyses carried out as part of the 1985–1986 National Health Sector Analysis by several Peruvian public and private organizations, funded by the US Agency for International

Development (USAID). While it is impossible to calculate every possible measure of equity—for instance, data on the likelihood of a cure or spontaneous recovery are lacking—a range of indicators are available.

4.3.2.6. Distribution of Health-Related Resources

When comparing different countries, it is common to look at the percentage of the population with access to safe water or sewerage connections or to calculate the population to healthcare resources ratio, such as physicians or hospital beds. This analysis can also be done within a country, as shown in Table 4.1. The comparison reveals that physicians are highly concentrated, especially in Lima, where over a quarter of the population has two-thirds of all physicians in Peru. Nurses are more evenly distributed but still tend to be concentrated in the same areas as physicians. Hospital beds are slightly more evenly distributed, and access to safe water is even more so. Generally, expensive resources appear more concentrated than cheaper ones (physicians versus nurses, and sanitation versus water supply). As measures of equity, these relatively simple indicators—which only require the place of residence as demographic data—have three significant drawbacks.

Table 4.1. *Measures Related to Equity in Healthcare, Peru (1982): Healthcare Resources and Sanitation Services (Percentages of National Total)*

DEPARTMENT	POPULATION	RESOURCES PHYSICIANS	RESOURCES NURSES	RESOURCES HOSPITAL BEDS	RESOURCES HOSPITAL TOTAL	DWELLINGS WITH WATER	DWELLINGS WITH SEWERAGE
Amazonas	1.5	0	0.1	0.3	2.4	0.6	0.4
Ancash	4.8	1.2	3.4	2.7	5.1	4.5	3.7
Apurimac	1.9	0.1	0.5	0.7	2.2	0.5	0.2
Arequipa	4.2	5.3	8.2	6.8	4.3	5.7	6
Ayacucho	2.9	0.2	1.3	0.9	2.6	1.5	0.7
Cajamarca	6.1	0.5	0.6	0.9	6.3	2	1.4
Callao	2.7	6.3	4.5	4.9	2.3	4.4	5.3
Cuzco	4.9	1	2.2	2.9	5.4	2.6	2.1
Huancavelica	2	0.1	0.4	0.7	2.4	0.6	0.4
HuÃ¡nuco	2.8	0.6	0.6	1.5	2.9	1	0.9
Ica	2.5	2.8	3.8	3.7	2.5	3.1	2.4
JunÃn	5	1.5	4	4.5	5.3	4.3	3.1
La Libertad	5.6	4.9	5.5	4.9	5.5	6.5	6.1
Lambayeque	4	2.6	5.4	3.8	3.53.5	4.5	4.3
Lima	28.1	66.6	50.7	48.4	26.4	45.1	52.8
Loreto	2.6	0.8	0.7	1.5	2.2	2	1.8
Madre de DiÃ³s	0.2	0.1	0.1	0.2	0.2	0	0.1
Moquegua	0.6	0.7	0.2	1.1	0.2	0.7	0.7
Pasco	1.2	0.6	1.2	1.7	1.3	0.8	0.6
Piura	6.6	2.3	2.7	3.2	6.1	5.2	4.2

Puno	5.2	0.5	1.5	1.6	6.4	1.5	0.8
San MartÃn	1.9	0.2	0.5	0.8	1.7	0.9	0.3
Tacna	0.9	0.6	1.3	1.4	0.9	1.5	1.4
Tumbes	0.6	0.2	0.3	0.3	0.50.5	0.10.1	0.1
Ucayali	1.2	0.3	0.3	0.6	1	0.4	0.3
National total	100	100	100	100	100	100	100
Gini coefficient of inequality		0.51	0.38	0.34		0.32	0.41

Source: https://documents1.worldbank.org/curated/en/840211468779068549/pdf/279270PAPER0Health0economics.pdf.

First, they can only be compared geographically; one cannot determine their distribution based on other demographic factors, like income, without knowing who consults the doctors. Second, the idea that needs are dispersed equally is implicit. Regarding sanitary facilities, this is probably a fair assumption, but it is dubious when it comes to health requirements. Given the potential for significant regional variations in the incidence or prevalence of health issues, an equitable allocation of resources would be uneven rather than uniform. Third, it is assumed that the facilities or resources under analysis meet the needs of the general public. Once more, this is a more realistic assumption for sanitation facilities, even though the effects of safe water on health can vary greatly based on the pattern of illness in an area and the population's hygiene habits. The assumptions surrounding healthcare are even more dubious: in many cases, medical intervention may not be required; several physicians may be involved in teaching or research; patients with more complex issues may seek treatment from other departments, etc. Therefore, even though these metrics hint at equality in resource distribution and, by extension, in healthcare spending, it is incorrect to believe that they are the only or best measures of system equity.

4.3.2.7. Probabilities of Need and Treatment

A primary shortcoming of the resource in comparison to. The morbidity and utilization data from a large sample of the Peruvian population in the 1984 survey, provided in Table 4.2, can be used to circumvent the population comparisons in Table 4.1. With one notable exception, the likelihood of presenting with a disease or symptom during the two-week reference period was roughly one-third among the urban population in the mountainous central region of the nation.

Table 4.2. *Measures Related to Equity in Healthcare in Peru (1984): Morbidity and Medical Attention*

AREA	PREVALENCE (%) OF SYMPTOMS			TOTA	PERCENTAGE SEEKING MEDICAL ATTENTION WITH SYMPTOMS			
	ALL KINDS	RESPIRATORY DISEASE	PARASITIC INFECTION		ALL AGES	UNDER 1 YEAR	1-4 YEARS	OVER 4 YEARS
Coast	*34.89*	*16.11*	*0.21*	*12.67*	*30.86*	*51.41*	*30.68*	*28.64*

Urban	34.87	16.34	0.20	13.36	31.54	55.74	32.69	29.96
Lima	36.57	17.68	0.15	14.88	33.49	59.43	35.87	31.62
Slums	37.32	16.85	0.19	14.14	32.05	64.84	32.85	29.78
Rural	35.00	14.38	0.28	7.50	18.76	27.14	16.52	18.71
Mountains	30.05	11.95	0.16	5.53	15.89	24.13	15.47	15.49
Urban	21.50	9.88	0.11	7.38	28.20	41.33	25.63	28.09
Rural	33.75	12.84	0.18	4.73	12.49	19.32	12.33	12.10
Jungle	36.03	12.06	1.78	7.65	18.39	27.33	17.20	17.94
Urban	33.72	11.59	1.36	10.36	25.59	42.63	22.34	24.97
Rural	37.35	12.32	2.02	6.11	14.69	18.42	14.46	14.41
National total	33.31	14.20	0.36	9.60	24.18	38.89	23.83	23.35
Urban	32.51	14.93	0.26	12.15	30.77	52.64	30.90	29.46
Rural	34.62	13.01	0.53	5.45	14.01	20.55	13.51	13.69

Source: https://documents1.worldbank.org/curated/en/840211468779068549/pdf/279270PAPER0Health0economics.pdf.

However, the unconditional probability of obtaining medical care (which includes going to the pharmacy but does not include home care) varied from less than 5% in rural mountainous areas to nearly 15% in Lima. As a result, in the rural mountains, the conditional probability P(T/S) varied from over one-third in Lima to 25%. Given that many illnesses and symptoms only require home care, equity in healthcare may not always imply certainty of attention. In this case, the Peruvian healthcare system exhibits stark regional disparities.

A few more aspects of these approximations are worth taking into account. The term "geographical dimension" can signify various things. To highlight the distinctions between urban and rural areas, the data in Table 4.2 are arranged based on the survey area. P(T/S) is more than twice as high in urban areas as it is in rural areas throughout the entirety of Peru. An alternative way to present the results would be to use the Ministry of Health's "health regions," as Table 4.3 does. While the health regions roughly correspond to departments or combinations of departments, neither of these classifications matches the departmental boundaries used in Table 4.1.

Table 4.3. *Measures Related to Equity in Healthcare in Peru (1984): Consultations, Hospitalizations, and Expenditures (Percentages of National Total)*

HEALTH REGION	POPULATION			MINISTRY OF HEALTH	
	TOTAL	WITH SYMPTOMS	CONSULTATIONS	HOSPITALIZATIONS	PATIENT-RELATED EXPENDITURES
Ancash	4.92	7.26	3.25	7.25	3.57

Arequipa	4.33	2.19	7.63	5.98	6.07
Cajamarca	4.48	5.08	1.57	1.38	1.80
Chiclayo	7.30	7.71	3.62	3.40	2.79
Cuzco	7.00	2.64	3.64	5.70	4.42
Huancayo	7.07	3.95	4.01	5.46	7.30
Hu6nuco	4.75	4.52	2.67	4.64	2.65
Ica	3.40	2.58	4.04	5.16	4.55
Iquitos	3.01	2.95	1.88	2.84	2.06
Lima	32.12	35.81	52.79	41.25	46.71
Moyobamba	2.00	3.30	2.18	2.20	2.51
Piura	7.44	10.28	4.29	4.81	3.90
Puno	5.09	5.26	1.36	2.13	2.81
Tacna	1.51	1.39	1.880	2.27	3.03
Trujillo	5.59	5.08	5.33	5.51	5.83
National total*	100.0	100.0	100.0	100.0	100.0

**Excluding the Ayacucho health region; percentages have been adjusted to 100% over the rest of the country.*

Source: *https://documents1.worldbank.org/curated/en/840211468779068549/pdf/279270PAPER0Health0economics.pdf.*

4.3.2.8. Differences by Illness and by Age

The overall morbidity's relative homogeneity conceals more significant differences for particular conditions or symptoms. Between less than 10% and more than 17% of the population suffered from respiratory diseases, while parasitic infections were incredibly common in the jungle, particularly in rural areas, despite being insignificant overall. For various causes like these, conditional probabilities of treatment can be computed independently. Table 4.2 demonstrates that P(T/S) varies significantly by age, as younger children are far more likely than older children to receive medical attention. Presumably, this is due to the increased likelihood of a severe illness during the first year of life. However, it seems that inequality is worse in how infants are treated. For instance, there is a larger disparity between urban and rural areas in the likelihood of providing care for infants than for other age groups. Therefore, increased service coverage or utilization does not always translate into increased equity or decreased inequality.

4.3.2.9. Equity in Vaccination Coverage

A large portion of the variation in the likelihood of receiving medical care may be explained by the differences in the danger or severity of illnesses and symptoms, as the comparison between older children and infants highlights. Not every one of these variations can be taken as evidence of unfairness. It might be prudent to examine equity in relation to a single, clearly defined need or condition in order to account for this source of variation. For all children under five, this is done in Table 4.4, where vaccination against the six target diseases of the Expanded Program on Immunization is done first by vaccine type and then based on the mother's educational attainment. This analysis is among the few conducted thus far that employ a socioeconomic classification; in the future, the survey data will enable classification by educational attainment as well as by income or a proxy variable for it.

A comparison of the four vaccine types demonstrates unequivocally that coverage inequality rises as overall coverage declines. The urban/rural difference for the BCG vaccine is less than 2:1; it reaches roughly 2:1 for the measles vaccination and nearly 4:1 for tetanus, whooping cough, poliomyelitis, and diphtheria protection. The country's mountain and jungle regions follow a similar national pattern. In the comparatively favored coastal region, the disparity is significantly smaller. Naturally, inequality decreases as national coverage approaches 100%; however, the significant disparity that arises in rural areas with low coverage reflects the extremely inadequate protection against these diseases in those areas.

Table 4.4. *Measures Related to Equity in Healthcare in Peru (1984): Vaccination Coverage (%) of Children Under 5*

AREA			BY TYPE OF VACCINE		
	BCG	POLIO	DPT	MEASLES	ALL TYPES
Coast	84.02	54.29	52.24	67.08	46.43
Urban	87.40	58.07	56.01	70.05	50.14
Lima	90.31	62.49	60.22	73.96	53.88
Slums	91.24	58.35	55.50	74.42	50.02
Rural	62.44	30.14	28.13	48.10	22.71
Mountains	49.99	18.31	17.94	39.31	12.99
Urban	77.16	41.56	41.86	59.70	30.29
Rural	39.42	10.11	9.51	32.13	6.89
Jungle	57.06	32.42	31.23	50.44	27.63
Urban	84.20	61.46	60.01	74.02	55.82
Rural	43.16	17.48	16.42	38.30	13.13
National total	67.62	37.81	36.51	54.40	31.31
Urban	85.36	55.47	53.87	68.56	47.14
Rural	44.34	14.66	13.75	35.82	10.57

BY MOTHER'S EDUCATION

	NONE	SOME PRIMARY	COMPLETE PRIMARY	SECONDARY	HIGHER
Coast	31.59	41.97	50.60	60.23	69.66
Urban	37.19	46.70	53.29	61.28	69.56
Lima	37.37	59.16	55.10	62.67	69.45
Slums	38.29	66.99	59.30	65.23	62.01
Rural	23.47	27.76	32.70	42.38	81.09
Mountains	10.778	14.18	25.68	35.81	51.39
Urban	27.02	30.51	30.57	39.30	50.37
Rural	9.32	10.70	23.05	27.88	58.50
Jungle	16.42	23.94	40.18	60.52	79.70
Urban	36.08	44.58	56.08	66.74	83.43
Rural	15.04	17.33	29.29	43.85	50.00
National total	16.17	26.62	42.23	55.73	65.28
Urban	34.36	43.46	50.23	58.49	65.47
Rural	11.82	15.05	26.79	36.02	61.01

Source: https://documents1.worldbank.org/curated/en/840211468779068549/pdf/279270PAPER0Health0economics.pdf.

When vaccination coverage is compared across educational levels, a somewhat similar pattern becomes apparent. Geographic inequality decreases as vaccination coverage increases along with educational attainment. It is also true that there is more disparity between educational groups the lower the coverage is in a given geographic area. Therefore, the rural mountainous areas, where overall protection is very low, exhibit the most marked socioeconomic inequality, while Lima exhibits the least amount of inequality. Except for urban slums, children of less educated mothers—presumably from low-income families—are the last to be reached. Better educated mothers are more likely to take their children to get vaccinated, without the need for a public campaign to encourage them to do so, and are better able to pay a private physician for service if necessary. This pattern likely reflects parental demand for vaccination rather than just differences in availability. Despite their extreme poverty, Tables 4.2 and 4.4 also demonstrate that Lima's slum dwellers do not constitute a disproportionately disadvantaged population regarding access to healthcare.

4.3.2.10. Summary Measures of Inequality

Tables 4.1, 4.2, and 4.4 place special emphasis on all the variations between geographic areas or socioeconomic classes because these variations could have a significant impact on determining the degree of equity or inequality in a healthcare system as well as the areas where its disparities are concentrated. To make general conclusions about whether a distribution represents a more or less equitable situation than another, summary measures of inequality can also be computed. However, all of these metrics omit data, and a given statistic condenses a distribution aligns with assumptions that may or may not be relevant when assessing equity. The Gini coefficient is frequently used for this purpose because of its simple geometric interpretation; the Central Reserve Bank's analysis for Peru is one example. The Lorenz curve, which ranks the groups from lowest to highest values of resources per capita, is first drawn. It relates the cumulative population across groups to the cumulative resource or utilization measure studied. This process yields the coefficient. Based on Table 4.1, the Lorenz curve corresponding to the physician departmental distribution in Peru is displayed in Figure 4.2. It shows, for instance, that while 70% of the nation's population lives in the departments with the highest physician shortage, only roughly 28% of physicians work in these areas.

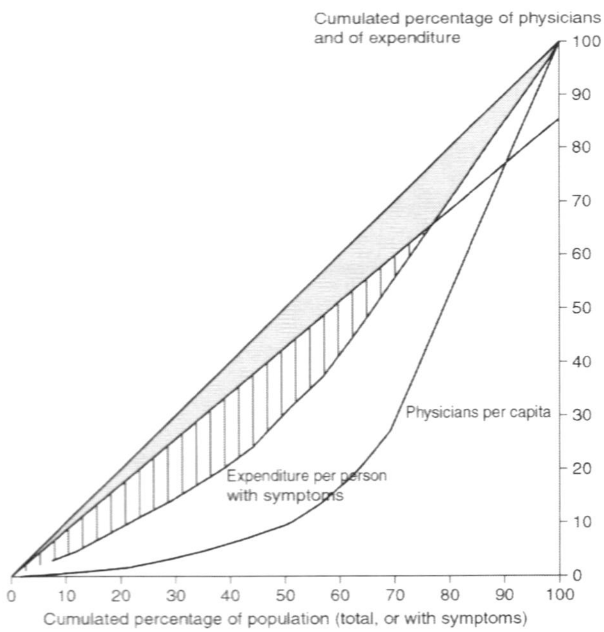

Figure 4.2. *Lorenz curves of inequality of the distribution of physicians relative to population (by department) and of Ministry of Health Patient related expenditure relative to population with symptoms.*

Source: https://documents1.worldbank.org/curated/en/840211468779068549/pdf/279270PAPER0Health0economics.pdf.

The ratio of doctors to the population is perfectly equal, as indicated by the diagonal line. The area under the diagonal divided by the area between it and the Lorenz curve is the Gini coefficient, a measure that rises from 0 to 1 as inequality rises. This measure is higher for physicians than for any other health-related resource taken into consideration, as Table 4.1 demonstrates. Inequality can also be represented by the Lorenz curve without the need to compute the Gini coefficient or any other summary statistic.

4.3.3. Financial Measures of Equity

Health services are provided by doctors, nurses, medications, vaccines, and other resources and supplies; however, none of these factors by itself is a sufficient indicator of the resources used in the medical field.

The cost of providing health services is the best overall indicator of the resources allocated to those services. Two questions about equity are brought. The first is about the same amount of money spent on all population groups; the second is about how different groups contribute to the same amount of money, either through taxes or through direct payment (fees for services).

These issues are especially crucial for the equity of the Ministry of Health Services, which is normally funded in large part by general government revenues and aims to serve populations that are too impoverished to pay for private healthcare and are unlikely to be covered by social security's medical benefits.

4.3.3.1. Equity in the Distribution of Expenditure

Differences in the likelihood of getting sick or needing care, the likelihood of getting care, and the cost of that care per patient can be used to isolate variations in the per capita healthcare spending. From 1982–1984, estimates of the overall costs by health region in Peru have been created. These estimates can be divided into two categories: costs associated with specific patients and costs related to maintenance and preventive care. The costs associated with the former can then be contrasted with those of the general population, the population that is ill or exhibiting symptoms and in need of care, or the population that receives care. A portion of these 1984 estimates is categorized by health region in Table 4.3. Cost per capita, the first of these metrics, is frequently employed as a gauge of equity, but like the metrics in Table 4.1, it is hampered by the unproven presumption that needs are always proportionate to the population. On the other hand, a uniform cost per consultation would not make the health system equitable if the likelihood of receiving care differed significantly among population groups. This is the other extreme of the cost per consultation, which leaves out much that is crucial for equity. Therefore, the expense per person in need of assistance appears to be the best indicator of equity in healthcare spending; ideally, this indicator would exclude people with symptoms that are too mild to warrant medical attention.

4.3.3.2. Expenditure and Morbidity

Table 4.3 suggests that patient-related expenses are allocated more fairly in Peru than some of the resources that support those expenses. For instance, two-thirds of Peru's doctors work in the Lima health region, which is home to roughly one-third of the nation's population, a slightly higher proportion of those who are ill or have symptoms, and less than half of all spending is related to individual treatment. Figure 4.2 confirms this perception, which contrasts the Lorenz curves for medical costs per capita and per sick person. The former distribution is by far more equitable in practice; the disparity in the distribution of physicians certainly exaggerates the unfairness of the healthcare system in Peru. For example, costs per consultation vary over a range of only 2:1 in most health regions, and even those differences may depend on regional variations in the incidence of specific diseases or conditions, some of which cost more to treat than others. Differences in unit costs contribute to overall inequality, but their impact is small compared to differences in the likelihood of receiving treatment. These findings support the notion that differences in receiving medical care when ill are the primary cause of healthcare disparities in Peru.

4.3.3.3. Inequality Without Inequity

Since equality and equity are not the same thing, inequality does not always imply inequity, as was previously mentioned. Assume, for instance, that although Peruvian health regions' costs per consultation in 1984 ranged from 8,845 to 23,843 soles, appropriate care could be provided for a unit cost of 15,000 soles. In other words, higher unit costs indicate inefficiencies, the use of overqualified labor, etc. Then, for only 85% of the total amount spent, all the patients who were seen could have received quality medical care. Figure 4.2 illustrates, where inequality is represented by the ted area and real inequality is represented by the hatched area. The former is primarily caused by variations in the likelihood of receiving care as well as some inequality in unit costs under 15,000 soles, indicating, on average, subpar care in some regions. The latter is solely attributable to average spending levels in certain health regions surpassing that threshold. Although the 15,000 sole unit cost was arbitrarily chosen and is merely used as an example, the claim that not all inequality reflects actual healthcare inequity is broadly applicable. This comparison makes sense in the same way as when one draws a "poverty line" in the income distribution and considers it unfair that some people earn less than that line while ignoring income disparities among those who make more than that.

4.3.3.4. Equity Is Getting What You Pay for

The question of how those expenses are funded is still not addressed when comparing costs or expenditures to the population or medical needs. Equity is typically understood by medical professionals to mean meeting needs, and payment concerns are only considered as potential roadblocks to receiving medical care. This is not the same as the consumer's or patient's satisfaction because the latter may not feel that his needs as identified by a doctor align with his demand for medical attention. One could also argue that equity necessitates the fulfillment of desires or demands. To economists, however, equity means something different: that is, there should be a net subsidy (expenditure less tax contributions) to population groups with low incomes and a net contribution by groups with high incomes, or that the distribution of healthcare expenditures should be less unequal than the distribution of income. The amount and direction of net subsidies then become a question of equity. Research with this perspective frequently concludes that public healthcare spending is more equitable than some other forms of public social spending, such as spending on education, and that it is progressive when compared to the distribution of income. That is to say, the impoverished typically gain more from public healthcare than they do from paying taxes, but they might lose money on some other areas of government spending. While studies in several other Latin American nations have been finished, this analysis has not yet been carried out for Peru.

It is crucial to remember that although they might not always coincide, these two ideas of financial equity in healthcare—expenditure relative to need and expenditure relative to payment—may. Following one criterion, but not the other, it will be equitable if a specific population group makes no contributions and receives little to nothing. When evaluating the equity of a public health service system in the presence of private fee-for-service healthcare, this question assumes special significance. The answers to these questions determine which indicators to construct and how to interpret the available data. Is the public system equitable if it provides access to those who cannot afford private care while ignoring those who can and do buy medical attention from private providers? Or does equity require the public system to reach and subsidize those poor consumers who currently pay for private services because they are more accessible or thought to be of higher quality than public services?

The concept of equity is too intricate to be boiled down to a single metric; analyzing it necessitates a wealth of data as well as some degree of subjective assessment regarding the specific types of inequality that actually qualify as inequity. On the other hand, a wide range of indicators that are relevant to equity or aid in measuring it can be created. The empirical analysis of the Peruvian case highlights the challenges in assessing healthcare equity as well as the potential applications of administrative, financial, and household data in forming general conclusions and pinpointing the locations and factors associated with inequity. This is far more important than determining a single, comprehensive metric for gauging the equity of a specific healthcare system.

To construct relatively full assessments of equity, population-based data must be used; information typically available to a Ministry of Health alone cannot be used to compare medical consultations and expenditures to population, morbidity, or perceived needs for assistance.

Since these population data are expensive and rarely collected, it is easier to study equity in a cross-sectional analysis rather than analyzing year-over-year variations. However, changes in the distribution of resources and effort over time can provide a good indication of whether a system is becoming more or less equitable, given a baseline assessment of how equitable the system is and where its main problems are. It is more crucial to understand the range of variation in the probabilities selected for analysis than it is to compute complex statistical measures like summary coefficients of inequality. For any such endeavors to be fruitful, they must consider the multiplicity of health conditions and the ways in which people respond to them, as well as the various demographic characteristics that can be used to assess equity.

4.4. Equity in Distribution

For a long time, health policymakers have faced a significant challenge in ensuring an equitable distribution of resources within the health system. Studies that have been done have typically focused more on equality than equity. We have tried to look at equity and equality in the distribution of resources in this chapter.

For researchers, planners, and policymakers in the health sector, concerns about fairness in the allocation of health resources are thought to present the biggest obstacles. By definition, equity refers to the equitable distribution of resources among individuals while taking their needs into account. The majority of research conducted in Iran has evaluated the population-level resource distribution geographically. That is a distribution that disregards the requirements of the populace. These studies show that although human resources and non-cardiac intensive care beds have been distributed fairly among Iran's provinces, kidney transplant beds and neonatal intensive care units have not. The Gini coefficient is one of the most useful metrics used globally to assess the degree of equality and inequality in access to healthcare resources. To remove the scale of equity in distributed resources, however, additional indicators have also been used, such as the Robin Hood and concentration index. Within health systems, hospital beds and specialists are regarded as two of the most valuable resources. Most of the time, an inefficient allocation of these complementary resources can result in the waste of medical resources and additional costs for patients. The World Health Organization (WHO) has highlighted the importance of paying attention to the equity principle in the distribution of health resources due to the significance of the issue, as one of the leading indicators in health systems (i.e., access) is satisfied with a fair allocation. These issues are primarily observed in developing nations because of deficiencies in the health system's information infrastructure. End-stage renal disease (ESRD) and chronic kidney diseases (CKD) are two of the most serious illnesses that not only endanger patients' physical health but also can put a great deal of strain on the financial constraints of health systems. High-risk patients may be in a situation where they are unable to receive appropriate referrals or diagnosis, which may be the consequence of an uneven distribution of kidney-related specialties (ESRD). Stated differently, the distribution of related resources has a significant impact on the management and control of these diseases. Management and control would be simpler the more equitable the distribution.

Therefore, implementing integrated medical practices and ensuring equitable access to complementary needed resources are essential for managing and controlling the risk factors increasing chronic kidney failure as well as improving the quality of care provided to dialysis patients. Iran has 335 nephrologists, 3,775 hemodialysis beds, and 18,545 hemodialysis patients, according to recent statistics. According to statistics, the annual growth rate of Iranian hemodialysis patients is approximately 12%.

Furthermore, CKD is almost 20 times more common in Iran than ESRD. To slow down the number of patients requiring kidney replacement treatments through earlier diagnosis and to help improve the quality of care given to hemodialysis patients, it is necessary to pay attention to equity as a rational and moral principle in the distribution of resources, whether physically or humanely, among the provinces. This will ultimately lessen the pressure on scarce resources.

The concentration index, Robin Hood, Lorenz curve, and Gini coefficient are a few of the commonly used metrics that are frequently applied to analyze equity and equality in the distribution of health resources.

While the distribution of two distinct variables is evaluated in the computation of the concentration index, the Lorenz curve compares the distribution of a particular variable with an equal distribution of the same variable. The best information available indicates that no such study using this methodology has been carried out in Iran.

Therefore, the purpose of this study was to assess the equity in the geographic distribution of hemodialysis beds and nephrologists concurrently in Iran using the need indicator (i.e., the number of patients receiving hemodialysis in population deciles) using the Lorenz curve, Gini coefficient, concentration, and Robin Hood index.

This will help policymakers make decisions to address the situation of complementary resource allocation and close the disparity in access to healthcare resources.

4.4.1. Geographical Units of Analysis

Iran is divided into 30 provinces, and each province's medical services are often overseen by a medical science university. We used each province as an analysis unit in this study. As a result, the Iranian Health Ministry provided all of the 2011 data, which included the number of hemodialysis patients, beds, and nephrologists by province. Next, we determined the data parameters (e.g., the number of patients and nephrologists per 10,000 people and the number of beds).

4.4.2. Measuring Equality and Equity

To evaluate equality in the distribution of beds and nephrologists at the population level, we employed the Gini coefficient. Its values span from maximum inequality (value = 1) to perfect equality (value = 0). We employed Brown's suggested formula, which is as follows, in the current study.

$$G = 1 - \sum\nolimits_{i=0}^{k-1} (y_{i+1} + y_i)(x_{i+1} - x_i)$$

where; G is the Gini index; y_i is the cumulative percentage of hemodialysis beds and nephrologists in its province; x_i is the cumulative percentage of beds and nephrologists to population in its province; and k is the total number of provinces.

The Lorenz curve was created by plotting the cumulative percentage of the proportion of beds and nephrologists on the (y) axis against the cumulative percentage of the sorted population on the (x) axis. This was done twice in ascending order, first based on the bed-to-population ratio and then again based on the nephrologists-to-population ratio. In the following phase, we ranked the population according to the number of hemodialysis patients in each province in descending order on the (x) axis. We also placed the cumulative percentage of hemodialysis patients, beds, and nephrologists on the (y) axis to provide the feasibility of comparing the distribution of beds and nephrologists with patients at the same time on a single graph. This allowed us to assess the status of equity in the distribution of hemodialysis beds and nephrologists for hemodialysis patients. After that, we constructed three concentration curves by plotting the corresponding points on the (x) and (y) axes, and we finally computed the concentration index. It is the area between the concentration curve and the 45° line. The variable's value would vary from −1 to +1 depending on whether it is disproportionately concentrated on the richest or poorest individuals. In a proportionate distribution, its value would be 0 (zero). The separation between the patient distribution concentration curve and the other two concentration curves (i.e., nephrologists and beds) is called the "equity gap" (Figure 4.3).

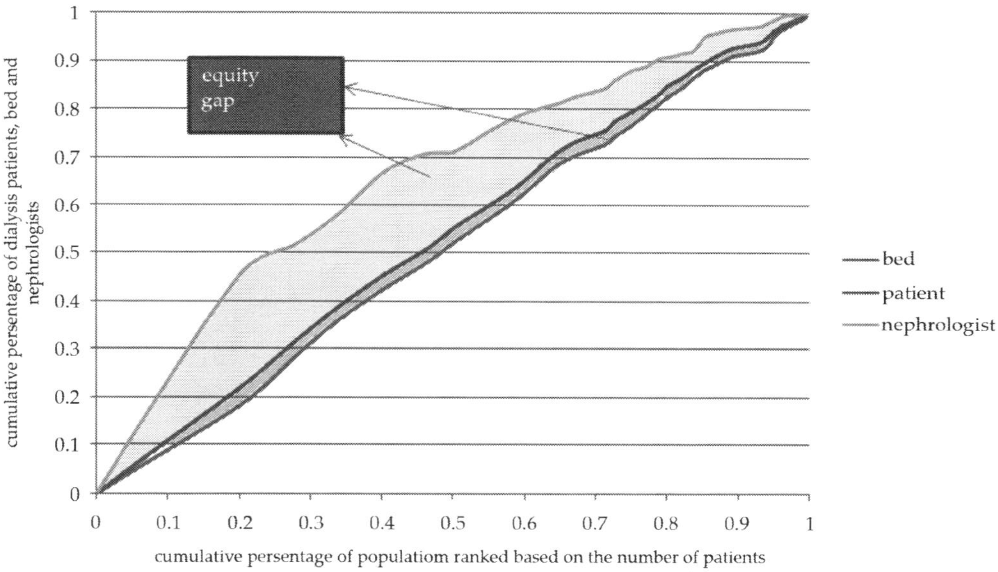

Figure 4.3. *Concentration curve of distribution of hemodialysis patients, hemodialysis beds, and nephrologists.*

Source: https://www.ncbi.nlm.nih.gov/pmc/articles/PMC4499072/bin/IJPH-42-1299-g003.jpg.

Additionally, we used the Robin Hood indicator to measure the degree of inequality in the distribution of hemodialysis beds and nephrologists. Specifically, we compared the actual need with the resources allocated in each population decile, subtracted the need from the extra resources allocated, and finally added up all of the extra resources allocated. We believed that the additional resources should be distributed to population deciles that are in need. Excel and STATA (version 11) were used to calculate the indicators.

$$R = 1/2 \sum_{i=1}^{n} |A - N|$$

where; R is the Robin Hood index; i is the number of deciles; n is the total number of deciles; A is the access in idecile (%); and N is the need in idecil (%).

4.4.3. Findings Related to Geographical Distribution of Hemodialysis Patients

Iran had 18,585 patients receiving hemodialysis in 2011. Ilam Province had the fewest hemodialysis patients, with 85, while Tehran had the greatest number of patients, with 3,991. Put differently, the province of Tehran accounted for 21% of these patients. Generally, 50% of hemodialysis patients were found in 5 provinces: Khuzestan, Tehran, Fars, Isfahan, and Khorasan Razavi. There were 25 dialysis patients for every 1,00,000 people on average. There was a significant variation in the number of patients per 1,00,000 people, ranging from a minimum of 9 in Sistan and Balochistan Province to 34 in Bushehr Province. Additionally, Table 4.5 demonstrates that 55% of the population represents 55% of patients, and 75% of the population represents 80% of patients. The hemodialysis patient distribution's Gini coefficient was 0.06 at the population level (Table 4.6).

Table 4.5. *The Number of Hemodialysis Patients, Nephrologists, and Hemodialysis Beds and Their Cumulative Percentage in Each Province*

ID	Province	Population	N Patient	N Neph	N Bed	PCP	BCP	PACP	NCP
1	Tehran	14,795,116	3,991	151	666	0.20	0.18	0.22	0.45
2	Khorasan Rezavi	5,940,766	1,811	21	378	0.28	0.28	0.31	0.51
3	Fars	4,528,514	1,348	22	289	0.34	0.36	0.39	0.58
4	Esfahan	4,804,458	1,240	30	247	0.40	0.42	0.45	0.67
5	Khuzestan	4,471,488	972	13	201	0.46	0.48	0.50	0.71
6	West Azerbaijan	3,016,301	904	2	168	0.50	0.52	0.55	0.71
7	East Azerbaijan	3,691,270	896	14	188	0.55	0.57	0.60	0.76
8	Mazandaran	3,037,336	788	11	163	0.59	0.62	0.64	0.79
9	Gilan	2,453,469	769	5	154	0.63	0.66	0.69	0.80
10	Golestan	1,687,086	454	3	97	0.65	0.69	0.71	0.81
11	Kermanshah	1,905,793	441	5	78	0.67	0.71	0.73	0.83
12	Kerman	2,947,346	413	6	84	0.71	0.73	0.76	0.84
13	Qom	1,127,713	367	5	61	0.73	0.75	0.78	0.86
14	Hamedan	1,699,588	360	7	82	0.75	0.77	0.80	0.88
15	Kordestan	1,467,585	330	3	87	0.77	0.79	0.81	0.89
16	Markazi	1,392,435	328	5	84	0.79	0.81	0.83	0.90
17	Bushehr	9,43,535	322	1	52	0.80	0.83	0.85	0.91
18	Hormozgan	1,558,878	318	3	73	0.82	0.85	0.87	0.92
19	Ardabil	1,242,956	304	2	72	0.84	0.87	0.88	0.92
20	Yazd	1,065,893	280	9	64	0.85	0.88	0.90	0.95
21	Qazvin	1,212,464	280	3	37	0.87	0.89	0.91	0.96
22	Lorestan	1,758,226	272	3	64	0.89	0.91	0.93	0.97

23	Sistan and Baluchestan	2,733,205	242	2	44	0.93	0.92	0.94	0.97
24	Zanjan	983369.3	226	3	47	0.94	0.93	0.95	0.98
25	Semnan	6,24,482	210	2	67	0.95	0.95	0.96	0.99
26	Chaharmahal	892909.3	203	2	51	0.96	0.97	0.97	0.99
27	South Khorasan	676794.1	150	1	32	0.97	0.98	0.98	1.00
28	North Khorasan	838780.8	148	0	33	0.98	0.98	0.99	1.00
29	Kohgiluyeh and Boyer-Ahmad	669139.6	93	1	23	0.99	0.99	1.00	1.00
30	Ilam	566332.4	85	0	36	1.00	1.00	1.00	1.00
Total		**74,733,230**	**18,545**	**335**	**3,722**	–	–	–	–

Abbreviations: N Neph: Number of nephrologists; PCP: Population cumulative percentage; BCP: bed cumulative percentage; PACP: patient cumulative percentage; and NCP: nephrologists' cumulative percentage.

Source: https://www.ncbi.nlm.nih.gov/pmc/articles/PMC4499072/.

Table 4.6. *Distribution of Healthcare Resources and Hemodialysis Patients Along with Their Dependent Indices*

Resources	Index	Value
Hemodialysis bed at the population level.	Gini coefficient	0.03
Nephrologists in the population level.	Gini coefficient	0.38
Hemodialysis beds concerning need.	Concentration index	–0.02
Nephrologists concerning need.	Concentration index	–0.31
hemodialysis beds with regard to need.	Robin Hood index	0.24
Nephrologists with regard to need.	Robin Hood index	0.02
Hemodialysis Patients in population level.	Gini	0.06

Source: https://www.ncbi.nlm.nih.gov/pmc/articles/PMC4499072/.

Findings related to the distribution of hemodialysis beds – there were 3,722 hemodialysis beds available in total. With 666 (or 17.9%) hemodialysis beds, Tehran had the most, while Kohgiluyeh and Boyer-Ahmad Province had the fewest, with only 23 (or 0.6%) beds. Both Table 4.5 and Figure 4.4 demonstrate how almost proportionately beds are distributed among the population. The Gini coefficient was 0.3. There were five beds for every 1,00,000 people, with Semnan having the highest proportion (10.8 beds) and Sistan and Balochistan having the lowest ratio (1.6 beds). To determine the current state of hemodialysis bed distribution based on the need indicator, we also tracked the distribution of beds for patient count. Thus, to achieve this goal, we computed the concentration index. The value was –0.02. According to Table 4.5, 50% of the population has access to 52% of the beds, but 55% of the patients are in the same percentage of the population.

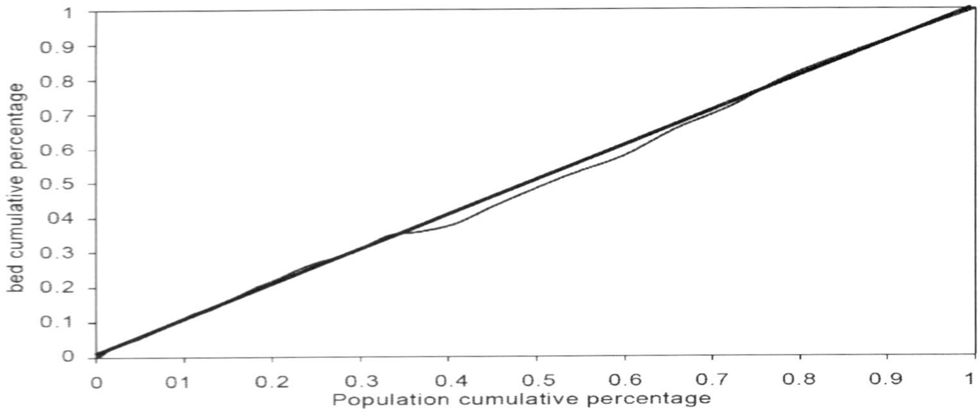

Figure 4.4. *Lorenz curve of hemodialysis beds distribution in population level.*

Source: https://www.ncbi.nlm.nih.gov/pmc/articles/PMC4499072/bin/IJPH-42-1299-g001.jpg.

4.4.4. Findings Related to the Nephrologist Distribution

There were 335 nephrologists in total. Elam and North Khorasan had no nephrologists, while Tehran had the greatest concentration of 151. In Tehran, nephrologists accounted for nearly 45% of the workforce. There were 0.45 nephrologists for every 1,00,000 people. Additionally, there were 55 dialysis patients for every nephrologist. Lorenz and concentration curves for the cumulative distribution of nephrologists are displayed in Figure 4.5, first for the population as a whole and then concerning patients (i.e., according to necessity).

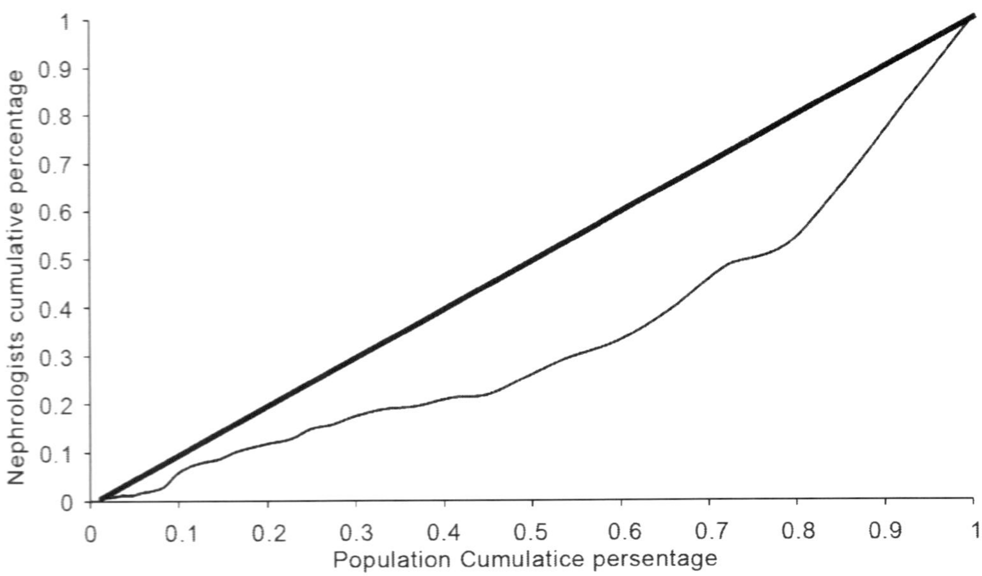

Figure 4.5. *Lorenz curve of nephrologists' distribution in population level.*

Source: https://www.ncbi.nlm.nih.gov/pmc/articles/PMC4499072/bin/IJPH-42-1299-g002.jpg.

According to Table 4.5, 25% of the population, which includes 22% of patients, account for 45% of nephrologists, while 50% of the population, which includes 52% of patients, have access to 71% of nephrologists. These statistics demonstrate a significant disparity in the distribution of nephrologists across population deciles. The distribution of nephrologists is accompanied by a great deal of inequality, as confirmed by the calculation of the Robin Hood index (25%) (Table 4.7).

Table 4.7. *Access and Need (%) to Nephrologists Among the Population Deciles for Calculation of Robin Hood Index*

Deciles	Access (%)	Need (%)	Difference (%)
1	21	10	+11
2	24	11	+13
3	6	10	–4
4	8	9	–1
5	11	10	+1
6	5	10	–5
7	6	11	–5
8	7	10	–3
9	7	10	–3
10	5	9	–4

Robin Hood index = 11 + 13 + 1 = 25% (0.25)

Source: https://www.ncbi.nlm.nih.gov/pmc/articles/PMC4499072/.

In the current study, we first used the Lorenz curve and Gini coefficient to examine the distribution of hemodialysis beds and nephrologists at the population level, i.e., without taking the needs of the population into account. The distribution of hemodialysis beds among population percentiles is largely equivalent, as evidenced by the results, which showed that the Gini coefficient for hemodialysis bed distribution at the population level was 0.03. Amerion et al. have verified this equality in the distribution of ICU, post-ICU, and NICU beds. Additionally, other research showed that there was inequality in Iran's kidney transplant bed distribution. According to the findings of a Chinese study, hospital beds were distributed fairly when the Gini coefficient was taken into account as a determining factor. However, the distribution of nephrologists, one of the most valuable human resources associated with kidney failures, did not follow the same pattern as the distribution of hemodialysis beds. Both the Robin Hood index, which is 0.25, and the Gini coefficient, which is 0.38, were used to support this claim. Our findings are consistent with an Albanian study's finding that there was moderate inequality in the distribution of general practitioners. But the pattern was reversing. On the other hand, the evaluation of physician distribution in the United States using the Gini coefficient between 1970 and 1998 showed that inequality was on the rise.

What is noteworthy, though, is that there is no value placed on judging how to distribute healthcare resources in an equitable manner while ignoring the needs of the populace. To put an end to this, we then distributed resources by population needs. That is, the number of people receiving hemodialysis. We distributed both of the aforementioned resources (i.e., hemodialysis patients' distribution) against hemodialysis beds and nephrologists. The distribution of beds and nephrologists does not precisely match the distribution of hemodialysis patients.

We reasoned that we could have concluded that these complementary resources had been distributed fairly if concentration curves for beds and nephrologists had been placed on concentration curves for patient distribution. However, the results of Robin Hood and the concentration index calculations showed there is some inequality in the distribution of hemodialysis beds, particularly among nephrologists. Nonetheless, the disparity in the distribution of nephrologists across the provinces was significantly larger than the number of hemodialysis beds. The concentration index for nephrologists and beds was −0.32 and −0.02, respectively. According to these coefficients, the distribution of nephrologists is 16 times more unequal than that of beds. This discrepancy between the distribution of resources and hemodialysis patients is known as the "equity gap."

One of the outcomes of improper distribution is difficult access to necessary services. The distribution of nephrologists was inconsistent with the hemodialysis patients, according to the results. This access barrier may lead to inadequate diagnosis and referrals. Research has indicated that although hemodialysis is 12% common in Iran, chronic kidney disease (CKD) is 20 times more common. This claim thus aligns with the reality that the health system and society will face greater pressures if policies aimed at allocating resources are not manipulated.

Therefore, equity-oriented approaches to resource allocation must be given top priority to manage and control the increasing trend of ESRD patients due to the high cost of hemodialysis and the severe budgetary constraints that health systems face (Asada et al., 2005; Beauchamp et al., 2001).

4.5. Equity in Health Financing

To guarantee that everyone has access to necessary health services without experiencing financial hardship, equity in health financing refers to the equitable and just distribution of financial resources for healthcare among individuals and populations. It covers a range of topics related to healthcare financing, such as how money is raised, gathered, and distributed to satisfy the various healthcare requirements of the populace.

To advance the goal of health for all and universal health coverage (UHC), equity in health financing must be achieved. Inequalities in healthcare access and financial protection resulting from geographic disparities, socioeconomic inequality, and other social determinants of health must be addressed. Countries can work toward lowering health inequalities and improving health outcomes for all by making sure that healthcare financing mechanisms are progressive, transparent, and sensitive to the needs of vulnerable and marginalized populations.

Key principles and strategies for promoting equity in health financing include:

1. **Progressive Financing:** Ensuring that the burden of healthcare financing is distributed based on individuals' ability to pay, with higher-income individuals contributing a larger share of their income towards healthcare costs.
2. **Universal Coverage:** Establishing mechanisms, such as social health insurance or tax-funded healthcare systems, to ensure that everyone has access to essential health services, regardless of their socio-economic status.
3. **Financial Protection:** Implementing measures to protect individuals and households from catastrophic health expenditures and impoverishment due to healthcare costs, such as

subsidies, exemptions, or waivers for low-income groups.

4. **Redistribution:** Using health financing mechanisms to redistribute resources from wealthier to poorer populations and from healthier to sicker individuals to address health inequities.
5. **Participation and Accountability:** Engaging communities, civil society organizations, and other stakeholders in the design, implementation, and monitoring of health financing policies to ensure transparency, accountability, and responsiveness to the needs of marginalized groups.

Countries can get closer to realizing the goal of health for all, in which everyone has access to high-quality, reasonably priced healthcare services and no one is left behind because of financial hardship or social disadvantage, by placing a higher priority on equity in health financing.

Social justice views influence the questions of what constitutes an equitable distribution of the costs associated with supporting the health system and its benefits. The libertarian and egalitarian points of view are arguably the two most prevalent in the discussion of health financing. According to the egalitarian perspective, public financing should take precedence, with health services being provided based on need and financial contributions being made based on income. Health service coverage is not correlated with financial contributions.

The private financing of health services and the distribution of those services based on ability and willingness to pay are the extremes of the libertarian perspective. Any donations to the underprivileged are contingent upon individual acts of generosity. A less extreme form that guarantees a safety net for the impoverished while maintaining a preponderance of private funding and minimal public involvement is known as sufficientarian liberalism. They are able to achieve a respectable standard of living, complete with some degree of healthcare coverage, thanks to this safety net.

The participation of government funding for safety nets is implied by this libertarianism, albeit not to the same extent as in the egalitarian perspective. The impoverished are unable to pay for the services they require, or cannot pay for them entirely, so the rest of society must provide funding for a sufficient range of services for them. But after that, the laws of the market take over.

There is disagreement over which metric should be the focus of any equity concern: health outcomes, service utilization, use given need, or a notion of access to essential services. Here, we use the fundamental ideas behind the UHC concept, which suggest that equity in access to necessary services and affordable coverage should be the main focus. Benefit-wise, the UHC concept echoes the egalitarian principle of allocating health services based on need. The issue is not just whether these services are covered, but also whether they are effective, which is a crucial aspect of their quality. These two aspects are typically combined under the umbrella term of effective coverage.

The notion of need-based service distribution has consequences for the burden of care as well. Primarily, revenue-generating schemes that require patients to pay out-of-pocket (OOP) should not prevent those who cannot afford them from accessing healthcare services. On the burden side, however, there are other ways in which the connection between egalitarian principles and the UHC concept is less clear-cut and complex. UHC merely requests protection from financial hardship resulting from having to make out-of-pocket payments. There are two commonly recognized definitions of financial hardship resulting from out-of-pocket payments (OOPs): first, OOPs that cause someone to fall into poverty or further into it, and second, OOPs that have disastrous effects on households without necessarily impoverishing them. Catastrophic effects can include severe asset depletion, excessive borrowing to cover healthcare costs, and foregone consumption of essential goods and services like food, housing, clothing, and education. Therefore, UHC suggests that everyone should have access to affordable coverage with necessary services and that no one should face financial hardship from out-of-pocket expenses. However, there is no mention of the equity of other financial contributions to the system, such as taxes and insurance premiums.

However, moving away from OOPs to shield people from financial hardship depends on financing arrangements that align with egalitarian viewpoints, according to the practical application of UHC principles. Decoupling financial contributions from service utilization is necessary to protect against financial hardship because health products and services can have high direct costs, which affect most income groups in addition to the poor. Although any kind of prepayment and pooling can theoretically lead to decoupling, this has only been accomplished at a large scale, i.e., by providing mandatory prepayment and pooled funding for the whole population. In actuality, this entails associating financial contributions with the ability to pay in some manner, since many impoverished people will not be able to contribute financially.

UHC is still a ways off for the majority of nations, and only a small number of them can afford universal coverage that includes all health interventions that can increase life expectancy or improve its quality while guaranteeing everyone's financial security. This calls into question equity in the pursuit of UHC. As we've seen, the idea of UHC entails equality in long-term access to necessary services and affordable coverage, but it says nothing about the role that equity plays in getting there. According to the broad definitions of equity and fairness, those who are less fortunate in terms of need and means of support should be given some preference, i.e., those with the greatest illnesses and the poorest finances. Indeed, this is also in line with the sufficientarian perspective, which holds that the poor should have access to adequate health services; however, this is subject to the qualification that UHC requires governments to gradually advance toward the full realization of UHC outcomes.

The WHO Consultative Group on Making Fair Choices on the Path to UHC proposed a set of principles to identify inequalities and policy choices that are unfair, drawing on the ideas of equity, fairness, and the values and principles inherent to the concept of UHC.

Based on the earlier arguments, these are defined as:

1. **Benefits:** Effective coverage of services is according to need. On the path to UHC, priority is given to cover those with the greatest health needs.
2. Burden: Financial contributions are based on the ability to pay and are independent of service use. On the path to UHC, priority is given to covering (under such financing arrangements) those with the least ability to pay.

These ideas align with progressive universalism, which maintains that the poorest people should gain at least as much as the rich do on the route to universal healthcare. It's critical to understand that these principles are not absolute and that, as will be discussed later, they necessitate trade-offs with social goals other than equity and fairness. However, there is leeway for interpretation in these principles. Fair contributions based on financial capacity, for instance, could be understood as equitable contributions for all health funding from an egalitarian standpoint or, from a sufficientarian's perspective, as the amount of money needed to cover the impoverished essential medical needs only. According to the principle of contributions based on ability to pay, which is commonly referred to as progressive contributions, the rich either pay more than the poor or a larger percentage of their income than the poor. Furthermore, opinions on how much more the wealthy should pay will differ even after this issue is resolved.

Furthermore, trade-offs might be necessary to separate the principles for benefits and burdens. Moreover, within each component, policymakers will have to make additional trade-offs: in terms of benefits, for instance, whether to increase coverage or improve the quality of available services; or, should they prioritize expanding the range of high-quality services available for those with the greatest health needs, or expanding financial protection to those with the least ability to pay? To provide answers, it is necessary to evaluate how policy options will lessen unfair disparities in addition to how much they will advance UHC overall, that is, across all of its dimensions and outcomes.

The distinction made between benefits and burden also stands in contrast to some recent research examining whether fiscal policies generally, including those about health, enhance equity. The distribution of pretax gross income is compared with the distribution of post-tax final household income in order to examine the effect of fiscal policy on "final" income. Final income is calculated by deducting taxes, social security contributions, and levies from gross income, then adding any cash or in-kind government benefits that each household receives (e.g., child allowances, unemployment or illness benefits, and the use of government-funded health or educational services). Fiscal policies that accomplish this kind of redistribution are regarded as more equitable than those that do not, insofar as the poor receive a larger portion of final income than gross income (Brown et al., 1994; Calman et al., 1994).

A Closer Look

Health Equality

Health equity, also referred to as health equality, encompasses the principle of fairness and justice in health outcomes, access to healthcare services, and opportunities for health improvement among all individuals and populations. It emphasizes the elimination of health disparities that are avoidable, unfair, and unjust, irrespective of socio-economic status, race, ethnicity, gender, age, or other social determinants of health. Health equity goes beyond simply providing equal access to healthcare; it also addresses the underlying social, economic, and environmental factors that contribute to health inequities.

Health equity ensures that all individuals have equal access to high-quality healthcare services, regardless of their socio-economic status, geographic location, or demographic characteristics. This includes access to preventive care, primary care, specialty care, medications, and other health services needed to maintain and improve health.

Health equity recognizes that health outcomes are influenced by a wide range of social, economic, and environmental factors, such as income, education, housing, employment, neighborhood conditions, access to healthy food, and exposure to environmental pollutants. Efforts to achieve health equity involve addressing these social determinants and creating conditions that promote health and well-being for all.

Health equity aims to eliminate disparities in health outcomes and healthcare access that exist between different population groups. This includes reducing disparities in disease prevalence, morbidity, mortality rates, and life expectancy, as well as addressing disparities in healthcare utilization, quality of care, and health insurance coverage.

Achieving health equity requires creating healthcare systems that are inclusive, culturally competent, and responsive to the needs of diverse populations. This involves providing culturally and linguistically appropriate care, promoting diversity in the healthcare workforce, and engaging communities in decision-making processes related to healthcare delivery and policy development.

Policies and interventions aimed at achieving health equity may include expanding access to affordable healthcare coverage, investing in healthcare infrastructure in underserved areas, implementing strategies to address social determinants of health, promoting health literacy and education, and advocating for policies that reduce discrimination and promote social justice.

Overall, health equity is a fundamental principle of public health and healthcare systems, emphasizing the importance of ensuring that everyone has the opportunity to achieve their highest level of health, regardless of their background or circumstances. By addressing health inequalities and promoting health equity, societies can create healthier, more equitable communities where everyone can thrive.

Summary

- Equity in health represents the ethical principle of fairness and justice in the distribution of healthcare resources, opportunities, and outcomes among populations.
- Health equity means ensuring everyone has the chance to be as healthy as possible. However, factors outside of a person's control can prevent them from achieving their best health.
- Health disparity is a difference that affects a person's ability to achieve their best health. Examples of health disparities include race, gender, education, income, disability, geographic location, and sexual orientation.
- Health equity and health equality aim to improve outcomes and increase access to services, especially for underserved populations and marginalized groups.
- Social determinants of health are the conditions where people live, learn, work, play, and worship that affect a wide range of health risks and outcomes.
- Racism prevents millions of people from attaining their highest level of health, and consequently, affects the health of our nation.
- The fundamental idea of equity is of equal treatment for all the population. The intention is to ensure good health for all, and as far as possible, equally good health, to be pursued through preventive or curative treatment.
- Physicians, nurses, drugs, vaccines, and other resources and supplies are used to produce health services, but none alone is an adequate measure of resources used in healthcare.
- Equitable distribution of health system resources has been a serious challenge for a long time among health policymakers.
- Equity in health financing refers to the fair and just distribution of financial resources for healthcare among individuals and populations, ensuring everyone has access to essential health services without suffering financial hardship.

References

1. Aghighi, M., Heidary Rouchi, A., Zamyadi, M., Mahdavi-Mazdeh, M., Nourozi, S. H., et al. (2008). Dialysis in Iran. *Iran J Kidney Dis, 2*(1), 11–15.
2. Ameryoun, A., Meskarpour-Amiri, M., Dezfuli-Nejad, M. L., Khoddami-Vishteh, H., & Tofighi, S. (2011). The assessment of inequality on geographical distribution of non-cardiac intensive care beds in Iran. *Iranian J Public Health, 40*(2), 25–33.
3. Asada, Y. (2005). Assessment of the health of Americans: The average health-related quality of life and its inequality across individuals and groups. *Popul. Health Metr., 3*(1), 7.
4. Beauchamp, T. L., & Childress, J. F. (2001). *Principles of Biomedical Ethics* (5th ed.). Oxford University Press, USA.
5. Berndt, D. J., Fisher, J. W., Rajendrababu, R. V., & Studnicki, J. (2003). Measuring healthcare inequalities using the Gini index. In *System Sciences, Proceedings of the 36th Annual Hawaii International Conference on* (p. 10). IEEE.

6. Brown, M. C. (1994). Using Gini-style indices to evaluate the spatial patterns of health practitioners: Theoretical considerations and an application based on Alberta data. *Soc Sci Med, 38*(9), 1243–1256.
7. Brown, R. L., & Prus, S. G. (2006). Income inequality over the later-life course: A comparative analysis of seven OECD countries. *Annals of Actuarial Science, 1*(2), 307–317.
8. Calman, K. (1994). The ethics of the allocation of scarce health care resources: A view from the center. *J. Med. Ethics., 20*(2), 71–74.
9. Daniels, N., Kennedy, B. P., & Kawachi, I. (1999). Why justice is good for our health: The social determinants of health inequalities. *Daedalus, 128*(4), 215–251.
10. Feinberg, J. (1995). Justice. In W. T. Reich (Ed.), *Encyclopedia of Bioethics* (pp. 802–810). Macmillan.
11. Graves, N., Halton, K., & Lairson, D. (2007). Economics and preventing hospital-acquired infection: Broadening the perspective. *Economics, 28*(2), 178–184.
12. Health Metrics Network. (2008). *Framework and Standards for Country Health Information Systems*. Geneva: World Health Organization. Retrieved from: https://iris.who.int/handle/10665/43872.
13. Horev, T., Pesis-Katz, I., & Mukamel, D. B. (2004). Trends in geographic disparities in the allocation of health care resources in the US. *Health Policy, 68*(2), 223–232.
14. Jimenez, E. (1986). The public subsidization of education and health in developing countries: A review of equity and efficiency. *The World Bank Research Observer, 1*(1), 111–129.
15. Kennedy, B. P., Kawachi, I., & Prothrow-Stith, D. (1996). Income distribution and mortality: Cross-sectional ecological study of the Robin Hood index in the United States. *BMJ, 312*(7037), 1004–1007.
16. Khan, S., & Amedia, C. A. (2008). Economic burden of chronic kidney disease. *J. Eval. Clin. Pract., 14*(3), 422–434.
17. Lai, D., Huang, J., Risser, J. M., & Kapadia, A. S. (2008). Statistical properties of generalized Gini coefficient with application to health inequality measurement. *Soc Indic Res, 87*(2), 249–258.
18. Mahdavi-Mazdeh, M., Zamyadi, M., & Nafar, M. (2008). Assessment of management and treatment responses in hemodialysis patients from Tehran province, Iran. *Nephrol Dial Transplant, 23*(1), 288–293.
19. Matsumoto, M., Inoue, K., Bowman, R., & Kajii, E. (2010). Self-employment, specialty choice, and geographical distribution of physicians in Japan: A comparison with the United States. *Health Policy, 96*(3), 239–244.
20. McIntyre, D., & Mooney, G. (2007). *The Economics of Health Equity*. Cambridge University Press.
21. Mobaraki, H., Hassani, A., Kashkalani, T., Khalilnejad, T., & Ehsani Chimeh, E. (2013). Equality in distribution of human resources: The case of Iran's Ministry of Health and Medical Education. *Iranian J. Publ. Health, 42*(Supple 1), 161–165.
22. Munga, M. A., & Mæstad, O. (2009). Measuring inequalities in the distribution of health workers: The case of Tanzania. *Hum. Resour. Health, 7*(1), 4.
23. Musgrove, P. (1983). Equity in health system services—Concepts, indicators, and interpretation (summary in English). *Boletin de la Oficina Sanitaria Panamericana, 95*(6), 525–546.

24. Nishiura, H., Barua, S., Lawpoolsri, S., Kittitrakul, C., & Leman, M. M., et al. (2004). Health inequalities in Thailand: Geographic distribution of medical supplies in the provinces. *Southeast Asian J Trop Med Public Health, 35*(3), 735–740.

25. O'Donnell, O., Van Doorsslaer, E., Wagstaff, A., & Lindelow, M. (2008). *Analyzing Health Equity Using Household Survey Data: A Guide to Techniques and Their Implementation*. World Bank Publications.

26. Pan American Health Organization. (1982). *Health For All by The Year 2000: The Plan of Action for The Regional Strategies*. Washington D.C., PAHO. (Official document no. 179).

27. President's Commission for the Study of Ethical Problems in Medicine and Biomedical and Behavioral Research. (1983). *Securing Access to Health Care: The Ethical Implications of Differences in The Availability of Health Services. Volume 1: Report*. Washington D.C., US Department of Health and Human Services.

28. Ranasinghe, P., Perera, Y. S., Makarim, M. F. M., Wijesinghe, A., & Wanigasuriya, K. (2011). The cost in the provision of hemodialysis in a developing country: A multi-centered study. *BMC Nephrol, 12*, 42.

29. Rashidian, A., Yousefi Nouraie, R., Azemikhah, A., Heydarzadeh, M., & Changizi, N., et al. (2008). Perinatal care regionalization and geographical distribution model in the Islamic Republic of Iran. *Hakim, 11*(2), 1–1.

30. Rawls, J. (1985). Justice as fairness: Political not metaphysical. *Philosophy & Public Affairs, 14*(3), 223–251.

31. Richard, J. B., Aldigier, J. C., Le Mignot, L., Glaudet, F., Said, B., et al. (2008). Equity of accessibility to dialysis facilities. In *Studies in Health Technology and Informatics* (Vol. 150, pp. 777–781).

32. Shahabi, M., Tofighi, S. H., & Maleki, M. R. (2010). The nurse and specialist physicians' manpower distribution by population and its relationship with the number of beds at public hospitals in Iran's 2001–2006. *Journal of Health Management, 13*(41), 7–14.

33. Theodorakis, P. N., Mantzavinis, G. D., Rrumbullaku, L., Lionis, C., & Trell, E. (2006). Measuring health inequalities in Albania: A focus on the distribution of general practitioners. *Hum. Resour. Health, 4*, 5.

34. Theodorakis, P., & Mantzavinis, G. (2005). Inequalities in the distribution of rural primary care physicians in two remote neighboring prefectures of Greece and Albania. *Rural Remote Health, 5*(3), 457.

35. Thomas, Vinod and Wang, Yan and Fan, Xibo, Measuring Education Inequality: Gini Coefficients of Education (January 2001). Available at SSRN: https://ssrn.com/abstract=258182.

36. Thornicroft, G., & Tansella, M. (2002). Balancing community-based and hospital-based mental health care. *World Psychiatry, 1*(2), 84.

37. Xu, J., Wu, N., Jin, S., Wang, F., & Wang, Y., et al. (2010). Analysis of inpatient bed allocation equity and utilization in the city community health service center of China. *J. Huazhong Univ. Sci. Technolog. Med. Sci., 30*(2), 141–144.

Chapter

5

FINANCING AND INSURANCE IN HEALTHCARE

Contents

Introduction

There are numerous ways to finance the cost of medical care. In certain nations, government-run healthcare programs may provide the majority of coverage, with residents being granted automatic access to care. In other situations, a large number of medical expenses are covered by mandated health insurance programs (provided by public or private organizations). A variable amount of household payments (either as stand-alone payments or as part of co-payment arrangements) and different types of voluntary health insurance meant to replace, supplement, or enhance automatic or mandatory coverage also make up the remaining portion of healthcare spending.

Healthcare financing arrangements primarily consist of government programs and mandatory health insurance in all OECD countries except one. When combined, they represented nearly 75% of all healthcare spending in the OECD in 2015 (Figure 5.1). Around 80% or more of all health spending in Denmark, Sweden, and the UK was funded by the federal, regional, or local government. More than 75% of all medical expenses in Germany, Japan, France, and the Slovak Republic were covered by mandatory health insurance. Less than half of all medical expenses were only covered by the government or required health insurance in the United States. On the other hand, voluntary health insurance accounted for a substantial amount of health spending (35%).

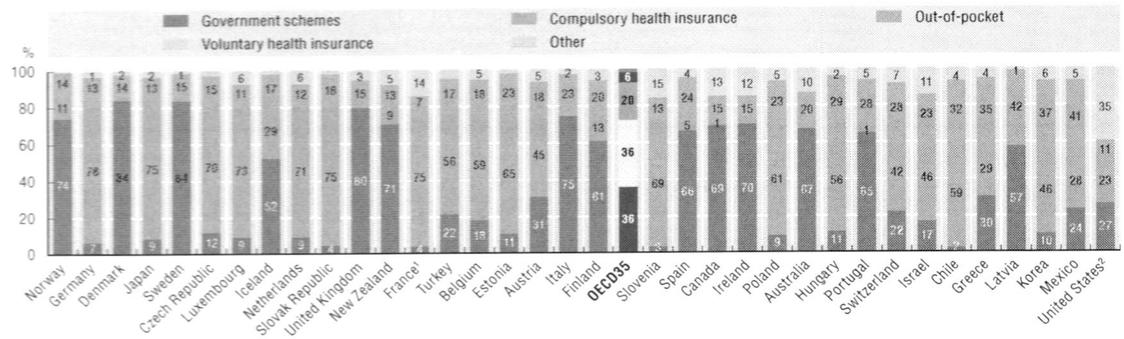

Figure 5.1. *Health expenditure by type of financing, 2015 (or nearest year).*

Source: https://www.oecd-ilibrary.org/docserver/health_glance-2017-46-en.pdf?expires=1714576412&id=id&accname=guest&checksum=916091D55FD3775F27AB7160BFC83A7B.

Governments use their overall budgets to fund a wide range of public services. Healthcare thus faces competition from a wide range of industries, including housing, education, and the military. The amount of public money allotted to health is influenced by several variables, such as the kind of system in place and the population's demographic make-up. Political decision-making and economic factors can also cause relative budget priorities to change every year. In 2015, the percentage of total government expenditure in the OECD allocated to health through government programs and mandatory insurance was approximately 15% (Figure 5.2). Over 20% of public spending in Germany, the United States, Switzerland, Japan, and New Zealand went toward healthcare. Conversely, in Latvia and Greece, healthcare received less than one euro for every 10 spent by governments or mandated health insurance.

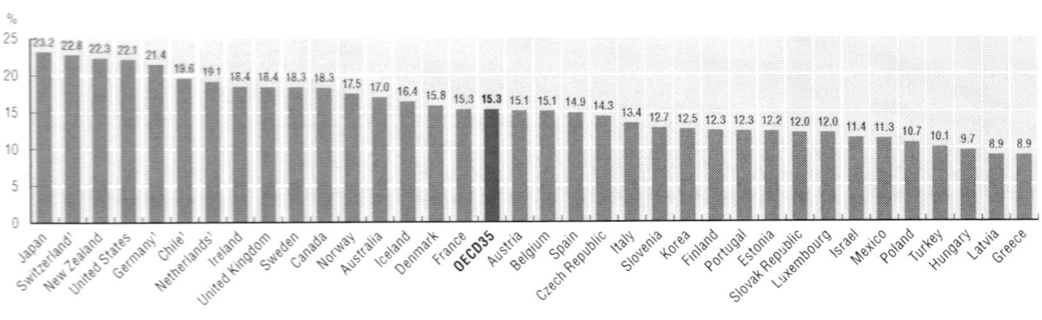

Figure 5.2. *Health spending by government schemes and compulsory health insurance as a share of total government expenditure, 2015 (or nearest year).*

Source: https://www.oecd-ilibrary.org/docserver/health_glance-2017-46-en.pdf?expires=1714576412&id=id&accname=guest&checksum=916091D55FD3775F27AB7160BFC83A7B.

After state-run programs and mandated health insurance, private funds are typically the primary source. Approximately one-fifth of all health spending in 2015 was directly financed by private households on average across the OECD. In Greece (35%), Korea (37%), Mexico (41%), and Latvia (42%), this percentage is higher than one-third, whereas in France it is less than 10%. The percentage of household healthcare costs that have been paid has decreased significantly in certain OECD countries over the past few decades as a result of the introduction of universal health coverage. In recent times, there has been a noticeable rise in certain European countries, but overall, the percentage of out-of-pocket spending has remained consistent (Figure 5.3). Due to the implementation of reforms to balance public budgets that shifted some financing responsibilities to patients, the share of health spending payable by households has increased in Greece (+6.2 percentage points (pp)) and Spain (+4.7 pp) since 2009. Conversely, during the same time, this share has decreased in Chile (–2.3 pp) and Mexico (–6.0 pp).

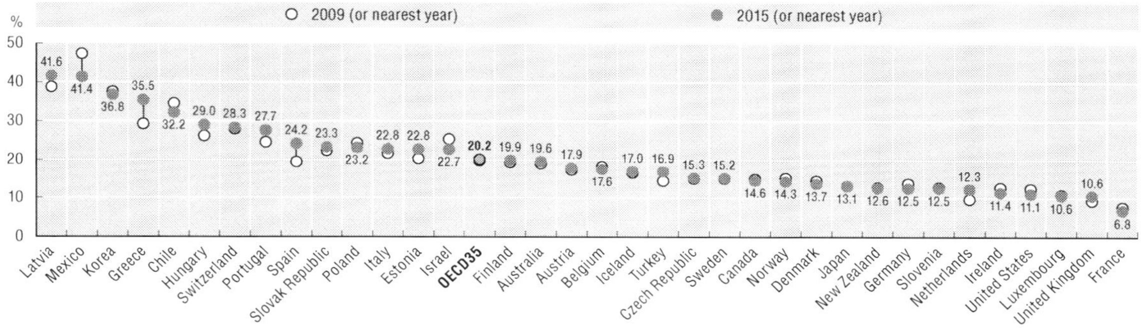

Figure 5.3. *Change in out-of-pocket expenditure as a share of expenditure on health, 2009 to 2015 (or nearest years).*

Source: https://www.oecd-ilibrary.org/docserver/health_glance-2017-46-en.pdf?expires=1714576412&id=id&accname=guest&checksum=916091D55FD3775F27AB7160BFC83A7B.

Orientation and Directional Terms:

Term	Definition	Illustration
Coinsurance	The percentage of a medical bill the insured must pay after deductibles and co-payments are met.	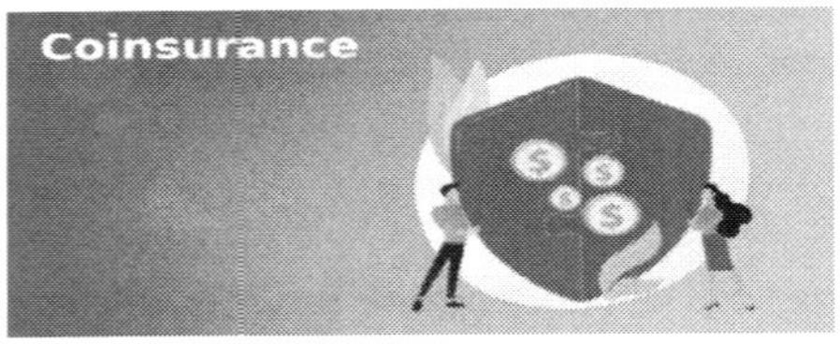
Community rating	Insurance premiums are based on the pooled risk of a community. All individuals in the community pay the same premium, regardless of claims experience or personal level of risk.	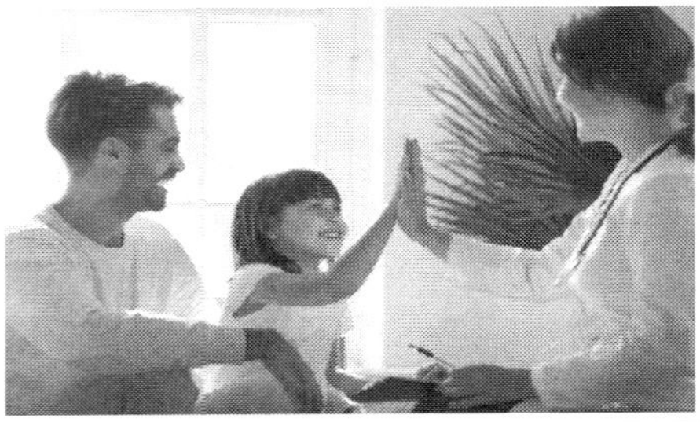
Co-payment	The insured must pay a specified amount for each received service that can vary by service.	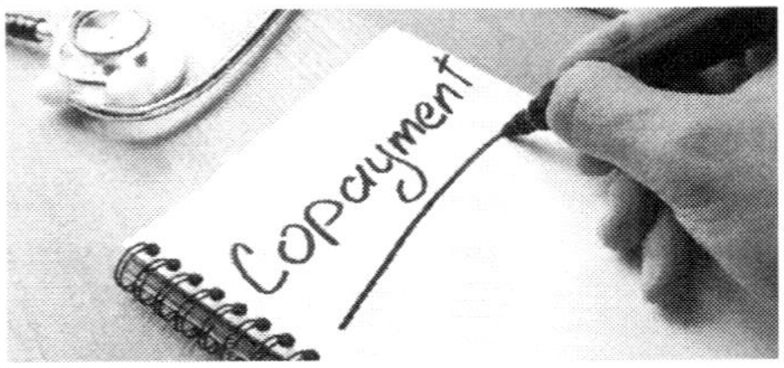
Deductible	The insured must pay a fixed amount of a healthcare charge before the insurer begins payment for all or part of the remainder of the costs.	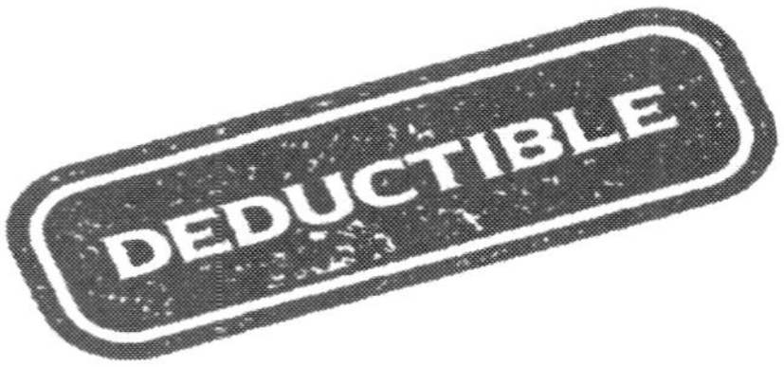
Experience rating	Insurance premiums are based on the claims experience or risk level, such as age, of each insured group.	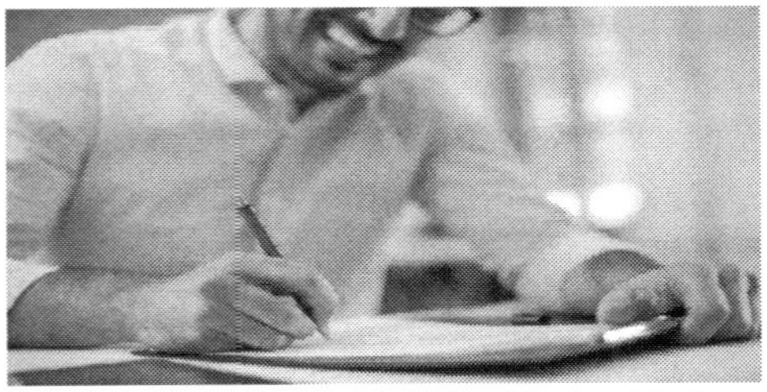
Financial intermediary	An agency collecting money to pay providers on behalf of patients.	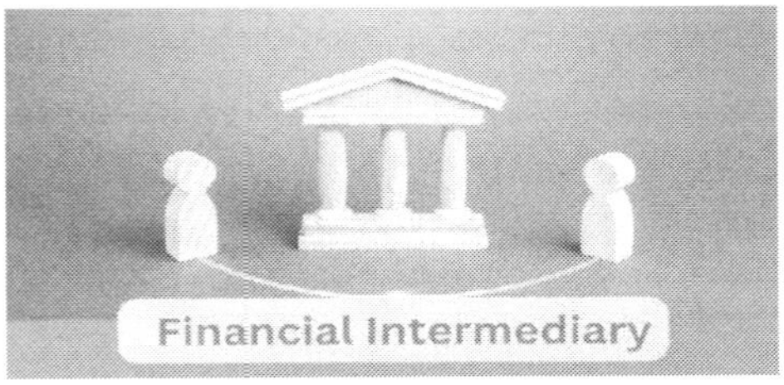

5.1. Financing of Healthcare

The financing schemes (financial arrangements through which people pay for and obtain health services, e.g., social health insurance), financing agents (organizations managing the financing schemes, e.g., social insurance agency), and types of revenues (e.g., social insurance contributions) can all be used to analyze healthcare financing. Here, the term "financing" refers to financing plans as those defined by the System of Health Accounts, which include government programs, both required and optional health insurance, as well as private funds from organizations, private companies, and households. Private health insurers may provide mandatory health coverage, sometimes with no requirement to sign contracts with specific people (e.g., in Chile and Germany). Cost-sharing plans and unofficial payments made to healthcare providers are examples of out-of-pocket expenses that patients bear on their own.

According to the System of National Accounts, total government spending comprises capital expenditures that are payable to the federal, state, and local governments as well as social security funds, interest, intermediate consumption, employee compensation, social benefits, social transfers in kind, subsidies, and other current expenses. For those nations where private insurers provide mandatory health insurance, the proportion of spending from government financing programs and mandatory insurance plans to overall government spending is somewhat inflated.

In the United States, expenditures made by private health insurance companies are classified as voluntary health insurance, even though since 2014, the Affordable Care Act (ACA) has made it mandatory for people to obtain health insurance or face penalties.

5.1.1. Definition of the Health Sector

To facilitate data collection and, in particular, to compare health systems between nations or eras, a clear definition of the services and activities that make up the health sector is required. The inability to clearly distinguish between elements of the health sector and non-health sector is demonstrated by the following pairs of items. Which ought to be a part of the health sector's definition?

- Health services Environmental services (e.g., water, sanitation, environmental pollution control, occupational safety, etc.);
- Hospitals, social welfare institutions;
- Education and training, pure medical research;
- Medical social work; social work;
- Formally trained medical practitioners; traditional medical practitioners.

National borders defining the health sector differ significantly, and various definitions have been created for various objectives. Since there are more deficiencies in some areas (such as education) than in developed countries, the definition is typically broader in developing countries (e.g., environmental health) and heavy reliance on the conventional medical field. As a helpful general guideline, all funding and expenses whose main goal is to improve health should be included (regardless of outcome).

5.1.2. Definitions of Financing

The process of generating money to pay for healthcare products and services is known as financing. There are several ways to pay for this, including out-of-pocket expenses, private insurance, and government funding. Ensuring that everyone, regardless of financial situation, has access to the healthcare they require is the aim of healthcare financing.

The function of a health system is to mobilize, accumulate, and distribute funds to meet the individual and community health needs of those enrolled in the health systems.

The whole process of healthcare finance involves:

- Where the money came from;
- How it was collected;
- Pooled;
- Redistributed to the third-party payers;
- Finally used to pay the providers for their services.

5.1.3. Health System Financing

Raising money for the health system involves gathering funds from primary and secondary sources, putting them in fund pools, and allocating them to provider operations. The function of health system financing within the overall health system is located in Figure 5.4. Three primary tasks comprise the health system's financing function. The raising of money, either directly from people seeking medical attention or indirectly through governments or donors, is referred to as revenue collection. The act of pooling funds so that contributors to the fund share risks to finance the healthcare of a specific population is known as fund pooling. The process of giving money to healthcare providers is known as purchasing.

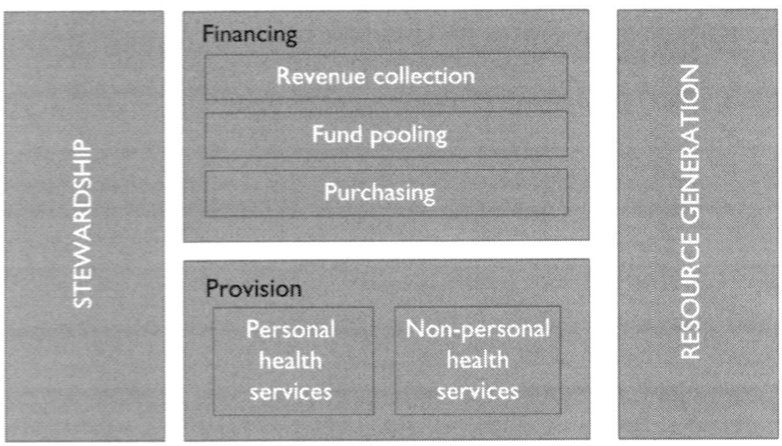

Figure 5.4. *Functions of the health system.*

Source: Lorna Guinness & Virginia Wiseman. Introduction to Health Economics (2nd edn.). McGraw-Hill. Open University Press.

In the end, household finances provide the majority of the funding for the health system, whether via taxes, insurance, or out-of-pocket expenses. Therefore, at its most basic level, healthcare financing is the transfer of money from patients to healthcare providers in return for services. Payment for health services can be made in two ways, as shown in Figure 5.5.

- Out-of-pocket payments: this is the simplest and earliest form of transaction between patient and provider;

- Third-party payments: where providers are paid by an insurance company or a government.

This section addresses the primary form of financing—that is provided by third parties. It is appropriate to consider out-of-pocket expenses in greater detail beforehand, as they represent a substantial portion of the cost of healthcare.

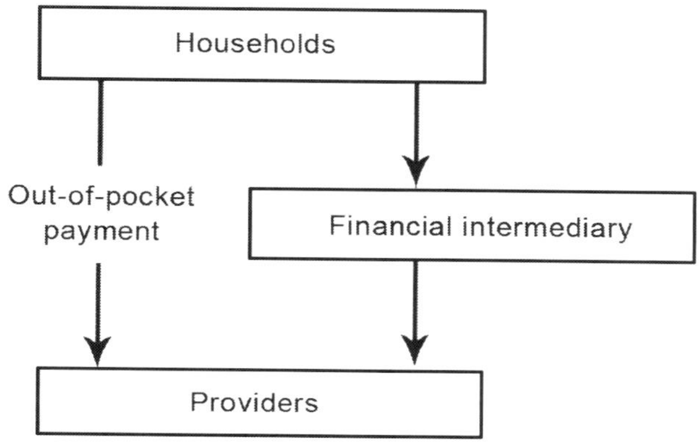

Figure 5.5. *The flow of funds in healthcare provision.*

Source: Lorna, G., & Virginia, W. Introduction to Health Economics (2nd edn.). McGraw-Hill. Open University Press.

5.1.4. Sources of Healthcare Financing

To pay for medical supplies and services for the people they cover, health finance programs must generate income. Various forms of income, though, can have a strong relationship with the financing plan. Finance schemes can generally receive government transfers, social insurance premiums, and required or voluntary prepayments (e.g., insurance premiums), as well as additional domestic and foreign income received as development assistance.

In actuality, a health financing scheme's revenues and expenses in a given year are usually unequal, resulting in a fund surplus or deficit. In reality, the majority of nations merely examine the revenue composition for each scheme and apply the resulting shares pro rata to the costs associated with each financing scheme, thereby matching revenues and costs.

The various healthcare payment schemes in each of the OECD member countries rely on a combination of different revenue streams. For instance, budgetary allocations for government programs are normally derived from total government revenues (e.g., from value-added tax, corporate and income taxes, etc.). Typically, employers' and employees' social contributions pay for social health insurance. But these programs might also get different percentages of their income from transfers from the government. Prepayments, which can be required or voluntary and usually take the form of regular premium payments made by an insurance contract, are the primary sources of funding for private health insurance. Only a household's income is used to cover out-of-pocket expenses. Certain health finance programs (e.g., non-profit organizations or enterprise schemes) may also get donations or extra money from real estate or investments. Transfers from overseas may also be made to resident financing schemes as a part of bilateral agreements with foreign governments or other development partners. In contrast, the vast majority of OECD nations do not consider these transfers to be relevant.

The way a nation finances its healthcare system is closely linked to the makeup of its revenue stream. Therefore, governmental transfers rank highest among all revenue sources when examining the overall revenue structure in, say, Denmark, where healthcare activities are primarily funded by local government schemes (Figure 5.6). In many countries, the government plays a larger role than that of a mere buyer of health services. This makes it possible to draw important conclusions about how financing functions in various health systems by comparing the structures of financing schemes with the types of revenues that these schemes receive. For instance, in Japan, government transfers to the various programs in place account for 42% of all income for financing healthcare, even though the government bears only 9% of the total cost of healthcare.

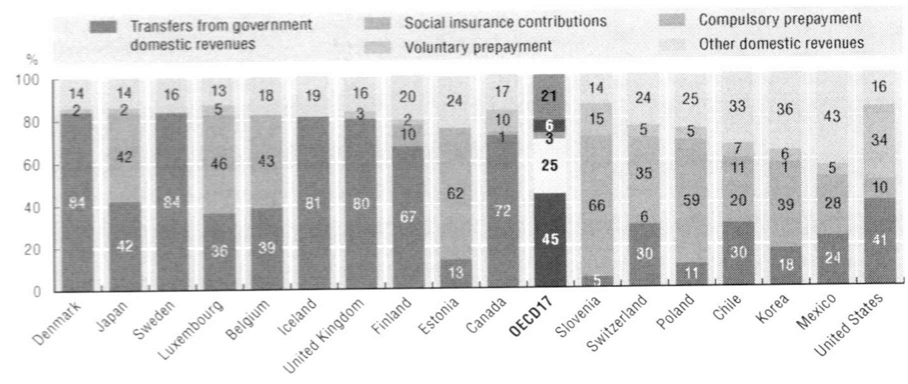

Figure 5.6. *Health financing sources by type of revenue, 2015 (or nearest year).*

Source: OECD, (2017). Health at a Glance 2017: OECD Indicators. OECD Publishing, Paris. http://dx.doi.org/10.1787/health_glance-2017-en.

By focusing solely on the breakdown of revenues for mandatory health insurance, which in the majority of OECD nations consists of social health insurance (SHI) (Figure 5.7), the role that governments play as a source of funding becomes more evident. Governmental transfers are a source of income in all of the examined countries, although their relative importance varies greatly. Government transfers account for more than 40% of SHI's income in Japan. While the shares are less than 5% in Estonia, Poland, and Slovenia, they are comparable in Chile and Finland. In those nations, social contributions account for almost all of the funding that SHI funds spend.

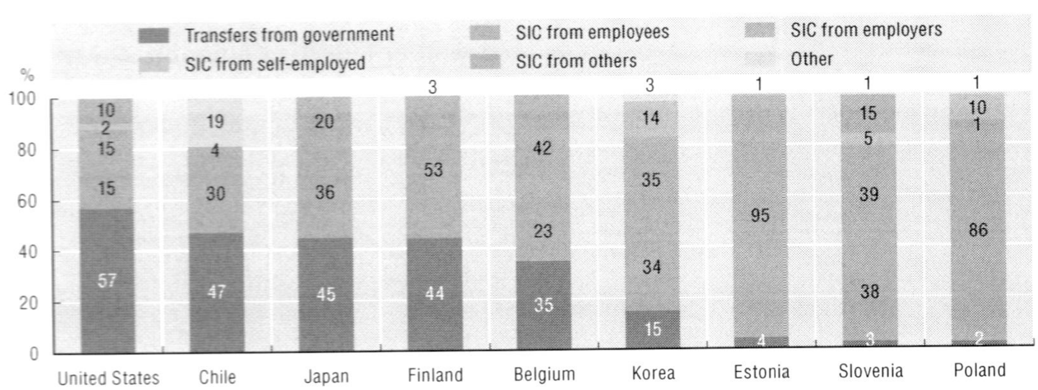

Figure 5.7. *Financing sources of compulsory insurance by type of revenue, selected countries, 2015 (or nearest year).*

Source: OECD, (2017). Health at a Glance 2017: OECD Indicators. OECD Publishing, Paris. http://dx.doi.org/10.1787/health_glance-2017-en.

Yet, a closer examination of this revenue stream reveals significant variations. In Poland, the majority of social contributions are made by employees, but in Estonia, employers are responsible for financing.

In response to financial shocks and contracting labor markets, few nations intend to lessen their reliance on wage-based contributions and are actively seeking to diversify their sources of income. The composition of revenues and the structure of health financing vary little from year to year, but there are some trends that can be seen over a longer period of time (Figure 5.8). For instance, during the past 10 years, Belgium's social contributions as a percentage of total revenues have decreased from over 50% to roughly 43%. Governmental transfers have grown in significance concurrently. The latter also holds for the US, where during the same period, the share from government transfers rose from 34% to 41%. In contrast, the share derived from social contributions has increased in Korea, but government transfers have stagnated.

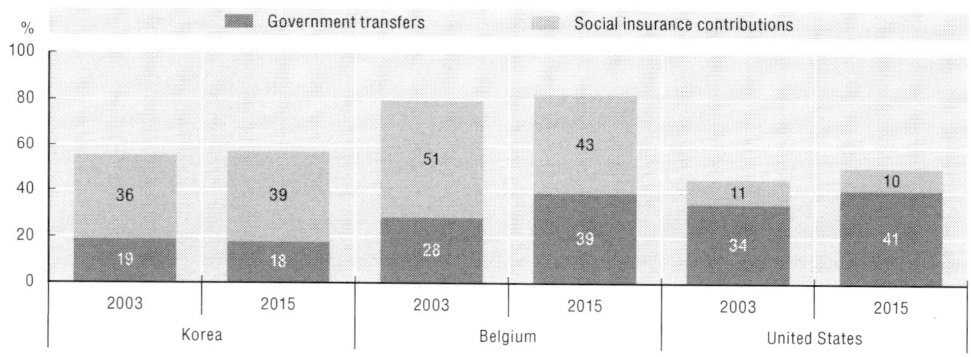

Figure 5.8. *Share of government transfers and social insurance contributions in all revenues of financing schemes, selected countries, 2003–2015.*

Source: OECD, (2017). Health at a Glance 2017: OECD Indicators. OECD Publishing, Paris. http://dx.doi.org/10.1787/health_glance-2017-en.

5.2. The Evolution of Health Service Finance

Comparing nations reveals that they have distinct methods for covering the cost of healthcare. For instance, the methods used by Sweden and France to finance physicians and hospitals are very different. While many African nations frequently receive government funding, social insurance systems are present in Latin America.

These discrepancies can be mostly attributed to historical factors. Understanding the historical background will help you realize how political and cultural influences have influenced healthcare financing today. It will clarify the reasons behind the variations in approaches to health finance across nations, allowing you to draw more insightful conclusions from your cross-national comparisons and assess the advantages and disadvantages of the healthcare system in your nation.

5.2.1. From Private to Social Health Insurance to Universal Coverage

Governments or charitable organizations funded services for segments of the public for whom they believed they owed a duty of care before the creation of contemporary healthcare systems. For instance, there were hospitals for the underprivileged in medieval Europe, China, India, and Arabia.

Private (or voluntary) health insurance was introduced in Europe in the 18th century for the wealthier classes. Private insurance originated in Europe and expanded to North and South America during the 1800s. While this was happening, Otto von Bismarck (1815–1898) established social (or mandatory) insurance for industrial workers in Germany in 1883, expanding on earlier voluntary programs. Payroll-based social insurance programs gradually spread throughout Europe, Asia, and now Africa.

5.2.2. Achieving Universal Healthcare Coverage

Different countries have employed strategies to ensure that everyone has access to healthcare: universal coverage can be attained by expanding social insurance or by providing government-funded healthcare to the entire populace.

In 1938, the Soviet Union expanded coverage through government provision; the post-World War II Soviet bloc nations emulated this model. In 1948, the UK opened up coverage to everyone. To provide health services for the entire population, William Beveridge recommended social reforms, of which the British NHS was created as a key component. Compared to Europe, private insurance now plays a bigger role in the USA. However, even in the USA, government-funded healthcare is crucial for the underprivileged (Medicaid), the elderly (Medicare), and members of the armed forces (Medicare). The 2010 healthcare reforms seek to bring healthcare to everyone in the country.

Low-income nations' health finance systems have been greatly impacted by their colonial past. In French colonies, the model was supplied by larger companies that were compelled to provide services for their employees. In British colonies, government-funded services for the armed forces and civil services served as the foundation for additional healthcare expansion. Hospital funding was also partially provided by missionaries and philanthropic groups.

These nations endeavored to expand services "as far as economic growth and available resources allowed" during the post-colonial era (Anderson et al., 2010; Armstrong et al., 2010).

5.3. Understanding the Financing Function

Raising and allocating funds for medical care is the fundamental, straightforward, but essential function of health financing. It can, however, accomplish far more. It can ensure that money is allocated appropriately and provide providers with financial incentives to guarantee that everyone has access to high-quality personal and public healthcare.

To facilitate interactions between healthcare providers and the general public, health financing is essential. It determines a number of factors, such as who pays for care, when they pay, how much they pay, who they pay and receive services from, and what kinds of services they can receive. It is a fundamental duty of health systems to enhance efficient service delivery and cost protection to facilitate the advancement of UHC.

To systematically unpack this function, we have broken health financing down into three sub-functions which, together, describe the flow of monetary resources through the health system:

- Revenue raising;
- Pooling resources;
- Purchasing goods and services.

5.3.1. Where Financing Fits into the Health System Performance Framework

One of the four primary functions of the health system, financing is connected to all of the other primary functions via a variety of channels. For example, finance plays a critical role in operational aspects of governance by establishing strategic directions and providing enough funds to support policy implementation. The financing function incentivizes providers to prioritize the provision of specific services and incentivizes them to do so at the highest possible level of quality and/or efficiency.

As eligibility for services is dependent on whether a person has made a financial contribution to the health system or whether an implicit contribution has been made on that person's behalf, the financing function is also in charge of guaranteeing appropriate population coverage.

Health workers may leave for health systems that pay more if there is a weak finance function, and there won't be enough money to build new facilities or buy medications. To put it plainly, funding is essential to the effectiveness of every aspect of the health system.

While financing has a significant impact on the overall performance of a health system, it usually does so through interactions with the other three functions. For instance, financial compensation encourages providers to provide high-quality healthcare, so financing influences health outcomes indirectly through other processes like service delivery. The degree to which households face financial hardship as a result of using health services is another clear connection between financing and financial protection. Several aspects of health financing systems can lead to variations in financial protection.

These include the necessity for the health system to produce enough financial resources to ensure access to high-quality services and the significance of co-payment design in determining exposure to out-of-pocket (OOP) payments; in the absence of these, individuals will likely seek care privately and may incur significant costs.

Nevertheless, to prevent unmet needs rather than financial hardship from use, financial protection depends on other factors, such as the availability of services. It should go without saying that even though funding is essential to the health system's operation, it is only one component of an intricately linked system.

5.3.2. Conceptualizing Financing

Researchers studying health policy and academia have given the financing function a lot of attention, including the WHO. Kutzin's groundbreaking 2001 framework for a general health financing system is shown in Figure 5.9. The framework illustrates the connections between revenue collection, pooling, procurement, and provision, and the movement of funds among these entities.

This framework's main contribution to the field of health financing has been to shift the focus from identifying health financing systems according to their institutional features—such as whether they are tax- or social health insurance-based, which are essentially meaningless classifications despite being widely used—to the sub-functions of those financing systems.

Consider a hypothetical tax system where payroll taxes play a major role in public financing. This system would be similar to the classic social health insurance system in that it heavily depends on the labor market for funding, demonstrating how little information is captured by the tax versus social health insurance distinction. Alternatively, transfers from general tax revenues could provide the majority, if not all, of the funding for a social health insurance-based system. The truth lies halfway between these erroneously divisive labels in a lot of nations. Most importantly, there is no clear indication of how money is raised, consolidated, or disbursed in either the tax or social health insurance titles.

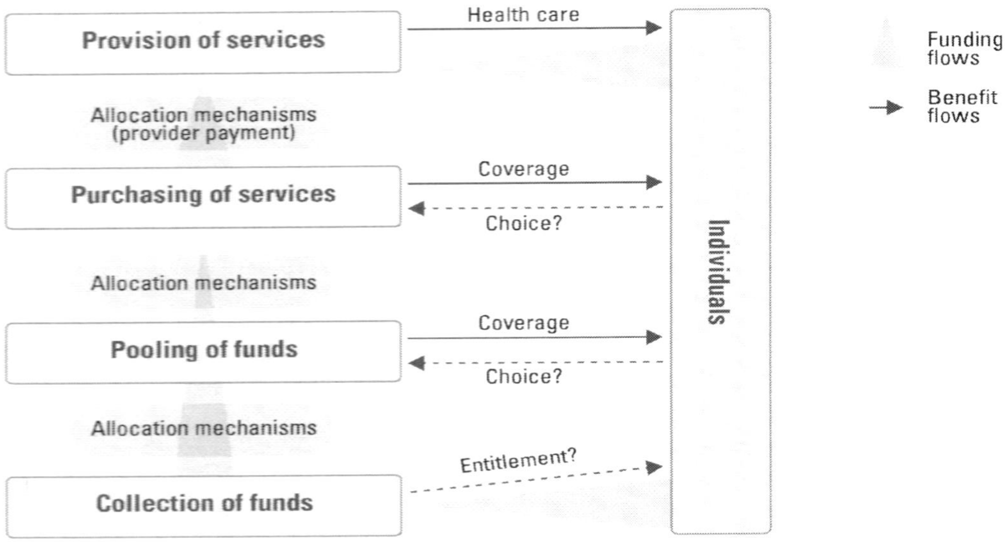

Figure 5.9. *Health financing framework (Kutzin).*

Source: Jonathan, C., Julia, S., & Matthew, J. Financing. Health system performance assessment: A framework for policy analysis. World Health Organization. https://www.ncbi.nlm.nih.gov/books/NBK590186/.

The Kutzin framework in Figure 5.9 also illustrates how the three primary financing sub-functions—fund collection, fund pooling, and service purchase—are connected by the gray triangles that depict the flow of funds through the health system. A variety of policy choices regarding who is covered, what is covered, and how much of the cost is covered are also taken into account by the framework; some of these are covered in more detail in the sub-function on governance of health financing.

5.3.3. Sub-Functions of Health Financing

Figure 5.10 illustrates how the fundamental components of health financing fit together. These functions are widely recognized.

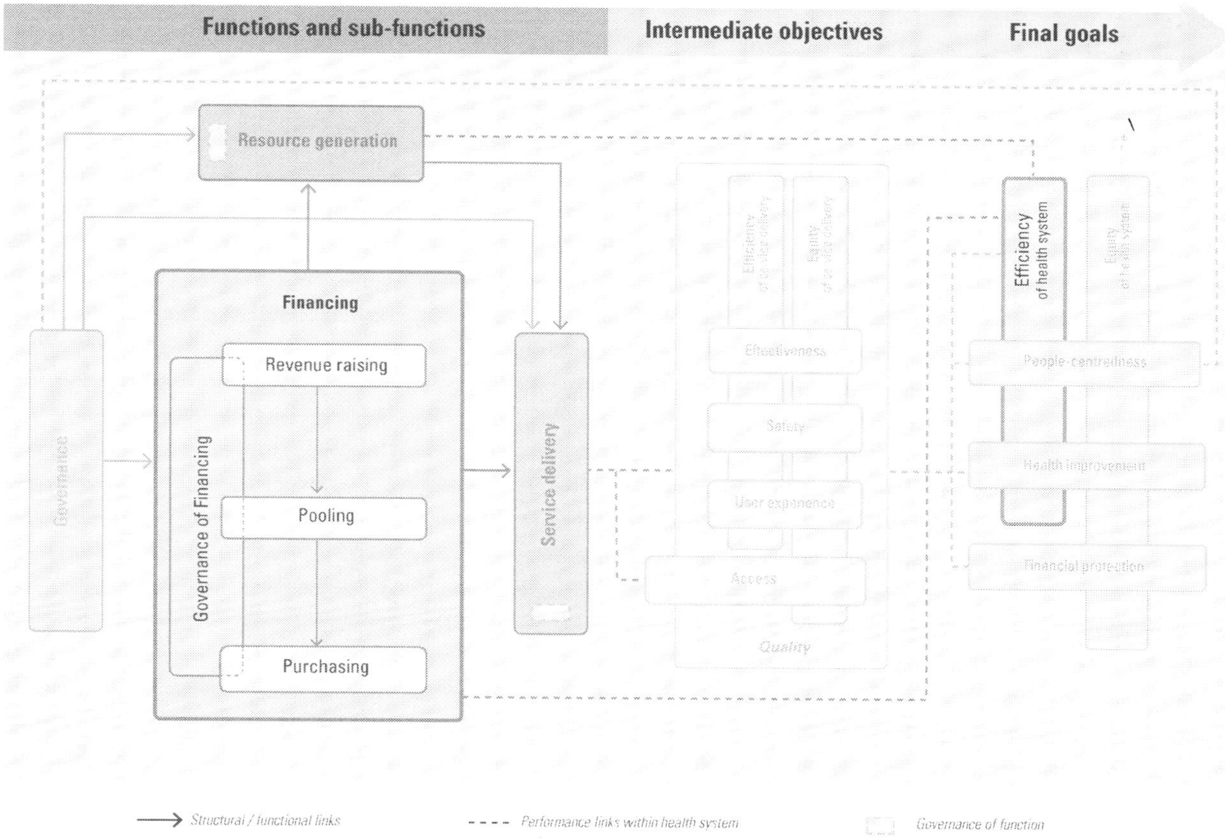

Figure 5.10. *Financing sub-functions.*

Source: Jonathan, C., Julia, S., & Matthew, J., (n.d.). Financing. Health system performance assessment: A framework for policy analysis. World Health Organization. https://www.ncbi.nlm.nih.gov/books/NBK590186/.

5.3.3.1. Revenue Raising

The methods used to bring funds into the health system are referred to as revenue raising. Except funds from outside sources, the population in the majority of these countries provides all or most of the system's funding. At the point of service utilization, revenue is obtained either by OOP payment or through pre-paid funds that may include taxes and/or insurance contributions. The way funds are raised for the health system is partially determined by whether third-party payers are private, operating under profit or non-profit-making models, or public or quasi-public, making them required.

The funding for the health system in a public, or quasi-public, scheme comes from social health insurance contributions, which is essentially a form of earmarked taxation, or from taxes that may or may not be expressly designated for health. Additionally, money may come from outside sources like donors and be directed through the Ministry of Finance into the health system. While other systems do not associate eligibility with having made pre-paid contributions, many settings impose eligibility for care as a condition of paying taxes or contributions. There are still many different potential sources of funding when considering taxation. Corporation taxes, income taxes, payroll taxes, property taxes, and consumption taxes are a few of these.

Funding for a private scheme, whether for profit or not, comes from premiums paid by employers and/or households. These can be experience-rated, where premium levels vary by individual based on expectations regarding their specific risk, or community-rated, where everyone in a given geographic area must pay the same premium level. Tax laws may indirectly impact private insurance revenues if pre-tax premiums are paid, thereby subsidizing private insurance. Private health insurance plans can be community-based or offered by major private insurers.

One could also classify out-of-pocket payments as a type of revenue raising. However, instead of building up resources that can eventually be combined and used to pay for care, they are utilized to pay for it at the time of use.

5.3.3.2. Pooling Resources

The accumulation of pre-paid money that can be used to buy goods and services for a population is known as pooling. It's critical to distinguish between revenue raising and pooling as two distinct aspects of health financing. When we talk about revenue raising, we're talking about the sources of funding, or who puts money into the system. This can tell us a lot about how fairly the load is distributed. The pooling structure determines the degree to which prepaid funds can be redistributed across a specific population; pooling concentrates on who gains from health spending.

Not just insurance plans, but all health finance systems depend on pooling. Certain systems may consist of a single pool that unifies funds from various sources of revenue generation, while other systems may have several pools. Additionally, if there are several pools, each one may have its unique methods for collecting revenue, or they may all come from different sources of income generation. Regional pools, for example, receive funding from both national and regional sources.

To ensure that each pool has an allocation suitable for the population it covers, some form of equalization formula or resource allocation may be employed. Allocations can be made from one pool to another, such as the allocation from a central pool to competing or geographically based pooling organizations, using a risk adjustment process that accounts for differences between populations that are expected to correlate with healthcare costs, such as age, health status, or socioeconomic characteristics. Allocations can also be made from the initial source of funds to the pooling agency, such as private insurers that implement collection and pooling together.

The populations and benefits covered by each pool are frequently key differentiators. While people can select which pool to join in some health systems, in others, membership in the pool is required or decided for them automatically. The legal requirement for certain individuals, groups, or the entire population to join the pool is compulsory participation. Next, the covered population makes mandatory contributions themselves or on their behalf. The basis for eligibility is non-contributory and stems from citizenship, residency, or other factors like low income. Automatic participation is usually predicated on legal or constitutional obligations. Usually, the only source of automatic entitlement is general budget revenues. There is no clear connection between explicit contributions and entitlements, even though many people with non-contributory entitlements pay taxes in one way or another. On the other hand, people who voluntarily prepay and sign up for a program are not required to do so by law. The efficiency and redistributive capacity of pools are significantly impacted by the way individuals are added to or assigned to them. Examples of the different kinds of pooling organizations and how money is allocated to them are given in Table 5.1.

Table 5.1. *Examples of Pooling Organizations and Mechanisms for Allocating to or Among Them*

Pooling Organizations	Allocation Mechanisms
• Ministry of Health Central • Decentralized units (provincial, district health authorities)	• Government (central or local) revenues. • Historical patterns related to infrastructure. • Needs-based weighted capitation formula. • Subsidize premium payment for the participation of those who are otherwise uninsured.
• Local government health department • Area health boards • Social health insurance fund(s) • Private insurance companies • Employers as "self-insuring" firms • Member-owned "mutual" insurers	• Earmarked: compulsory contributions • Percentage of salary or income • Risk-adjusted allocation to insurers, usually with consumer choice of insurance fund • Opting out, with or without risk adjustment
• Fundholding providers and provider-based	• Voluntary contributions • Individual risk-rated or community-rated premium

Source: Irene, P., Dheepa, R., Marina, K., Agnes, S., & Josep, F., (n.d.). Health System Performance Assessment: A Framework for Policy Analysis. World Health Organization. https://www.ncbi.nlm.nih.gov/books/NBK590192/pdf/Bookshelf_NBK590192.pdf.

5.3.3.3. Purchasing Goods and Services

Payers who use funds to cover healthcare costs on behalf of a population are referred to as purchasing or commissioning. These monies may be combined or used to cover direct out-of-pocket expenses at the point of service.

Procurement is not the same as purchasing. While procurement is the process of obtaining inputs and includes commodities, such as medicines and laboratory supplies, and aspects of capital investment, such as medical devices, purchasing specifically refers to payment for services or items, such as medicines and other supplies used in the context of care provision. Purchasing is often seen as a more useful term than paying because it implies a potentially active approach that might involve:

- Choosing to purchase only from accredited providers;
- Purchasing only cost-effective services;
- Payment mechanisms that incentivize more, or less, provision.

When purchasing in a more passive manner, provider performance or attempts to affect the amount or caliber of health services are not taken into account when allocating funds, past budgetary allotments, or payments to providers. In the worst situation, a third-party payer might just pay back any invoice they receive without asking any questions. A shift toward more active, or strategic, purchasing suggests that financing is connected, at least partially, to a provider's performance or the health requirements of the community they serve.

As we have stated throughout this section, one could also consider OOP payments made at the point of service to be a component of purchasing. Payments made by specific service users at the time of use are referred to as "out-of-pocket." They cover all or part of the cost of services if there is no insurance. They can be formal or informal payments.

In cases where partial costs are covered, out-of-pocket (OOP) payments may be imposed as a percentage of the stated price of care – known as a percentage-based co-payment, a flat user charge regardless of the full price, or a combination of both. This is commonly seen in the purchase of medicines, where there may be a flat user charge or a dispensing fee along with a percentage-based co-payment based on the difference between the advertised price and a reference price. Some systems utilize deductibles, requiring a certain amount to be paid out of pocket before insurance coverage begins. These mandated OOP payments, which contribute to the actual cost of care and reflect decisions on how much should be covered, are considered part of the benefit package design. For instance, policymakers may choose to only cover a small portion of the cost of a low-value service and require users to cover the majority of costs OOP or limit coverage to a select group of individuals who are most likely to benefit. The inclusion of OOP payments in benefit design is emphasized in the WHO Health Financing Progress Matrix (HFPM).

OOP payments are frequently required in an almost futile attempt to rationalize patient demand for health services by sending price signals to them; in other contexts, they are also seen as a means of generating income. It's crucial to remember that our discussion of OOP payments as a kind of purchase does not contradict the idea that they can also be used to generate income. OOP payments, however, are best understood as an example of the purchasing sub-function since they are not pooled.

5.3.3.4. Governance of Health Financing

The flow of funds is naturally described by the three sub-functions of health financing mentioned above: how money is generated, gathered, and used to pay for medical services. However, several connected decisions and considerations impact whether or not the sub-functions can carry out their intended duties and do so to a sufficient standard. For instance, will funds be able to flow smoothly from government agencies to purchasers and providers, or are there structural barriers that prevent funds from being collected and distributed? Will the funds collected be adequate to cover the benefits promised? The sub-function known as "governance of health financing" refers to the decisions, regulations, and normative choices about health financing. More precisely, we view public financial management (PFM) and policies pertaining to benefits design and coverage as two crucial facets of the governance of health financing. While PFM outlines the regulations that control the distribution, utilization, and accounting of public monies, coverage policies are normative choices that are directly related to health financing.

Even though we only discuss the two specific governance elements that are directly related to the governance of financing, there are many more that are extremely important for both financing and other functions of the health system, like participation and transparency, especially concerning decision-making by different institutions.

5.3.3.5. Coverage Policies

Coverage policies specify who is covered, how the pooled public funds will be used, and whether there are any limitations or requirements for access. Every nation restricts health service entitlements in some manner. Decisions about coverage policies affect the finer points of benefit rationing, which in turn affects the efficiency of the health system and the advancement of UHC objectives. Because they represent decisions about entitlements, some may view coverage policies as a component of purchasing. However, it is arguable that decisions about coverage should be made by a higher level, like the central government, which may be less concerned with cost implications and more directly answerable to the people.

The well-known coverage cube (Figure 5.11) divides healthcare coverage into three dimensions: population coverage, service coverage, and financial coverage or financial protection. The yellow box in the middle represents pooled funds. This helps to show the intricate connections between the other aspects of financing and coverage policy. In the end, the health system's performance is determined by a plethora of coverage policy options within these dimensions, all of which are closely related to and reliant upon other elements of the financing function.

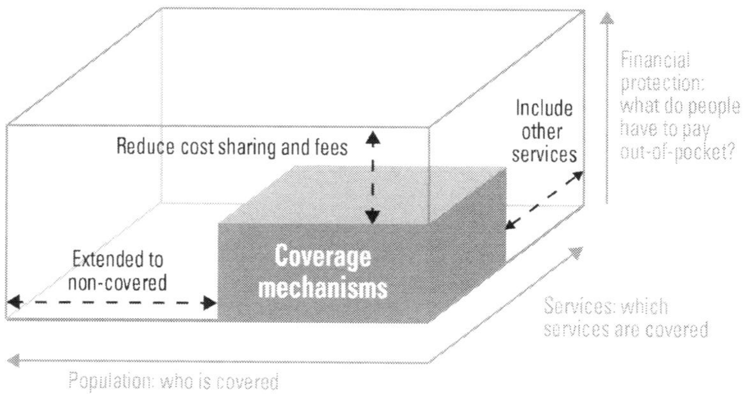

Figure 5.11. *UHC cube.*

Source: Irene, P., Dheepa, R., Marina, K., Agnes, S., & Josep, F., (n.d.). Health System Performance Assessment: A Framework for Policy Analysis. World Health Organization. https://www.ncbi.nlm.nih.gov/books/NBK590192/pdf/Bookshelf_NBK590192.pdf.

For instance, a health system might provide a full range of benefits that are theoretically available to the whole population. However, in reality, it won't be able to provide access to high-quality services if it doesn't generate enough money to pay for this coverage. This can occur in a few different ways: insufficient funding can lead to restricted benefit offerings or shortages of supplies; it can also result in unreasonably high out-of-pocket payments (OPPs) to cover the shortfall, either in the form of large co-payments or unofficial payments. Even in systems with universal population coverage, high user fees combined with no co-payment exemptions for low-income households make it difficult for people to get the care they need. However, a nation may spend a lot of money while excluding a sizable portion of its population from coverage due to factors like citizenship, age, or employment status.

Inequalities in funding distribution across pools may lead to disparities in service accessibility, even in cases where the entire population is theoretically covered for the same range of services. A purchasing function that isn't strong enough can result in excessively high costs and restrict the scope of benefits a health system can afford.

As these examples illustrate, coverage policies impact the rest of the financing function, and vice versa.

5.3.3.6. Public Financial Management in Health

The term "public financial management" describes the collection of guidelines and procedures that control how public monies are distributed, spent, and handled. It is crucial for the management of resources at the national and local levels, originating from all sources. The PFM system is important to the health system because it influences budgetary formulations that establish the amount and distribution of public funding for health, how well the budget is executed in terms of effectiveness and spending targeting, and financial transparency and monitoring. Health policymakers should have a thorough understanding of PFM and its operation to make sure they are prepared to frame and direct their conversations with ministries of finance.

PFM and health financing systems can support one another's goals and accomplish more effective and efficient use of public funds, improved financial accountability, and increased transparency if they are in alignment. For instance, a close relationship between PFM and health financing can guarantee that funding decisions take into account the goals and priorities of the health sector and that there are transparent lines of accountability for resource allocation. Policy-based budget formulation, in which the processes of formulating policies and budgets are closely related, and program-based budget classification, in which nations shift from budgeting based on input line items (e.g., hospital bed counts) to budgets based on programs, which can be connected to performance and strategic priorities and objectives, are two significant and pertinent concepts that highlight the significance of PFM to health financing.

5.3.4. Assessing the Performance of the Financing Function

The performance of each of the financing sub-functions can be assessed along several dimensions. Here, we examine a few of the key evaluation dimensions related to each sub-function (Figure 5.12) and, where necessary, provide quantitative and/or qualitative indicators to support our points. We examined possible indicators from a variety of tools to inform this:

- National Health Accounts, which feature in many other tools.

- Health system assessment approach: A how-to manual.
- Situation analysis of the health sector.
- Health system reviews (HiTs).
- WHO HFPM, which aims to collect timely information on the health financing sub-functions through a series of questions and ratings or categorizations.

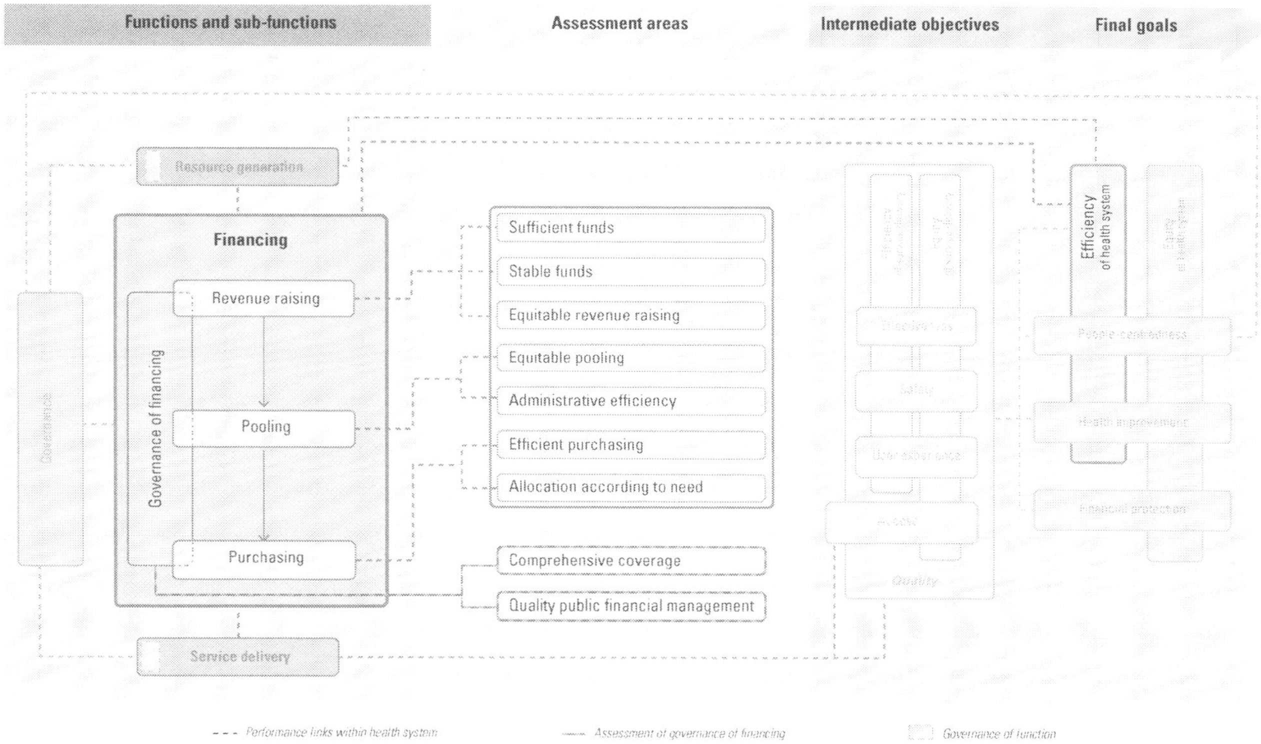

Figure 5.12. *Assessing financing.*

Source: Irene, P., Dheepa, R., Marina, K., Agnes, S., & Josep, F., (n.d.). Health System Performance Assessment: A Framework for Policy Analysis. World Health Organization. https://www.ncbi.nlm.nih.gov/books/NBK590192/pdf/Bookshelf_NBK590192.pdf.

Our main goals are to facilitate some level of performance assessment, generate an objective, mostly qualitative evaluation of each health financing sub-function's alignment to best practices, and foster communication with other nations regarding health system priorities.

5.3.4.1. Assessing the Performance of Revenue-Raising

A well-functioning sub-function of revenue raising should guarantee that the health system has enough resources to meet demand for healthcare; that these resources are steady, predictable, and resilient to shocks; and that they are collected fairly to prevent the sick and impoverished from bearing the brunt of the financing burden.

A variety of publicly accessible indicators can shed some light on these objectives. Information about the various funding sources and their relative sizes over time would be ideal. Though data on health expenses are readily available, precise information on revenues is typically lacking or nonexistent. This distinction is crucial because revenues can be generated through various mechanisms, and these can have varying effects, especially on equity and stability, when it comes to expenditures. For instance, various taxes and outside funding sources can be used to increase government spending on healthcare; however, not all of these funding sources will be consistent, reliable, or fair in all nations.

However, data on health spending can be found in every reviewed HSA and national report. Internationally comparable National Health Accounts data on health spending for nearly 190 countries between 2000 and 2017 can be found in the WHO Global Health Expenditure Database. A few pertinent National Health Accounts indicators are included in Table 5.2. These can be expressed in various ways, such as total spending or expenditure per capita, but they are typically expressed as a percentage of GDP or current health expenditure. It is crucial to remember that while these accounts can be instructive when paired with other data from the health system, they don't reveal much on their own. For instance, even though per capita spending is sufficient or comparable to comparator nations—as it is in Singapore—current health spending as a percentage of GDP may be relatively low in an extremely wealthy nation. However, nations like the USA, which devote a large portion of their financial resources to healthcare, could do poorly on metrics that track health outcomes and equity of access. This implies that these hefty costs are insufficient because of distributional problems and other inefficiencies. In other words, increased spending does not always translate into adequate revenue generation. One could search for signs of underfunding, such as lengthy wait times, limited benefits package, or other obstacles to receiving necessary services, to determine whether the revenue generated meets the expenditure needs. But in the HSAs we looked at, this information is either scarce or, at best, inconsistently available.

Table 5.2. *Measures from National Health Accounts*

Current health expenditure (CHE) as a percentage of gross domestic product (GDP)
Domestic general government health expenditure (GGHE-D) as a percentage of gross domestic product (GDP)
Domestic general government health expenditure (GGHE-D) as a percentage of current health expenditure (CHE)
Domestic general government health expenditure (GGHE-D) as a percentage of general government expenditure (GGE)
Out-of-pocket (OOP) expenditure as a percentage of current health expenditure (CHE)
Health expenditure from external sources (EXT) as a percentage of current health expenditure (CHE)
Domestic private health expenditure (PVT-D) as a percentage of current health expenditure (CHE)
Voluntary health insurance (VHI) Prepayments as a percentage of current health expenditure (CHE)

Source: Irene, P., Dheepa, R., Marina, K., Agnes, S., & Josep, F., (n.d.). Health System Performance Assessment: A Framework for Policy Analysis. World Health Organization. https://www.ncbi.nlm.nih.gov/books/NBK590192/pdf/Bookshelf_NBK590192.pdf.

For efficient planning and to avoid any shortages that jeopardize service delivery, stable funding is essential. Looking at the National Health Accounts indicators in Table 5.2 over several years could yield information at a very general level, such as whether there are significant variations. For instance, significant annual fluctuations in the domestic government's funding as a percentage of current health expenditures may indicate a problem with the stability of public finances. Furthermore, it is important to take into account National Health Accounts data on the portion of spending that originates from public sources, as there is substantial evidence that progress toward UHC in general and improved health outcomes, in particular, depend on public funding.

An alternative approach to evaluating the stability of revenues would be to examine historical economic fluctuations, such as shifts in unemployment rates, or demographic shifts, and any correlations between these factors and variations in revenues from specific sources. This method is more dependent on revenue data than expenditure data. For instance, as people age out of the formal labor market, population aging lowers the ability to raise funds from social insurance contributions, according to recent research (Figure 5.13). However, studies conducted in Slovenia have demonstrated that increases in unemployment can affect social contributions made to the Health Insurance Institute. The main takeaway from this is that revenues can be vulnerable to outside shocks to a specific revenue base in the absence of varied revenue streams.

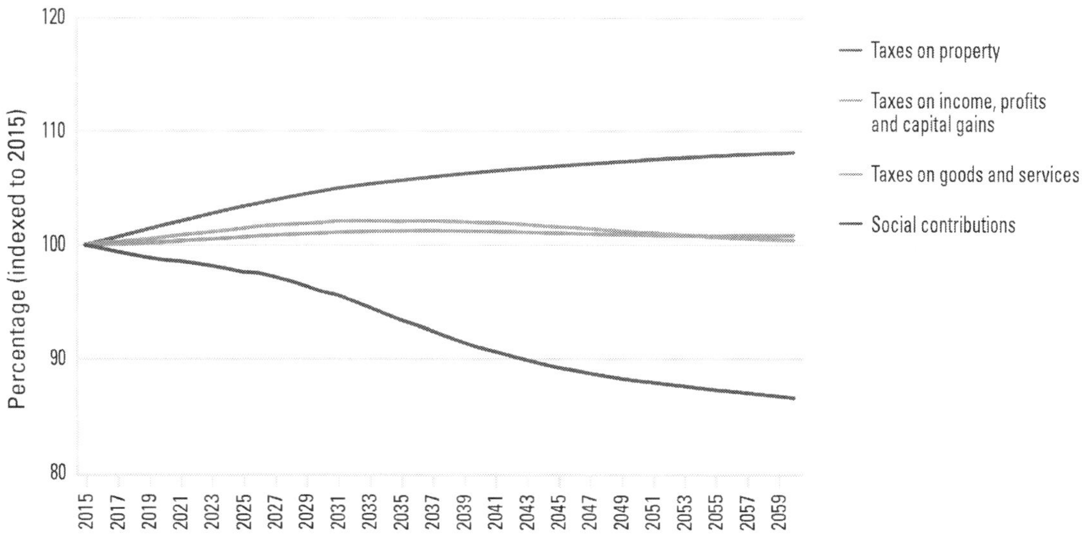

Figure 5.13. *How does population-aging affect revenue generation for health? – Japan case study.*

Source: Irene, P., Dheepa, R., Marina, K., Agnes, S., & Josep, F., (n.d.). Health System Performance Assessment: A Framework for Policy Analysis. World Health Organization. https://www.ncbi.nlm.nih.gov/books/NBK590192/pdf/Bookshelf_NBK590192.pdf.

Equity of financing addresses several important questions:

- Who pays for healthcare?
- To what extent is the funding of healthcare related to the ability to pay?
- Is the relationship proportional?

- Is the relationship progressive, in other words, do healthcare payments account for an increasing proportion of ability to pay as the latter rises?
- Is there a regressive relationship?

When evaluating equity of financing, particularly concerning revenue raising, a variety of metrics can be applied (Table 5.3). OOP spending as a percentage of overall spending offers some insights into the equity of revenue generation, even though in our framework we consider OOP spending as part of purchasing. This is because high levels of OOP payments imply that people are paying at the point of use following need rather than ability to pay. Generally speaking, when a health system depends on funding from out-of-pocket payments, it is much harder to guarantee equitable revenue generation. Additionally, there is a strong probability of disparities in access and final results if healthcare financing is dependent on direct out-of-pocket payments, as certain individuals may encounter financial obstacles to receiving care.

Table 5.3. *Indicative Measures for Revenue Collection*

OOP expenditure as a total health expenditure.
OOP expenditure as a total of total household consumption.
Kakwani indices: a measure of progressivity that can be calculated for each source of financing. The progressivity of the entire financing system can be subsequently established by weighting the progressivity (using the macro-weights) of the finance sources.

Source: Irene, P., Dheepa, R., Marina, K., Agnes, S., & Josep, F., (n.d.). Health System Performance Assessment: A Framework for Policy Analysis. World Health Organization. https://www.ncbi.nlm.nih.gov/books/NBK590192/pdf/Bookshelf_NBK590192.pdf.

Proper analysis of the financing burden distribution usually requires household-level data, not macro-level National Health Accounts data. If wealthier people allocate a larger percentage of their resources to health than poor people, then health financing is progressive. On the other hand, if the poor allocate a larger percentage of their resources to health, that is regressive. Fundamentally, data from household budget surveys can be used to examine how OOP health spending is distributed based on the socio-economic status of the household. This would entail contrasting the share of OOP in total household consumption between wealthy and low-income households. Alternatively, Kakwani indices, which can be weighted to take into consideration each funding source's contribution to the overall amount of health financing, can be used to examine the progressivity or regressivity of particular funding sources (Figure 5.14). Figure 5.14 illustrates the relative contributions of various forms of financing sources to financing's progressivity or regressivity. For instance, in Estonia, social taxes and personal income taxes are relatively progressive due to the higher rates paid by wealthier individuals; on the other hand, OOP spending is highly regressive because it disproportionately affects lower-income households.

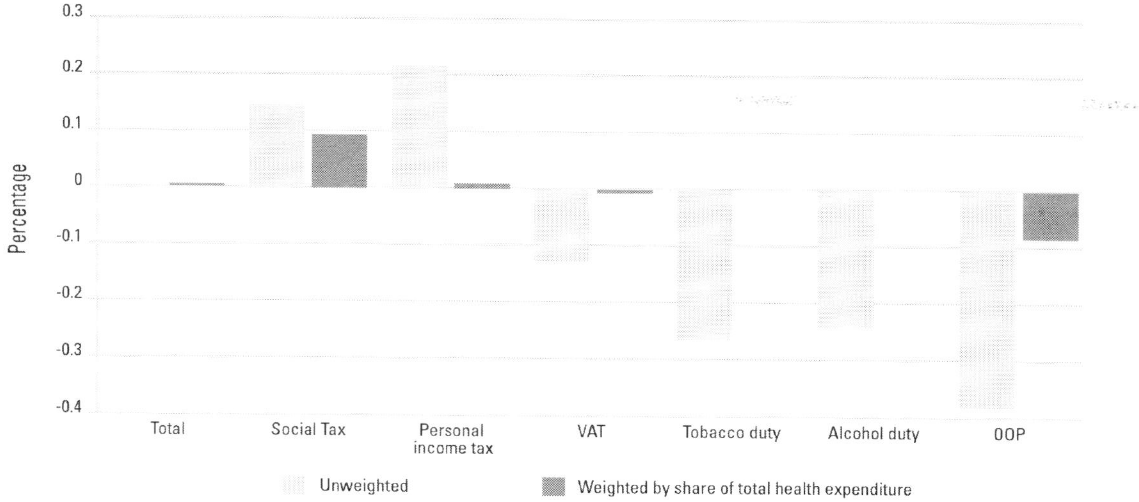

Figure 5.14. *Equity of financing using Kakwani indexes, Estonia.*

Source: Irene, P., Dheepa, R., Marina, K., Agnes, S., & Josep, F., (n.d.). Health System Performance Assessment: A Framework for Policy Analysis. World Health Organization. https://www.ncbi.nlm.nih.gov/books/NBK590192/pdf/Bookshelf_NBK590192.pdf.

5.3.4.2. Assessing the Performance of Pooling

The main goals of the pooling function are to guarantee fair resource distribution and to promote efficiency through economies of scale.

In the HSA tools we reviewed, the pooling of financial resources is taken into consideration using a combination of qualitative and quantitative data (Table 5.4). Perhaps because variations in the populations covered by the pools and the benefits basket are viewed as the most important aspects of pooling, pooling is sometimes referred to in HSAs along with the design of benefits and entitlement as a single sub-function. Because the choice to differentiate coverage or benefits by pool is normative, we view the design of benefits and entitlements—that is, coverage policies—as distinct from pooling. This distinction isn't very significant, though.

Table 5.4. *Indicative Measures for Pooling*

Indicative Measure
Per person expenditure, by the pool.
Population coverage, by pool.
Spending on administration, total and by pool.
The ratio of voluntary health insurance coverage as a percentage of the population, to voluntary health insurance expressed as a percentage of current health expenditure.
Pooling arrangement description.

Source: Irene, P., Dheepa, R., Marina, K., Agnes, S., & Josep, F., (n.d.). Health System Performance Assessment: A Framework for Policy Analysis. World Health Organization. https://www.ncbi.nlm.nih.gov/books/NBK590192/pdf/Bookshelf_NBK590192.pdf.

There exist multiple methods for evaluating the extent to which the pooling function is accomplishing its goals. First, using the HFPM approach as a guide, one can characterize the pooling arrangements qualitatively or quantitatively (Table 5.5). This can indicate the extent of fragmentation and if efficient mechanisms to redistribute resources across the population following need are likely to exist.

Table 5.5. *Measures for Pooling in the Health Finance Progress Matrix*

Indicative Measure from HFPM	Definition and Descriptive Information
Does your country's strategy for pooling revenues reflect international experience and evidence?	This question focuses on the country's policy, strategy and/or vision regarding pooling arrangements. Information you need to look at: • Available policy statements on fragmentation and how they try to mitigate it. • Policy statements on Voluntary Health Insurance.
Are multiple revenue sources and funding streams organized in a complementary manner, in support of a common set of benefits?	Look at different revenue sources and fund flows within a health system and how they may or may not complement each other. Promised benefits/entitlements and the way that funds flow to, or from, this is of great importance in the analysis of the issues raised by this question.

Source: Irene, P., Dheepa, R., Marina, K., Agnes, S., & Josep, F., (n.d.). Health System Performance Assessment: A Framework for Policy Analysis. World Health Organization. https://www.ncbi.nlm.nih.gov/books/NBK590192/pdf/Bookshelf_NBK590192.pdf.

If there are several schemes, it might be helpful to take into account the differences in resource distribution among pools more thoroughly in order to assess how well they mesh. This sheds some light on the possibility of differences in care access for individuals covered by various schemes. For instance, it would be easy to compare per capita spending by program. Data from Thailand are shown in Figure 5.15, which indicates that compared to other schemes, the majority of the population covered by the universal care scheme has fewer resources available per person. This suggests that better allocation mechanisms could lead to gains in equity.

In terms of efficiency, one could examine spending on administrative costs to gauge the extent of administrative waste resulting from fragmentation, aside from the obvious consideration that having fewer schemes is likely to achieve greater economies of scale. That being said, it is crucial to remember that a system shouldn't be rated as good or bad based only on its administrative costs; excessively low administrative costs may indicate a lack of funding, while excessively high administrative costs may indicate waste.

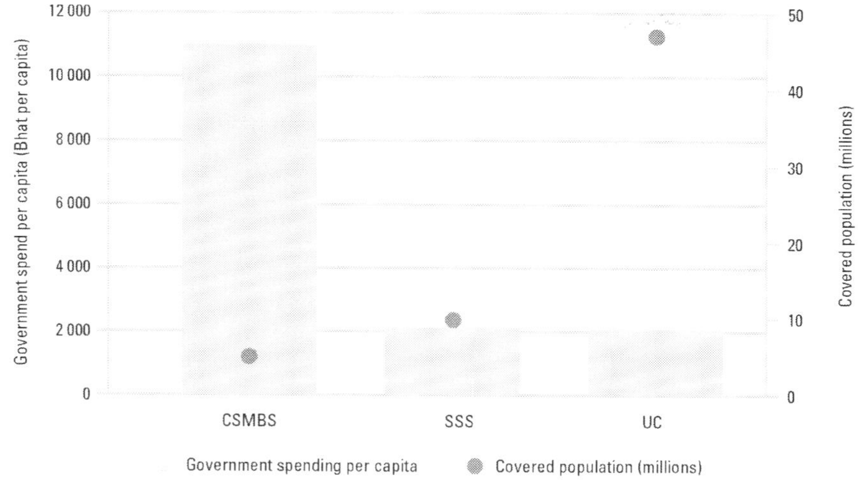

Figure 5.15. *Per person spending by scheme, Thailand.*

Source: Irene, P., Dheepa, R., Marina, K., Agnes, S., & Josep, F., (n.d.). Health System Performance Assessment: A Framework for Policy Analysis. World Health Organization. https://www.ncbi.nlm.nih.gov/books/NBK590192/pdf/Bookshelf_NBK590192.pdf.

5.3.4.3. Assessing the Performance of Purchasing

Similar to pooling, purchasing focuses on allocating resources to the most deserving parties while keeping costs as low as possible. Consequently, purchasing can have a significant effect on intermediate goals like quality and, eventually, health outcomes. However, few metrics directly address purchasing, making it difficult to evaluate this function (Table 5.6). Information on provider payment methods is included in the reviewed HSAs, and depending on the larger context, this information may help evaluate purchasing. For instance, it might be helpful to know whether fee-for-service payments are in place if there are any indications of overuse of specialized services, as this could lead to some supplier-induced demand.

Table 5.6. *Indicative Measures for Purchasing*

Indicative Measure	Definition
Payment mechanisms	Descriptive information about how different types of care are paid for.
Information on strategic purchasing	The extent to which health systems can choose who to purchase from, what to purchase, and at what price.
Price data	Data on prices paid for certain services, ideally used for comparison.

Source: Irene, P., Dheepa, R., Marina, K., Agnes, S., & Josep, F., (n.d.). Health System Performance Assessment: A Framework for Policy Analysis. World Health Organization. https://www.ncbi.nlm.nih.gov/books/NBK590192/pdf/Bookshelf_NBK590192.pdf.

Using patient vignettes—as in the case of Euro-DRG, a project that used data from hospital payment systems to group patient episodes with similar characteristics—it would make sense to compare costs for different types of care to evaluate purchasing using quantitative data. However, these kinds of data are not routinely available. Making sure that the populations and services are comparable enough to justify comparison is the main obstacle to price comparison. However, assuming price data are available, a strong purchasing sub-function should be able to achieve low costs while maintaining good outcomes, making it a good indicator of purchasing performance.

A few attempts have been made to gauge the degree of strategic purchasing by nations. These have included examining the role of performance metrics, public participation in purchasing, and the contracting process for providers. However, this kind of data is again not consistently accessible throughout national borders. The extent to which countries conduct health technology assessments to determine coverage decisions may be a pertinent piece of information, as these assessments can be helpful in negotiations with manufacturers to guarantee value for money. But having a health technology assessment procedure or agency by itself does not ensure that the purchasing sub-function is robust.

When it comes to provider payment strategies and whether resource allocation strategies take population health needs into account, the HFPM gathers insightful qualitative data (Table 5.7).

Table 5.7. *Measures for Purchasing and Provider Payment in the Health Financing Progress Matrix*

Indicative Measure from HFPM	Definition and Descriptive Information
To what extent is the payment of providers driven by information on the health needs of the population they serve?	This question is concerned with the way in which funds flow from purchasers to service providers. Information you might look at: · the type of allocation mechanisms used.
Are provider payments harmonized within and across purchasers to ensure coherent incentives for providers?	When multiple payment methods exist across different purchasing agencies (for instance, coverage schemes or health programs), or within one purchasing agency, these need to be coordinated and harmonized to ensure a coherent set of incentives for providers. Information you might look at: · the payment methods used in different schemes, and at payment levels/rates; and · cost-sharing mechanisms (user fees and co-payments) and whether these are harmonized across different schemes and programs.

Do purchasing arrangements promote quality of care?	This question considers whether, or not, purchasers are taking active measures to influence provider behavior and performance specifically to improve quality of care. The information needed centers on purchasing instruments that specifically promote quality of care, for example: • performance agreements. • policies or instruments for selective contracting. • better coordination of care through blending or bundling of payment methods, for example, capitated provider networks. • specific financial incentives. • the existence and use of standardized quality indicators across payers and providers.

Source: Irene, P., Dheepa, R., Marina, K., Agnes, S., & Josep, F., (n.d.). Health System Performance Assessment: A Framework for Policy Analysis. World Health Organization. https://www.ncbi.nlm.nih.gov/books/NBK590192/pdf/Bookshelf_NBK590192.pdf.

5.3.4.4. Assessing the Performance of Governance of Financing

This section addresses how to evaluate coverage policies and public financial management, two important aspects of the governance of financing.

5.3.4.5. Coverage Policies

A thorough quantitative evaluation of the design of coverage policies is intrinsically difficult since coverage policies will be mirrored in every facet of the healthcare system. Perhaps more helpful would be an explanation of the normative coverage information, such as what, who, and how much is covered, as well as an analysis of the process by which normative policy decisions are made. Nevertheless, information on the proportion of the populace that is enrolled in the public or statutory health system is typically accessible. There is a tendency for nations to declare that they have achieved UHC because they provide coverage to 100% of their population, given the prevalence of claims to the contrary.

Unfortunately, because they don't reveal anything about the depth or breadth of coverage, population coverage statistics by themselves are not a very helpful metric. It might be that co-payments for using public services are absurdly high, or that the entire population is covered by a very limited benefits package. In actuality, supply limitations may also restrict access. The main takeaway from this must be that although population coverage is necessary for a healthy health system to operate, it tells us very little about how well coverage policies are working. We do not advise using it as an assessment indicator because of this.

On the other hand, it is frequently challenging to find information regarding the entitlement and benefit design, or what is covered. Not every nation keeps a "positive list," and even those that do might limit it to pharmaceuticals. Due to variations in the depth of coverage for the same basket of services, there are also unavoidable variations between countries. For instance, two nations may have identical benefit packages, but one may pay the entire cost of the medication while the other pays only a portion of it. This emphasizes how crucial it is to take into account all three aspects of coverage at the same time: the proportion of the population covered, the services covered, and the portion of the costs of care that is covered.

The first two dimensions are difficult to measure, but the issue of how much of the cost of care is covered is frequently assessed in HSAs. In general, OOP expenditures as a percentage of total spending may provide insight into the extent of coverage (Table 5.8). As opposed to direct payments for care outside of the benefits basket, very few nations report on OOP expenditures that are solely for public or statutory services, such as cost-sharing or co-payments. Because of this, it is challenging to determine how much high out-of-pocket costs are a result of a limited set of benefits and entitlements, rising demand for private services (possibly as a result of low public sector quality perceptions), or high user fees for public services.

Table 5.8. *Indicative Measures for Coverage*

Indicative Measure	Definition
Out-of-pocket spending as a share of current health spending OR as a share of household consumption.	–
Catastrophic health spending incidence.	The percentage of the population, or households, who spend over some share of their ability or capacity to pay on healthcare OOP expenses.
Impoverishing health spending incidence.	The percentage of the population, or households, whose remaining resources after OOP spending leave them below the poverty line.
Co-payment design.	Descriptive information on how co-payments and related exemptions are designed in public/ statutory health system(s).
Indicative Measure from HFPM	**Definition and Descriptive Information**

Is there a set of explicitly defined benefits for the entire population?	Being explicit and clear about entitlements, and any related conditions of access, reduces uncertainty for the population. As uncertainty generally constitutes a barrier to accessing services, this is a positive move. Information you might look for includes explicit statements of benefits and entitlements, for example: • a defined list of guaranteed services (either positive or negative lists), or levels of care, for example, PHC. • a specific set of universal entitlements, that is, for all citizens. • services with co-payments and exemptions for certain priority groups.
To what extent are population entitlements and conditions of access defined explicitly and in easy-to-understand terms?	This question focuses on the population's awareness and understanding of its entitlements. For example, what it can access free, or with a limited co-payment, at the point of service. Information you might look at: • explicit statements that are concise and simple, and are widely communicated to the population. • any available survey that might capture aspects of this question.

Source: Irene, P., Dheepa, R., Marina, K., Agnes, S., & Josep, F., (n.d.). Health System Performance Assessment: A Framework for Policy Analysis. World Health Organization. https://www.ncbi.nlm.nih.gov/books/NBK590192/pdf/Bookshelf_NBK590192.pdf.

The financial protection indicator set is another crucial set of data. The degree to which the health system shields individuals or households from the cost of paying for medical care at the point of use is known as financial protection. To track progress toward UHC under the Sustainable Development Goals, this is one of the main metrics. All of the sub-functions have a significant impact on financial protection. Insufficient revenue raising is likely to be accompanied by insufficient resourcing, which means that many goods and services—if they are covered at all—cannot be fully or affordably provided without high-cost sharing. Inadequate resource pooling may result in resource imbalances that require some individuals to pay a large amount out of pocket while providing comprehensive coverage for others. Poorly thought-out purchasing practices (such as underpaying suppliers or sending out the wrong signals) may encourage unofficial payments or excessive billing, which would further burden households financially. Crucially, if coverage policies are not made to guarantee that individuals or services are not excluded from the system or if out-of-pocket payments are made at the point of use at exorbitant rates, financial protection may suffer. Furthermore, since financial protection accounts for how OOP spending affects households that have access to healthcare, it should be noted that it is not a metric that is only related to health financing. In other words, it represents realized access, which happens as a result of service provision. Similarly, if high OOP spending is necessary for care, this could affect people's access to services and lead to unmet needs.

Common indicators used to assess financial protection include the incidence of catastrophic health spending, which is the proportion of the population or households that spend more on healthcare than a predetermined percentage of their available resources (either their entire budget or a measure of their ability to pay); or the incidence of impoverishment due to health spending, which is the proportion of the population or households that fall below the poverty line as a result of out-of-pocket medical expenses. However, there are several ways in which the construction of these indicators can differ. This may lead to significant disparities in measurements and propose quite distinct policy recommendations. It is crucial to understand exactly what a given metric is measuring because of this.

Financial protection measurement captures the distribution of OOP spending across the entire population, which sets it apart from national indicators measuring OOP spending. Measuring OOP spending by itself might be deceptive. A nation with a high reliance on out-of-pocket spending (OOP) cannot be compared to one where the burden of OOP spending is borne solely by the extremely poor and underinsured. For example, if spending is made only by wealthy individuals who do not face hardship as a result. Therefore, the distributional impact and significant level of granularity of OOP expenses are added by financial protection metrics.

Understanding the performance of coverage policies can also benefit from additional, more qualitative data on the decision-making process. For instance, HiTs contain comprehensive information on the procedures used to determine which goods and services are included in benefit packages, as well as information on the legal foundation and eligibility requirements. There isn't much information of this kind in other HSA tools.

The HFPM compiles several indicative metrics for evaluating coverage policies (Table 5.8). The questions cover topics like eligibility requirements and benefit package design procedures. They also capture topics like accountability, transparency, equity, and utilization of need.

There will inevitably be an overlap between other methods or metrics for evaluating coverage policies and the other sub-functions. It could be helpful to look more descriptively at the use of co-payments for services covered in the benefits package and how those co-payments are designed. For example, one approach could be to consider whether the benefits covered vary across pools and the basis used to determine what is included in a benefits package – for example, is there a body that decides whether services or goods are reimbursed and if so, are its decisions binding? For instance, are there co-payments that are set at a fixed percentage or are there exemptions for vulnerable groups?

5.3.4.6. Assessing the Performance of PFM

Evaluating public financial management as a whole encompasses much more than just health financing performance. However, in order for a PFM system to function effectively, it must be open, effective, and generally help the health system run smoothly by making sure that resources are distributed to the appropriate locations in a timely and responsible manner.

Although some aspects of budget flow in pooling are covered in general in the HiTs, USAID, and Situation Analysis, PFM has not been thoroughly evaluated in the reviewed tools. The Expenditure and Financial Accountability tool is the ultimate resource. By assigning grades to 94 attributes spanning 31 essential public financial management components—categorized into seven main areas—this analyses the effectiveness of a PFM system. One can partially explain performance in the other three sub-functions using information of a PFM system. An essential part of PFM, for instance, is the capacity to plan and forecast over multiple years, which will eventually affect how predictable revenues are.

5.4. Increasing Healthcare Costs

Growing concern has been expressed regarding the rising costs of healthcare as health systems have changed and a greater percentage of the national population is covered by health insurance. Over the past 15 years, Figure 5.16 illustrates how the growth in overall health spending in OECD countries has exceeded GDP growth. When examining changes in healthcare costs, it is important to take political and microeconomic factors into account. Why are health services becoming more expensive? To this question, there are several interconnected answers.

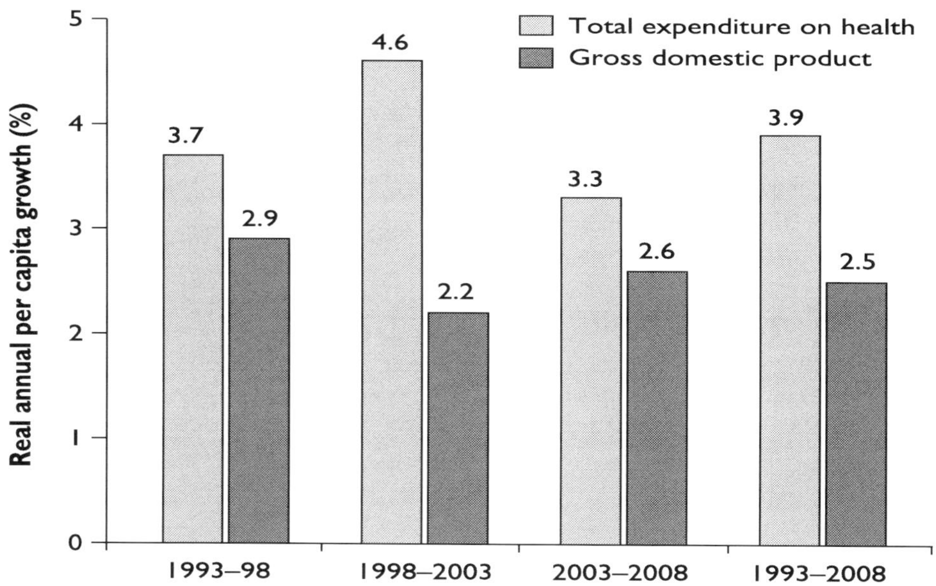

Figure 5.16. *Growth in total health expenditure and GDP 1993–2008.*

Source: Lorna, G., & Virginia, W., (n.d.). Introduction to Health Economics (2nd edn.). McGraw-Hill. Open University Press.

5.4.1. Demographic Factors

Healthcare costs are influenced by absolute population growth and relative changes within a population. Relative shifts can indicate that the population's distribution favors populations with greater healthcare needs, such as the elderly, the very young, and displaced populations.

5.4.2. Economic Factors

Changes in the economy impact the health sector as well as the expenses associated with providing healthcare. Typically, economic growth results in higher costs for health services, while economic recessions usually lead to lower costs. However, it's important to note that unemployment and poverty can lead to poor health outcomes and place additional burdens on health services. When analyzing cost increases, it's crucial to factor in inflation and consider supply-related influences such as the availability of healthcare providers and facilities, as well as changes in payment rates for healthcare workers.

5.4.3. Health Technology Advances

At the start of the 20th century, the options for effective health treatments were limited. As the years passed, the range of successful interventions grew significantly, including the development of antibiotics in 1938, open-heart surgery in 1954, hemodialysis in 1960, and computerized tomography in 1973. Technological advances played a significant role in the growth of health expenditure between 1960 and 2007, accounting for between one-quarter and one-half of the increase. More recently, the increased use of costly diagnostic tools such as MRI and CT scanners has driven up healthcare costs, with the number of MRI units per capita rising by over 100% across OECD member countries between 2000 and 2008.

5.4.4. Disease Patterns

What is the reason behind the observed shift in disease patterns in many low-income countries and how does it impact healthcare costs? First, the prevalence of new diseases such as HIV/AIDS rises with population age. Second, there is a correlation between treatment costs and the proportional rise in chronic illnesses and long-term sickness. Economic development will probably result in higher healthcare costs for a given country because infant deaths from communicable diseases are expected to decline in comparison to adult deaths from chronic diseases. One term for this trend is the "health" or "epidemiological" transition. Recall that non-communicable diseases accounted for 60% of all deaths worldwide in 2001. However, the distribution of these numbers varies by income level: non-communicable diseases accounted for only 36% of deaths in the world's poorest 20%, while they accounted for 87% of deaths in the richest 20%. This suggests that improving the health of the impoverished still places a high priority on low-cost, high-impact interventions against communicable diseases.

5.4.5. Evolution of the Health System

To explain how health systems have evolved over the past 60 years and how those changes have affected costs, some authors have proposed a three-stage model:

1. During the first stage, policies removed the existing financial barriers to healthcare. New funding arrangements increased population coverage and triggered the expansion of health services.
2. The subsequent increase in demand led to rapid growth of healthcare expenditure. Often spending grew faster than the

gross domestic product (GDP), and policy efforts were focused on cost control.

3. From the experience of ever-rising costs, it was realized that cost control alone is not effective. Policies of the third stage aim to improve the efficiency of service delivery and use.

5.4.6. Political Factors

Budgets for healthcare are invariably determined by political opinion. Before elections, there might be more "cash injections" or growth rates that deviate from the original projections due to competing priorities. Officially, money intended for healthcare may be redirected for other uses. Equity-related worries could make services more accessible and raise expenses. However, there could be significant financial losses if public officials, politicians, or healthcare providers are corrupted.

5.4.7. Some Popular Fallacies of the Current Debate

When estimating how aging will affect healthcare costs, use caution. According to recent research, regardless of age, the final year of life has the highest costs. Elderly individuals may tend to use fewer resources than younger ones. The rising expense of dying appears to be a bigger influence in high-income nations than the aging population's steady rise.

Additionally, you should know that, in contrast to popular opinion, early detection and prevention can ultimately result in higher costs. For instance, smokers have lower lifetime healthcare costs than non-smokers, which may indicate that smoking-related deaths are associated with lower costs for treating other diseases. Furthermore, paying retirement pensions at an earlier age saves money. Regarding the impact of new healthcare technologies, there is another misconception. Although new equipment may cost more at first, it might end up being more economical in the long run than the outdated technologies it replaces. Only when new technologies reduce costs or enhance services and/or results can they be justified. It is crucial to understand that the failure to apply the principles of economic evaluation, rather than technological advancement per se, is what drives up costs (Smith et al., 2009; Werblow et al., 2007).

5.5. The Changing World of Health Services Finance

Paying for healthcare is becoming a major concern in most, if not all, countries due to the rising costs of medical care. Governments attempt to contain spending through stricter regulations and other reforms because they are concerned about the political and economic fallout from the rising expense of healthcare. Numerous studies indicate that many nations have either been forced to implement reform due to significant political upheaval and economic hardship, as was the case with the former Soviet Union, or have been dissatisfied with how healthcare services are currently financed and delivered. There have been certain common themes among reforms, despite differences in their types and motivations:

- Separation of purchaser and provider responsibilities, whereby the underlying idea is that purchasers contract with those providers offering the best value for money and that this increases the efficiency of service delivery.
- Redefinition of the role of the state in responsibility for healthcare.
- Encouragement of the private sector.
- Encouragement of competition between providers.

- Alternative sources of funding: budget constraints and political change in many countries have resulted in the health sector and governments seeking out alternative ways of mobilizing resources.

When contemplating the final one, it is useful to differentiate between changes at the macro- and micro-levels. Modest adjustments have no bearing on the fundamental funding strategy. These modifications include the addition of co-payments and adjustments to the way providers are compensated. On the other hand, macro-level modifications entail a shift in the fundamental theory of financing. Examples of this include the transition from social insurance to a system primarily reliant on taxes in Italy and Spain, as well as the establishment of Thailand's tax-based universal coverage program. The former Soviet Union and Eastern Europe have seen some of the most significant recent changes. A significant number of former communist nations have switched from publicly funded programs to social insurance. Around 11 countries passed social insurance laws between 1991 and 1996. Significant transformations in certain low-income nations where increased utilization of patient fees and community funding has been pursued. The phrase "community financing" describes how local communities arrange their fundraising efforts rather than a specific type of financing mechanism. Rural communities work together toward goals other than health, like credit financing or crop insurance. In areas without free government services, there is a greater likelihood of developing community funding for healthcare.

5.5.1. Developing Methods to Pay Providers

Payment practices for healthcare providers have changed as funding systems have developed. Since it can be a crucial component of cost management, determining the best way to provide payment has long been a topic of political discussion. Doctors have founded their own insurance companies and engaged in takeovers and boycotts to obtain favorable conditions. Conflicts between the medical profession and financing agents are related to issues of whether:

- Doctors should be employed or act as independent contractors;
- Payments should be based on a salary, on the number of patients cared for (capitation), on the items of care provided (fee-for-service (FFS)), on the quality of their performance or on a combination of these options;
- Patients should pay healthcare providers directly and then claim reimbursement from government or insurance companies or payments should be made directly to the providers by the funders.

5.6. The Public–Private Distinction

The differentiation between public and private healthcare is a characteristic shared by all health systems. This differentiation pertains to both the funding and delivery of healthcare services. To determine if an organization is in the public or private sector, one uses the ownership concept. The term "public agency" does not only refer to government agencies; it also includes public bodies with statutory duties, such as social insurance companies. Organizations in the private sector can be classified as either for-profit or not-for-profit. The former group comprises the pharmaceutical industry and private healthcare facilities where a portion, occasionally the majority, of their earnings are distributed to the shareholders. Nonprofit organizations use any money left over to train employees and develop new facilities for their organization. The line separating "not-for-profit" organizations from "for-profit" organizations is less distinct because surplus funds from these organizations can also leave the company in the form of increased bonuses and salaries.

5.6.1. Public–Private Mix in Finance and Provision

Financial intermediaries may be set up in a monopolistic, oligopolistic, or competitive manner. A public organization like the government, a quango, or a health corporation typically acts as the financial intermediary in monopolistic systems. Finance can be governed by governmental organizations, private organizations like insurance companies, or a combination of these in an oligopolistic system (i.e., one with a limited number of large intermediaries). A competitive system would have a huge number of tiny private middlemen.

On the other hand, service delivery need not align with the financial institution. Hospital care, for example, is a large, vertically integrated health system in many European countries, where provision and financing are combined into one organization. Thus, both finance and provision are public as in the case of quadrant (1) [in Figure 5.17]. In many countries, general practice would fall into quadrant (2), such care being provided by self-employed doctors who, nevertheless, happen to receive almost all of their income from the public purse. Also, it is important to recognize that systems do not have to be vertically integrated in these ways: a third-party private payer, such as an insurance company, could also fit into segments (3) and (4). The fundamental idea is that neither public nor private funding must coincide with public or private provision. The financing of public services may come from private agreements (direct charges, private insurance, etc.) and private supply through public funding (e.g., potential direct payments from government organizations to private hospitals).

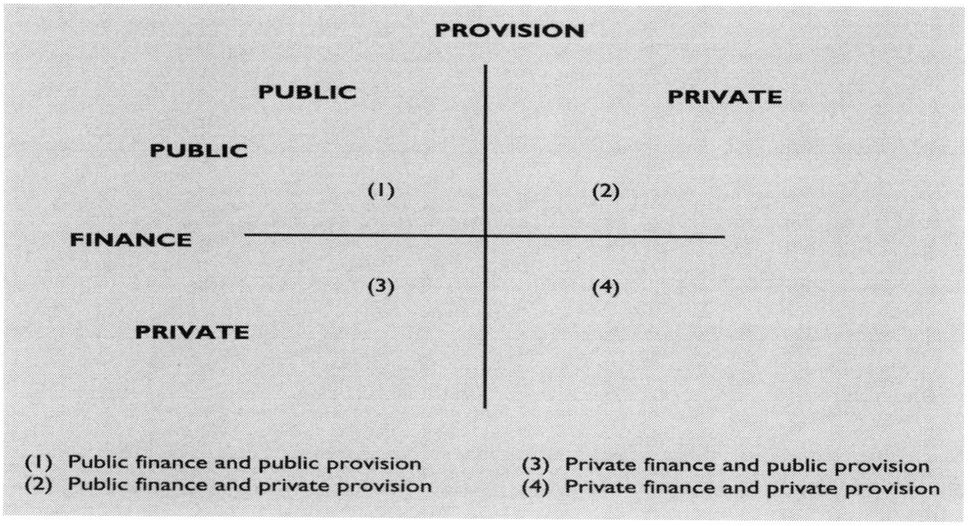

Figure 5.17. *Public–private mix in healthcare financing and provision.*

Source: Lorna, G., & Virginia, W., (n.d.). Introduction to Health Economics (2nd edn.). McGraw-Hill. Open University Press.

The case for government involvement in financing as opposed to healthcare delivery is stronger. Control over financial arrangements gives government agencies greater authority over the healthcare system to further societal goals. As the community's collective buyer of care, a public body can impose terms of provision on both public and private providers with equal authority. The provision of public services alone does not ensure that the targeted populations will use them; for example, hospitals may find that less sick, wealthy, or privately insured patients are more "attractive customers" than those who require more care (Murray et al., 2000; Sekhri et al., 2005).

5.7. Private Health Insurance

A collection of medical services paid for by a third party using non-income-related private payments known as premiums is known as private health insurance. It is optional to enroll in private health insurance. In the framework of healthcare financing systems, private health insurance is shown in Figure 5.18.

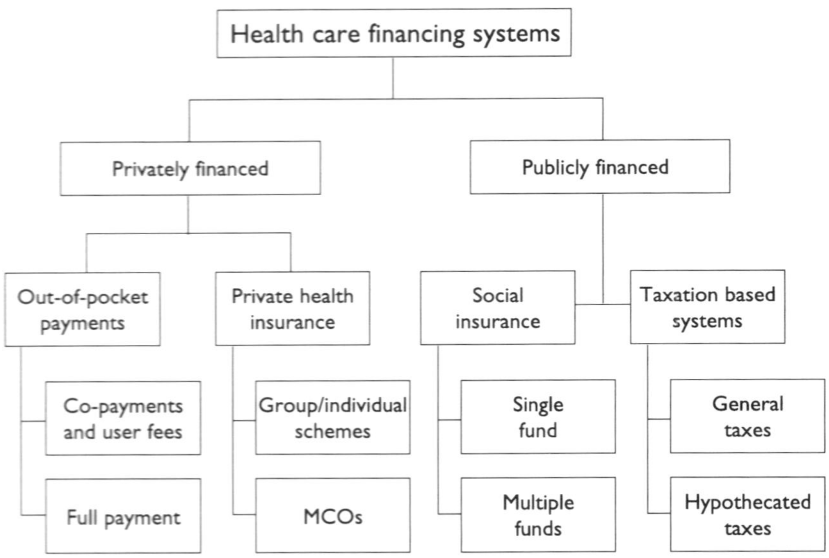

Figure 5.18. *Public and private methods of funding healthcare.*

Source: Lorna, G., & Virginia, W., (n.d.). Introduction to Health Economics (2nd edn.). McGraw-Hill. Open University Press.

5.7.1. The Mechanisms of Private Health Insurance

Voluntary premiums under private health insurance are paid to the insurance provider ahead of time to cover a portion of medical expenses in the event of illness. Insurance packages can be provided as managed care plans or as group or individual indemnity insurance schemes.

There are various types of private health insurance coverage, depending on the healthcare system:

1. **Principal:** If public health insurance coverage is not available, private health insurance will act as the person's principal coverage. This has been the case in the USA for individuals not eligible for public programs such as Medicare (above 65 or severely disabled), Medicaid (poor or near poor), and SCHIP (poor children). Principal coverage is also common in LMICs;
2. **Substitute:** If individuals can 'opt-out' of mandatory public insurance coverage, private health insurance can replace or substitute coverage. In Germany, employees with an income above a certain threshold can opt out of the social sickness fund system;
3. **Complementary:** If private health insurance covers co-payments incurred in the public system and not covered by public insurance, it is complementary. In France, Denmark, and Sweden, both complementary and supplementary private health insurance schemes are offered;
4. **Supplementary:** If private health insurance covers costs other than co-payments (e.g., drug costs) that are not covered by public insurance, it is supplementary. In Canada, private health insurance acts as supplementary coverage;
5. **Duplicate:** If private health insurance covers providers that are already covered by public insurance, it is considered duplicate coverage. In the UK, private health insurance offers duplicate and supplementary coverage.

5.7.2. Private Health Insurance, Efficiency, and Equity

Three main types of market failure affect the health insurance market: diseconomies of scale, moral hazard, and adverse selection. The efficiency and equity of the healthcare system are likely to be impacted if there is no government regulation of the private health insurance market.

5.7.2.1. Adverse Selection

Adverse selection occurs when customers choose plans that offer them the most utility because they have access to more comprehensive information about their own health status than insurers do. Certain governments have mandated that insurance companies underwrite premiums based on community characteristics, like age and gender composition, rather than using the health histories of individual policyholders to set the premium (i.e., community rating). Community rating has been introduced nationally in Australia and Ireland. However, without outlawing experience rating or occasionally using coercion (e.g., third-party car insurance), community rating cannot thrive in a market where prices are competitive. Customers who know they are less likely to become ill or for whom the cost of illness is low leave the insurance pool, leaving only those with relatively higher expected losses. This occurs when consumers with different expected losses are charged the same premium. This can then cause the premium to increase, which would cause more healthy people to drop out if the expense of the premium outweighs the advantages of having insurance. The market will collapse if this keeps happening unchecked.

5.7.2.2. Moral Hazard and Diseconomies of Scale

Moral hazard and diseconomies of scale have led to rising healthcare costs, but adverse selection is likely to result in unequal coverage, or none at all if the market collapses as a result. Insurance may also result in moral hazard for customers. For example, if insurance covers it, people might go to the doctor just to socialize.

Because there are typically numerous health insurance companies operating in the market, each with its insured pool, there are economies of scale present in the private health insurance sector. Because it is impossible to divide the fixed administrative costs and risks among a large number of clients, inefficiencies develop. High transaction costs are associated with marketing, processing claims, managing reimbursements, and detecting fraud in the insurance industry. Around 10% to 14% of total costs in unregulated markets are attributed to administration costs.

5.7.3. Combating Market Failure – The Insurer

Insurance companies and governments have difficulties in preventing moral hazard, which drives up costs and results in insufficient healthcare coverage, as well as consumers and providers who have incentives to practice adverse selection. Insurance companies employ a variety of cost-sharing strategies to reduce consumer moral hazard. These systems, which function as a financial barrier to prevent excessive service use, can be in the following forms:

- Co-payments are a flat fee paid by the insured patient each time they access a medical service;
- A deductible (also known as 'excess') is the amount a person pays before insurance coverage begins to have an effect;
- Co-insurance is a fixed percentage that the insured pays after the deductible is exceeded, up to the out-of-pocket maximum.

Individuals who have private health insurance usually have to pay the deductible prior to the start of the insurance coverage, as well as a co-payment for each medical consultation. Once the deductible is paid, co-insurance kicks in, requiring patients to contribute a predetermined portion (typically between 10% and 30%) of their medical expenses. When patients reach the maximum amount they must pay out-of-pocket, their co-insurance ends, and they are then fully covered by insurance up to the coverage limit. Such cost-sharing plans have the dual effect of discouraging people from seeking necessary medical care and preventing them from seeking potentially unnecessary medical care.

Improvements in underwriting can help manage adverse selection. Through the process of evaluating a customer's eligibility for health insurance and setting the premium based on risk, insurance companies attempt to better underwrite the risk. An adverse selection strategy could have negative consequences even though it might prevent the market's possible collapse. The sick can be denied access to affordable insurance due to underwriting, cherry-picking, and cream-skimming. Insurers can now use some of these strategies to lower supplier-induced demand and manage healthcare costs thanks to the creation of managed care plans.

5.7.4. Managed Care

In the USA, managed care organizations (MCOs) were primarily created in response to rising healthcare expenses. A "manager" steps in to oversee and keep an eye on the interactions between patients and doctors under a managed care system. The "manager" could be a software program designed to identify care that deviates from standard clinical practice, a trained utilization review nurse, or the medical director of the plan. The development and management of provider networks, the sharing and management of financial risk, the control of service utilization, the flow of information regarding received care, and the measurement of outcomes and quality are all central to managed care.

Managed care models can fall into one of three categories: health maintenance organizations (HMOs), point of service (POS) plans, or preferred provider organizations (PPOs).

1. **HMO:** The most restrictive form of managed care organization. HMOs are responsible for both the financing and the delivery of health services, acting both as a health insurer and a healthcare delivery management system. In a staff model (or closed-panel) HMO, physicians are directly employed by the HMO, whereas in a group model, the HMO contracts with physician group practices to provide services to its members. The insurance only covers care provided by physicians who are part of the HMO, and referrals are necessary for most specialist care.
2. **POS:** Similar to an HMO except that subscribers are allowed to see a non-HMO provider if they pay a significant out-of-pocket expense. The advantage is that subscribers are not locked into the HMO, though out-of-plan use remains low because of high cost-sharing.
3. **PPO:** A loosely organized MCO. The insurer negotiates contracts with a set of doctors and hospitals, which they consider the 'network,' to obtain care at a discount. Patients can decide whether to seek care in-network for a small co-payment, or obtain care out-of-network and pay substantially more.

The rising level of quality and cost control, from health maintenance organizations to traditional indemnity insurance, is depicted in Figure 5.19.

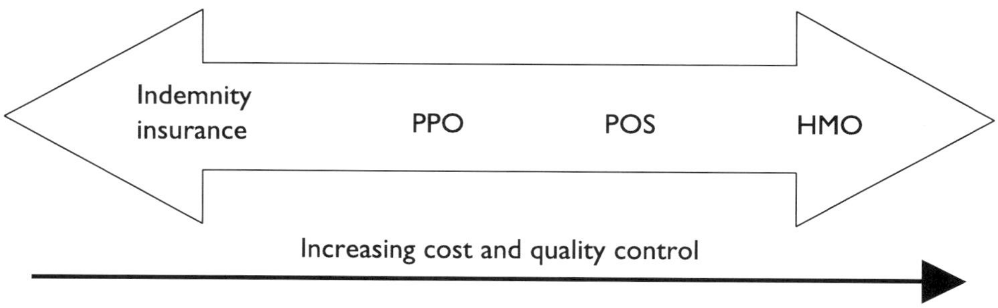

Figure 5.19. *The managed care continuum.*

Source: Lorna, G., & Virginia, W., (n.d.). Introduction to Health Economics (2nd edn.). McGraw-Hill. Open University Press.

5.7.5. Regulation of Private Health Insurance Markets

Governments have imposed restrictions on insurance companies' profits and premiums, as well as guidelines on benefit packages, to safeguard consumers and avoid coverage gaps. The majority of developed nations have expanded public insurance programs or offered tax-funded services to the underprivileged and elderly. Governments in numerous nations have mandated that employers with more than a particular number of workers provide health insurance options, or they have offered tax breaks to businesses that enroll their staff in private insurance.

The following measures merit attention:

1. **Prohibit Pre-Existing Condition Exclusions:** To make private health insurance accessible for those who are already sick, governments may forbid insurance companies to exclude such individuals with pre-existing conditions from being denied insurance. This was one of the main provisions of the USA health reform of 2010.
2. **Set a Minimum Package of Benefits:** To ensure that insurance companies will not take away certain benefits to save costs, many governments have developed a minimum standard of benefit packages that all private health insurance must provide. LMICs with private health insurance often face the challenges of regulating benefit packages.
3. **Risk Equalization:** In some countries, private health insurance companies are legally required to use community rating. Governments of these countries require insurers to pay or receive a payment that equalizes the risk profiles in order to avoid insurer risk selection or cream skimming.

Many LMICs have deregulated their private insurance markets in line with the current trend toward economic liberalization, or less government control and regulation. For instance, in Sri Lanka, this has led to a rise of insurance providers without significantly expanding population coverage. As you've seen, given the current market failures in private health insurance, some degree of government intervention is required to create an equitable and efficient health system (Bodenheimer et al., 2005; Colombo et al., 2004).

A Closer Look

Measuring the US Healthcare System: A Cross-National Comparison

Based on an analysis of OECD health data from 2008, the United States continues to differ markedly from other countries on several health system measures. Healthcare spending in the U.S. in 2006 was significantly higher than in other industrialized countries, both per capita and as a percentage of gross domestic product (GDP). The U.S. has a comparatively low number of hospital beds and physicians per capita, and patients in the U.S. have fewer hospital and physician visits than in most other countries. At the same time, spending per hospital visit is highest in the U.S., and American patients are among the most likely to receive procedures requiring complex technology. The nation now ranks in the bottom quartile in life expectancy among OECD countries and has seen the smallest improvement in this metric over the past 20 years.

Previous cross-national analyses of OECD data have examined several explanations for why the U.S. has higher health spending per capita. These include administrative complexity, the aging of the population, the practice of 'defensive medicine' under threat of malpractice litigation, chronic disease burden, healthcare supply and utilization rates, access to care, and resource allocation. These studies have consistently shown that, despite higher spending, the U.S. has, on many measures, lower healthcare utilization rates than most other OECD countries. The 2006 OECD data reveal similar findings—for example, in the high costs and low frequency associated with hospital discharges in the U.S. Some of these differences in average cost per discharge may be attributable to differences in patient case mix, the composition of the goods and services going into the treatment of a given medical condition, the prices paid by the hospitals for these goods and services, and the relative efficiency of hospitals. Furthermore, the administrative complexity in the U.S. healthcare system requires that American hospitals employ far larger staffs to handle billing requirements. While these issues require further investigation, one important difference may be the availability and use of technology in hospitals and other settings. U.S. providers have more access to expensive, high-tech medical technology in the treatment of patients and seem to perform more medical procedures involving sophisticated technology than do providers in other OECD countries.

Likewise, outpatient expenditures in the U.S. are also substantially higher than those in other OECD countries. One factor that could explain this large difference is that in the U.S., many expensive procedures are performed in outpatient settings, in contrast to most OECD countries, where they are more likely to be inpatient-based. For example, analysis of Medicare data shows that approximately half of beneficiaries receiving cardiac catheterization procedures, percutaneous transluminal coronary angioplasty, coronary bypass procedures, and knee replacements obtained them in outpatient settings. This heavy reliance on outpatient settings for medical procedures has two potentially negative consequences. First, it may be more difficult to ensure quality in the use of these technologies in the less tightly regulated ambulatory setting. Second, there is evidence that when physicians have a direct or indirect financial interest in outpatient facilities, the volume of these procedures tends to rise significantly.

Summary

- Healthcare financing can be analyzed from the point of view of financing schemes (financing arrangements through which health services are paid for and obtained by people, e.g., social health insurance), financing agents (organizations managing the financing schemes, e.g., social insurance agency), and types of revenues (e.g., social insurance contributions).
- Financing is the process of raising revenue to pay for healthcare goods and services. This can be done through a variety of means, such as government funding, private insurance, or out-of-pocket payments. The goal of healthcare financing is to ensure that everyone has access to the healthcare they need, regardless of their ability to pay.
- Function of a health system concerned with the mobilization, accumulation, and allocation of money to cover the health needs of the people, individually and collectively, in the health systems.
- Health system financing is the process by which revenues are collected from primary and secondary sources, accumulated in fund pools, and allocated to provider activities.
- Revenue raising refers to how money is brought into the health system. In most countries, apart from funds that come from external sources, the population is ultimately the source of all or most funds for the system. Revenue is collected through out-of-pocket payment at the point of service use, or through pre-paid funds including insurance contributions and/or taxes.
- Pooling refers to the accumulation of prepaid funds that can be used to purchase goods and services on behalf of a population. It is crucial to delineate pooling and revenue raising as two different functions of health financing.
- Purchasing, or commissioning, refers to payers using funds to pay for healthcare on behalf of a population. These funds can be pooled or include direct OOP payments at the point of service.
- Public financial management refers to the set of rules and mechanisms that govern the allocation, use, and accountability of public funds. It is important for the management of resources from all sources at national and subnational levels.
- Private health insurance is defined as a set of health services that are financed by a third party through private non-income related payments called premiums. Enrollment in private health insurance is voluntary.

References

1. Anderson, G., & Squires, D. (2010). Measuring the U.S. health care system: A cross-national comparison. *Issues in International Health Policy, 1412*(90), 1–9.
2. Armstrong, J., et al. (2010). Risk equalization in voluntary health insurance markets. *Health Policy, 98*(1), 1–49.
3. Bodenheimer, T. (2005). High and rising health care costs, part 3: The role of health care providers. *Annals of Internal Medicine, 142*(12, Part 1), 996–1002.

4. Colombo, F., & Tapay, N. (2004). Private health insurance in OECD countries: The benefits and costs for individuals and health systems. *OECD Health Working Papers, 15*, DELSA/ELSA/WD/HEA (2004)6.
5. Davis, C. (2010). Understanding the legacy: Health financing systems in the USSR and Central and Eastern Europe before transition. In J. Kutzin, C. Cashin, & M. Jakab (Eds.), *Implementing Health Financing Reform: Lessons from Countries in Transition*. Copenhagen: European Observatory on Health Systems and Policies.
6. Donaldson, C., et al. (2005). *The Economics of Health Care Financing: The Visible Hand*. Basingstoke: Palgrave Macmillan.
7. Drechsler, D., & Jutting, J. (2007). Different countries, different needs: The role of private health insurance in developing countries. *Journal of Health Politics, Policy and Law, 32*(3), 497–534.
8. Getzen, T. (2007). *Health Economics and Financing* (3rd ed.). Hoboken, NJ: John Wiley.
9. Gottret, P., & Schieber, G. (2006). Voluntary health insurance. In P. Gottret & G. Schieber (Eds.), *Health Financing Revisited: A Practitioner's Guide*. Washington, DC: The World Bank, 103–121.
10. Kongstvedt, P. (2007). *Essentials of Managed Health Care* (5th ed.). London: Jones & Bartlett.
11. Laing, W., & Buisson, W. (2003). *Private Medical Insurance: UK Market Report 2003*. London: Laing & Buisson.
12. Mathers, C. D., Lopez, A. D., & Murray, C. J. L. (2006). The burden of disease and mortality by condition: Data, methods, and results for 2001. In C. D. Mathers et al. (Eds.), *Global Burden of Disease and Risk Factors*. New York: Oxford University Press.
13. Mueller, M., & Morgan, D. (2017). New insights into health financing: First results of the international data collection under the System of Health Accounts 2011 framework. *Health Policy, 121*(7), 764–769.
14. Murray, C., & Frenk, J. (2000). A framework for assessing the performance of health systems. *Bulletin of the World Health Organization, 78*(6), 717–731.
15. Sekhri, N., & Savedoff, W. (2005). Private health insurance: Implications for developing countries. *Bulletin of the World Health Organization, 83*(2), 127–134.
16. Smith, S., Newhouse, J., & Freeland, M. S. (2009). Income, insurance, and technology: Why does health spending outpace economic growth? *Health Affairs, 28*(5), 1276–1284.
17. Werblow, A., Felder, S., & Zweifel, P. (2007). Population aging and health care expenditure: A school of 'red herring? *Health Economics, 16*(10), 1109–1126.

Chapter 6

ROLE OF GOVERNMENT IN HEALTH

Contents

Introduction

In recent years, health reform has become a top priority on the political agendas of countries worldwide. Developed industrial nations and many middle-income developing countries are concerned about the rapidly increasing costs of healthcare, a large portion of the population lacking health insurance, and the fear of diseases such as AIDS. Developing countries now recognize the importance of investing in health to improve worker productivity and achieve significant health improvements at minimal cost. The role of governments in advancing healthcare cannot be understated. Public health initiatives have successfully eliminated diseases like smallpox and contributed to the reduction of deaths from other vaccine-preventable illnesses in children. Government-provided clinical care has saved countless lives from infectious diseases and injuries. Additionally, improved prenatal and delivery services organized by governments have reduced the occurrence of serious complications for millions of mothers during pregnancy and childbirth.

Even with these astounding advancements, there are still serious health issues. The overall death rates in developing nations remain intolerably high; compared to established market economies, child mortality rates are roughly 10 times higher. Around 11 million fewer children would die annually if the death rates of children in developing nations were brought down to those of rich nations, according to a 1993 World Bank Development Report. Malnutrition-related diarrheal and respiratory illnesses account for nearly half of those avoidable deaths. In addition, tuberculosis alone accounts for 2 million of the 7 million adult deaths annually that result from diseases that are easily preventable or treated. The direct complications of pregnancy and childbirth account for over 4,00,000 deaths in women. In developing nations, maternal mortality ratios are typically 30 times higher than in high-income nations. The way health systems are currently managed and funded has several serious issues, and if answers are not found, the rate of progress in lowering the burden of early death and disability will slow.

Orientation and Directional Terms:

Term	Definition	Illustration
Public good	A public good is a good that is both non-excludable and non-rivalrous. Use by one person neither prevents access by other people, nor does it reduce availability to others. Therefore, the good can be used simultaneously by more than one person.	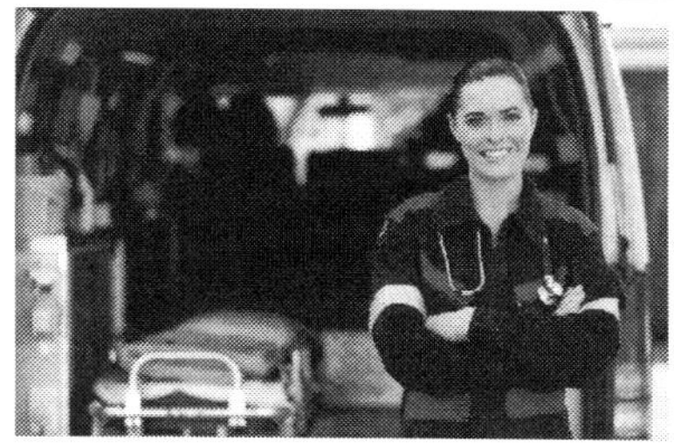
Public insurance	A program run by U.S. federal, state, or local governments in which people have some or all of their healthcare costs paid for by the government.	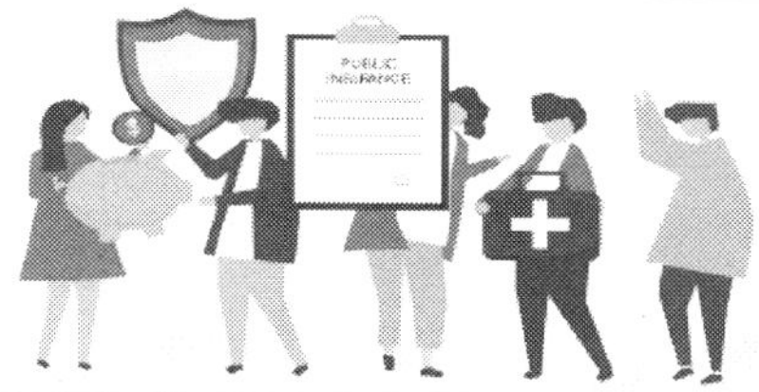
Health legislation	Health law is defined as a set of rules regulating the promotion and protection of health, health services, the equitable distribution of available resources, and the legal position of all parties concerned (namely, patients, healthcare providers, healthcare institutions, and financing) and monitoring bodies.	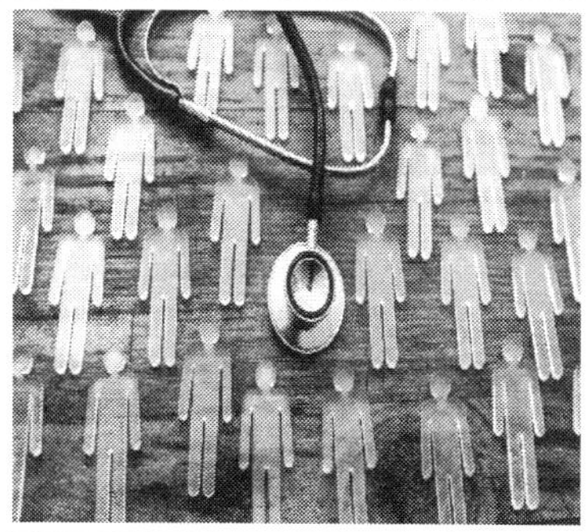
Health security	Health security is the actions needed to prevent and respond to acute threats that could endanger people's health across countries and borders. Many factors can jeopardize our health security – from new and emerging infectious diseases to the rise of antimicrobial resistance (AMR).	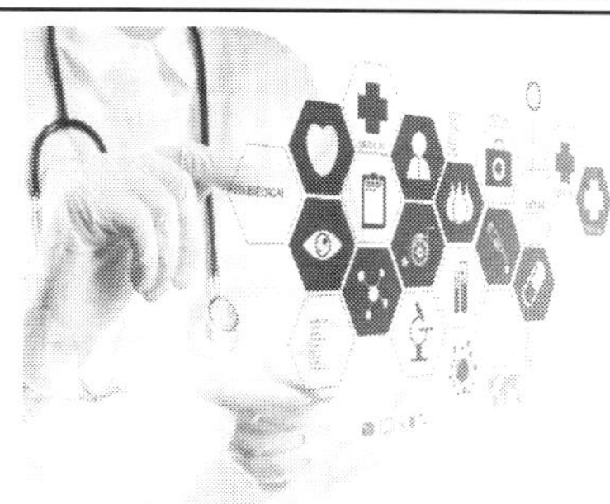
Marginal social benefit (MSB)	Marginal social benefit is the satisfaction experienced by consumers of a specific good plus or minus the overall environmental and social costs or benefits. For example, if positive externalities of consumption are present, marginal social benefits are larger than marginal private benefits.	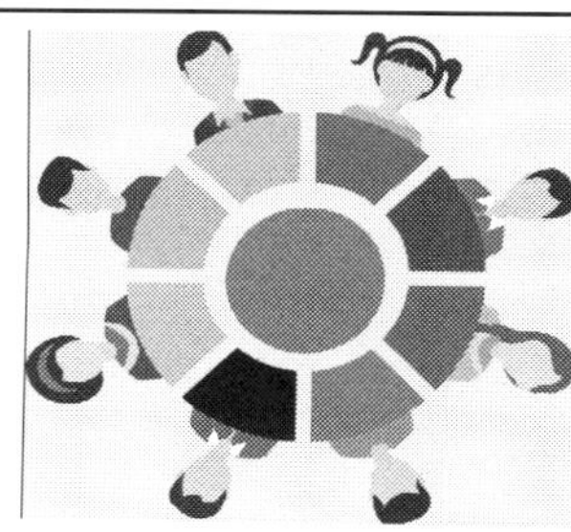

6.1. Problems of Health Policy

Countries will differ in what kind and degree of government involvement is appropriate, largely due to differences in income levels. Misallocation, inefficiency, and cost allocation are a few of the common policy issues faced by most nations:

1. **Misallocation:** The proper distribution of material, financial, and human resources is one of the most crucial applications of economics in the creation of health policy. This suggests the best possible division of financial resources among conflicting demands. This, in turn, necessitates accurately identifying the need. Public funds are occasionally allocated to health interventions that are not very cost-effective, like treating cancer, while critically important and highly cost-effective interventions, like treating tuberculosis and STDs, are not adequately funded.
2. **Inequity:** The impoverished receive subpar care and don't have access to basic health services. Government health spending disproportionately benefits the wealthy through subsidies to private and advanced public tertiary care hospitals.
3. **Inefficiency:** Much of the money spent on health is wasted because brand name pharmaceuticals are purchased instead of generic drugs, health workers are badly deployed and supervised, and hospital beds are underutilized.
4. **Cost Explosion:** A growing number of specialists, the availability of new medical technologies, and the expansion of health insurance linked to fee-for-service payments all combine to create a rapidly growing demand for expensive tests, procedures, and treatments, which is driving up healthcare costs in some middle-income developing nations much faster than income growth. Some contend that governments ought to increase their funding while permitting non-governmental organizations and the private sector to participate more in the provision of healthcare services, as both industrialized and developing nations reconsider how best to deliver healthcare in the coming century.

6.2. What Can Governments Do?

It makes sense for governments to get involved given the issues raised. The healthcare that would increase the productivity and well-being of the impoverished is sometimes out of their reach. Certain initiatives to advance health have significant positive knock-on effects or are pure public goods. Due to health insurance market failures, government intervention can increase welfare by enhancing the efficiency of those markets. Governments should carefully consider the extent of their involvement and spend prudently. The World Bank suggests four key measures to address the current shortcomings in the health systems of developing nations.

- Governments should finance a nationally defined package of essential public health and clinical care, especially for the poor, and ensure the widespread and efficient delivery of such a package.
- The public sector should devote far fewer resources or none at all to financing health services outside of the essential package which are of lower cost-effectiveness.

- Governments should promote types of health insurance that not only achieve broad coverage of the population but also build in payment mechanisms that control the cost of health services.
- Governments should encourage diversity and competition in the supply of health inputs, particularly drugs, supplies, and equipment, as a means of improving quality and driving down costs. They should also foster a competitive private sector to provide the full range of health services, including financial publicity.

6.2.1. A Basic Health Package

Government action in many areas of public health has already had an important payoff. The challenge now is to expand coverage of interventions with high cost-effectiveness:

- School-based health services;
- Information on family planning and nutrition;
- Programs to reduce tobacco and alcohol consumption;
- Regulation, information, and public investments to improve the household environment and AIDS prevention.

Governments should simultaneously assemble a package of fundamental clinical services, though this may differ from nation to nation based on regional requirements and economic status. A minimum package of health services that would reduce the burden of disease by slightly over 30% in low-income countries and be affordable for most developing countries at current health spending levels has been suggested by the World Bank Development Report (1993). The package includes 11 individual or clusters of interventions. These services, in addition to being cost-effective, target diseases that account for a significant portion of the disease burden in developing nations. The epidemiological profile of the nation (the distribution of disease burden across diseases) and the efficacy of the associated interventions will, however, largely dictate the precise contents of each country's essential package. The amount of money available for healthcare will determine the size of the package (the number of interventions cluster). Clustering interventions improves cost-effectiveness through at least three mechanisms:

- Synergism between treatments or prevention activities is common, particularly in pediatric care;
- Joint production costs can substantially reduce the amount of resources needed were interventions to be provided separately; and
- The optimal use of specialized resources, such as hospital beds, requires a screening process to refer the most severe cases from the first level of care to other facilities.

The interventions in an effective health cluster should be able to be administered to the same person at the same time using the same delivery method (hospital, health center, or outreach community health worker). An essential health package approach is a crucial measure that governments can be encouraged to implement. The expanded vaccination program, for instance, is incredibly effective because it comprises six vaccines given to the same people via the same delivery system, frequently at the same time.

6.2.2. Value for Money

One of the hardest choices developing countries have to make when it comes to health policy is how to best combine a range of medical services that will be paid for by public funds. Ideally, they would like to provide as many people with as much healthcare as they can. In actuality, though, they wind up focusing resources on urban hospitals that offer a plethora of services to a select few, leaving other population groups—especially those living in rural areas—with comparatively limited access. This distribution of public funds is both inefficient and unfair. Expensive treatments that only marginally extend life are prescribed, while large populations are denied low-cost services that significantly extend life, like immunization. The World Bank Development Report suggests that governments create and fund a national health package that includes fundamental clinical and public health services to significantly lower the burden of disease—defined as the present value of future streams of disability-free life lost due to illness, injury, or death—at reasonable costs. This implies that to reallocate resources in the most economical way possible, the government will need to assess the value of the interventions it offers.

Health interventions are what health services provide, regardless of how they are set up and funded. At the core of discussions about the ideal combination of interventions are disagreements over whether health services should prioritize "vulnerable groups" like children, expectant mothers, and the elderly, or the relative roles of hospitals and health centers. Customers want value for their money in the health industry, just like they do in any other. Because of this, the first step in creating a nation's essential health package is figuring out how cost-effective a health intervention is—that is, dividing the net health gain over doing nothing by the total cost. The developing nations that have improved health the most for a given amount of spending have focused their public funds on extremely economical interventions.

6.2.3. Redirecting Public Spending

The World Bank Development Report made it clear that health systems and policies require extensive and comprehensive reform. It demanded adjustments to insurance, cost recovery, and the ways in which healthcare is financed, as well as to the amount and makeup of government spending on health in both public and private organizations that provide healthcare services. Because an essential clinical package lowers poverty and has positive spillover effects, public financing of the package makes sense. The argument, however, is much weaker in favor of government funding of optional clinical health services that are not included in the essential national package. Governments would increase efficiency and equity if they reduced or eliminated public funding for these services.

Recovering hospital expenses, particularly from the wealthy and insured, is a crucial strategy for steering government spending away from non-essential care. Governments can impose fees for optional care provided in public hospitals due to a combination of limited private insurance and the ability of higher income groups to pay, even in low-income nations like Ethiopia, Kenya, Pakistan, and the Philippines where insurance may make up less than 5% of total health spending. There is always more room for cost recovery in middle-income nations, where insurance plays a bigger role.

Additionally, governments ought to gradually stop funding insurance that primarily benefits the wealthy. Given the public benefit nature of public health interventions and the necessity of several key clinical services, such as tuberculosis treatment, there are compelling efficiency arguments in favor of allocating government funding to them. In addition, there are equity grounds for financing the basic health package.

The poor are disproportionately affected by the disease burden the package addresses. This means that making public financing of this package with universal government finance leads to public subsidies to the wealthy, who can afford to pay for their own services, with the result that fewer government resources go to serve the poor.

Spending by the government on the impoverished is one approach to address this issue. Targeting is nearly inescapable in low-income nations where the cost of the minimum package exceeds current public health spending. Targeting might be relatively simple in nations where the wealthy prefer the higher quality and convenience of privately financed services, making them less likely to use government-financed services. A "district" hospital is the most advanced facility needed to provide the package's minimum elements; these hospitals act as health centers' initial point of referral. These hospitals provide emergency services, outpatient care, and basic surgery. They can typically accommodate between 100 and 400 beds and serve between 50,000 and 2,00,000 people; however, the minimal package necessitates having access to district hospitals and health centers across the nation. It takes one district hospital bed, zero to two doctors per 1,000 people, and two to four nurses for every doctor on average.

Governments can direct public spending to support the nationally defined essential package in several ways:

- In cases where services are funded and rendered by the government, funds can be reallocated to support the package by purchasing drugs, supplies, equipment, personnel, and facilities. Extending lower-level facilities is a necessary step in delivering the package in many countries. Governments can also completely stop funding inputs for less expensive services or drastically cut back on it. This could entail the conversion of specialized hospital physicians or the loss of wards. For instance, provincial governments in Canada, not specific hospitals, decide which cutting-edge diagnostic equipment to purchase.

In addition, the type of input that is available would have an influence on providers' treatment decisions rather than being micromanaged. For example, specialized personnel and supplies would be available to treat malaria in young children. One possible way to recognize and honor specific service providers, facilities, or districts that successfully reached a high population coverage rate with the package's services is through budgetary and salary incentives.

- In cases where services are privately rendered but publicly funded, governments should only pay for the essential services. This healthcare delivery model is expanding, but it is not common in developing nations. The regulatory framework needed to monitor these kinds of agreements is currently underdeveloped.

6.2.4. Controlling Costs

Governments still have to deal with the issue of rising healthcare costs, even in situations where subsidies for affluent people's optional clinical services are eliminated or universal public insurance is implemented and covers a wider range of services in the national package. These expenses have the potential to reduce investment in other economic areas or drive up labor costs, endangering a nation's ability to compete internationally. The causes of excessive healthcare expenses are numerous and hotly contested. The health services sector experiences slower productivity growth than other areas of the economy due to its labor-intensive nature. Part of the solution lies in the United States, where hospital amenities are better and underlying morbidity is higher than in other industrialized nations. However, two other forms of inefficiencies are also significant: excessive administrative expenses and needless use of an ever-expanding range of expensive technologies for surgical and diagnostic procedures.

There seem to be two fundamental aspects of the US health system that are closely related to these inefficiencies. Since neither healthcare providers nor patients have strong incentives to limit utilization or spending, open-ended free-for-all service compensation for healthcare providers promotes the development of new tools, medications, and procedures. The administrative costs of a complex system with numerous insurance companies and other payers, each with its processes, are significantly increased. These findings regarding the rise in health costs in developed nations are particularly pertinent to middle-income developing nations, as they face pressure to adopt new medical procedures from manufacturers, consumers, and medical professionals. They must make tough decisions about provider compensation policy. Paying a set amount per person (capitation) is one method of reducing healthcare costs. This is currently the practice of British national health services and health maintenance organizations in the United States. Another strategy that is employed in a number of developed nations is to allocate a set overall budget to each hospital or physician network. In nations with more developed insurance markets, insurers can also work together to agree on standard rates for doctors or set fixed costs for particular medical treatments.

6.2.5. Promoting Competition

Governments don't need to provide basic health services, even though they have a fundamental obligation to finance such services. Based on past experiences, it seems that competition and diversity produce better outcomes. People in need of health services in a competitive system have access to a range of providers, including public, private non-profit, and private for-profit organizations. Developing nations have a plethora of policy options at their disposal when it comes to how various providers—both public and private—impact allocative efficiency, technical efficiency, and the ability to serve the impoverished. A significant portion of healthcare in developing nations is provided by non-governmental organizations (NGOs), particularly to low-income households in the most impoverished nations. According to recent data from Africa, NGOs are frequently more effective. Essential services have deteriorated in governments that have either banned or severely restricted NGOs. If there are any such restrictions or impediments to NGO activity, they ought to be lifted. Beyond this, governments can work with NGOs to build positive partnerships to provide critical clinical services. Certain African governments, like those of Tanzania and Lesotho, permit religious mission hospitals in strategic locations to function as district hospitals. They then assign them the full range of clinical and public health services, as well as district-wide responsibilities like emergency transport maintenance, supervision of community activities and lower-level clinics, and health planning. The government reimburses part of the NGO's expenses in exchange.

Governments should employ traditional healers more frequently in regions like Asia and Africa where they continue to play a significant role in the healthcare system. Successful initiatives include the distribution of condoms in Zimbabwe and Uganda, the promotion of modern contraceptives in Kenya, and the use of healers in Thailand to screen for malaria and provide anti-malarial medications. In Bangladesh, efforts have also been made to enhance pregnancy outcomes by hiring traditional birth attendants.

Through decentralization and the application of managerial incentives, governments can simultaneously increase the equity and efficiency of their health programs and facilities, thereby enhancing their responsiveness to local needs. By transforming public hospitals into partially autonomous foundations or public businesses, governments can also increase efficiency. When it comes to handling their finances and obtaining donations for investments and running expenses, these foundations are not as constrained by public sector policies. Public health and a nationally defined package of essential clinical services would be financed by the government, leaving the remaining clinical services to be paid for privately or through social insurance within a framework of government-established policies. Governments can promote diversity and competition in the provision of health and insurance by adopting policies that:

- Encourage social or private insurance (with regulatory incentives for equitable access and cost containment) for clinical services outside the essential package.
- Encourage suppliers (both public and private) to compete to deliver clinical services and provide inputs, such as drugs, to public and privately financed health services. Domestic suppliers should not be protected from international competition.
- Generate and disseminate information on provider performance, essential equipment and drugs, costs and effectiveness of interventions, and accreditation and status of institutions and providers.

A large portion of the 20th century's dramatic improvements in health can be attributed to advances in science, which have sparked the development of preventive, curative, and diagnostic technologies and provided information that serves as the foundation for private and public policy. Investing in ongoing scientific research will increase the efficacy of each of the three recommended points of the approach.

6.2.6. Strengthening Household Capacity

Health within the household improves quickly as people rise out of poverty and pursue higher education. Beyond the home, a society's ability to provide health services is influenced by its national income and educational attainment and its capacity to learn and use new scientific knowledge.

6.2.6.1. The Role of Income

Income per capita is thought to have a significant correlation with life expectancy. People in a country are more likely to live long, healthy lives if their income per capita is higher. Income growth has a greater effect on impoverished populations because more money can be used to purchase needs like food and shelter, which have particularly significant positive effects on health. During the century, the relationship between life expectancy and income has improved as scientific and medical advancements have made it possible to achieve greater health for a given income. It is not only income per capita that matters, as poverty has a significant impact on health. The number of people living in poverty and the distribution of income are also important factors. Life expectancy in industrialized nations is largely determined by income distribution rather than income per capita, and it has been increasing more quickly in nations with better income distribution. Differences in life expectancy in developing countries are largely explained by variations in the prevalence of poverty and per capita public spending on health. Additionally, disparities in health between wealthy and impoverished neighborhoods and families can be observed, even within a single city, indicating the detrimental impact of poverty on health. Slow economic growth hurts health, as evidenced by the strong correlation between income level and health.

6.2.6.2. The Role of Education

Higher-educated households have better adult and pediatric health. Parental education is a significant predictor of the child's health. The benefits of a mother's education on her child's health are noticeable even before delivery and persist throughout the early years of life. Higher-educated women tend to delay marriage and parenthood, reducing the health risks associated with early childbearing. They also tend to use health services more efficiently and maintain better household hygiene. They are generally more adept at acting upon and obtaining health-related information.

An adult's personal habits and lifestyle have a significant impact on their health. There is a direct correlation between education and health because well-informed individuals make decisions that are better for their health. In Brazil, adults with only a primary education are roughly five times more likely to have high blood pressure than adults with post-secondary education. Educated individuals are quick to adjust their behavior when new health risks, such as AIDS, emerge or when new health information becomes available. For example, in the United Kingdom, the percentage of highly educated adult smokers decreased by 50% between 1958 and 1975, while the percentage of less educated smokers remained relatively stable.

The policy implications are obvious given the strong correlations between increased income, health, and education; governments should endeavor to promote economic growth, lower poverty rates, and increase access to education, particularly for girls, who represent one of the best avenues for enhancing women's capacity to care for their families. One of the most important things a government can do is to establish sound economic policies, as it is difficult to reduce poverty and subsequently improve health status without economic growth (Aaron et al., 1984; Baker et al., 1988).

6.3. Health Policy of Ethiopia

Ethiopia's health policy is founded on the primary healthcare approach, which includes family planning, nutrition, immunization, and health education as standard components. It also includes education on environmental and personal hygiene. The main goal of the health policy is to build over 500 new health centers to serve the underserved rural population with primary healthcare. The population of Ethiopia was estimated to be only 46% or fewer living within a reasonable distance from health facilities in 1990. A reasonable distance is defined as a radius of 10 kilometers from a person's place of residence. The estimated population-to-physician and population-to-nurse ratios were 30,700 and 15,000, respectively. Only 18% of people in rural areas and 78% of people in urban areas have access to clean water, and only 5.3% of people use latrines daily. The estimated daily calorie supply per capita is 76.0% of the recommended daily intake. It is obvious that the Ethiopian population is woefully underserved when it comes to even the most basic necessities of life, and there is still much work to be done to meet these needs even in the most basic way.

6.3.1. General Policy

This includes:

- Democratization and decentralization of the health services system.
- Development of the preventive and promotive components of healthcare.
- Development of an equitable and acceptable standard of health service system that will reach all segments of the population within the limits of resources.
- Promoting and strengthening of inter-Sectoral activities.
- Promotion of attitudes and practices conducive to the strengthening of national self-reliance in health development by mobilizing and utilizing internal and external resources to their maximum.
- Assurance of accessibility of healthcare for all segments of the population.
- Working closely with neighboring countries, regional and international organizations to share information and strengthen collaboration in all activities contributory to health development including the control of factors detrimental to health.
- Development of appropriate capacity building based on assessed needs.
- Provision of healthcare for the population on a scheme of payment according to ability with special assistance mechanisms for those who cannot afford to pay.
- Promotion of the participation of the private sector and non-governmental organizations in healthcare.

6.3.2. Priorities of the Policy

Information, Education, and Communication (I.E.C.) of health shall be given appropriate prominence to enhance health awareness and to propagate the important concepts and practices of self-responsibility in health.

Emphasis shall be given to:

- The control of communicable diseases, epidemics, and poor living conditions.
- The promotion of occupational health and safety.
- The development of environmental health.
- The rehabilitation of the health infrastructure.
- The development of an appropriate health service management system.

Appropriate support shall be given to the curative and rehabilitative components of health, including mental health. Due attention shall be given to the development of the beneficial aspects of traditional medicine, including related research and its gradual integration into modern medicine. Applied health research addressing the major health problems shall be emphasized. The provision of essential medicines, medical supplies, and equipment shall be strengthened.

Special attention shall be given to the health needs of:

- The family particularly women and children.
- Those at the forefront of productivity.
- Those hitherto most neglected regions and segments of the population including the majority of the rural population, pastoralists, the urban poor, and national minorities.

- Victims of man-made and natural disasters.

6.3.3. General Strategies

Establishing health committees at local levels to assist in identifying major health issues, budgeting, planning, implementing, monitoring, and evaluating health-related activities, as well as health councils with strong community representation at all levels, will help democratize the system. The main components of decision-making, healthcare organization, capacity building, planning, implementation, and monitoring will be transferred to the regions with clearly defined roles to achieve decentralization.

Intersectional collaboration shall be emphasized particularly in:

- Enriching the concept and intensifying the practice of family planning for optimal family health and planned population dynamics.
- Formulating and implementing an appropriate food and nutrition policy.
- Accelerating and provision of safe and adequate water for urban and rural populations.
- Developing safe disposal of human, agricultural, and industrial wastes and recycling.
- Measures to improve the quality of housing and work premises for health.
- Participating in the development of community-based facilities for the care of the physically and mentally disabled, the abandoned, street children, and the aged.
- Participating in the development of daycare centers in factories and enterprises, school health and nutrition programs.
- Undertakings in disaster management, agriculture, education, communication, transportation, expansion of employment opportunities and development of other social services.
- Developing facilities for workers' health and safety in production sectors.

Health Education shall be strengthened generally and for specific target populations through the mass media, community leaders, religious and cultural leaders, professional association's schools, and other social organizations for:

- Inculcating attitudes of responsibility for self-care in health and assurance of a safe environment.
- Encouraging the awareness and development of health-promotive lifestyles and attention to personal hygiene and healthy environment.
- Enhancing awareness of common communicable and nutritional diseases and the means for their prevention.
- In calculating attitudes of participation in community health development.
- Identifying and discouraging harmful traditional practices while encouraging their beneficial aspects.
- Discouraging the acquisition of harmful habits such as cigarette smoking, alcohol consumption, drug abuse, and irresponsible sexual behavior.

- Creating awareness in the population about the rational use of drugs.
- **Promotive and preventive activities shall address:**
  - Control of common endemic and epidemic communicable and nutritional diseases using appropriate general and specific measures.
  - Prevention of diseases related to affluence and aging from emerging as major health problems.
  - Prevention of environmental pollution with hazardous chemical wastes.
- **Human resource development shall focus on:**
  - Developing the team approach to healthcare.
  - Training of community-based task-oriented frontline and middle-level health workers of appropriate professional standards; and recruitment and training of these categories at regional and local levels.
  - Training of trainers, managerial and supportive categories with appropriate orientation to the health service objectives.
  - Developing appropriate continuing education for all categories of workers in the health sector.
  - Developing an attractive career structure, remuneration, and incentives for all categories of workers within their respective systems of employment.
- **Availability of drugs, supplies, and equipment shall be assured by:**
  - Preparing lists of essential and standard drugs and equipment for all levels of the health service system and continuously updating such lists.
  - Encouraging national production capability of drugs, vaccines, supplies, and equipment by giving appropriate incentives to firms engaged in manufacture, research, and development.
  - Developing a standardized and efficient system for procurement, distribution, storage, and utilization of the products.
  - Developing quality control capability to assure efficacy and safety of products.
  - Developing maintenance and repair facilities for equipment.
- **Traditional medicine shall be accorded appropriate attention by:**
  - Identifying and encouraging the utilization of its beneficial aspects.
  - Coordinating and encouraging research, including its linkage with modern medicine.
  - Developing appropriate regulation and registration for its practice.
- **Health system research shall be given due emphasis by:**
  - Identifying priority areas for research in health.
  - Expanding applied research

on major health problems and health service systems.

- Strengthening the research capabilities of national institutions and scientists in collaboration with the responsible agencies.
- Develop appropriate measures to ensure a strict observance of ethical principles in research.

- **Family health services shall be promoted by:**
  - Assuring adequate maternal healthcare and referral facilities for high-risk pregnancies.
  - Intensifying family planning for the optimal health of the mother, child, and family.
  - Inculcating principles of appropriate maternal nutrition.
  - Maintaining breastfeeding, and advocating homemade preparation, production, and availability of weaning food at affordable prices.
  - Expanding and strengthening immunization services, optimization of access and utilization.
  - Encouraging early utilization of available healthcare facilities for the management of common childhood diseases particularly diarrhea and acute respiratory infections.
  - Addressing the special health problem and related needs of adolescents.
  - Encouraging paternal involvement in family health.
  - Identifying and discouraging harmful traditional practices, while encouraging their beneficial aspects.
- **The referral system shall be developed by:**
  - Optimizing utilization of healthcare facilities at all levels.
  - Improving accessibility of care according to need.
  - Assuring continuity and improved quality of care at levels.
  - Rationalizing costs for healthcare seekers and providers for optimal utilization of healthcare facilities at all levels.
  - Strengthening the communication within the healthcare system.
  - Diagnostic and supportive services for healthcare shall be developed by:
  - Strengthening the scientific bases of healthcare.
  - Facilitating prompt diagnosis and treatment.
  - Guiding continuing care.
- **The health management information system shall be organized by:**
  - Making the system appropriate and relevant for decision-making, planning, implementing, monitoring, and evaluation.
  - Maximizing the utilization of information at all levels.

- Developing central and regional information documentation centers.

- **Health legislation shall be revised by:**
  - Up-dating existing public health laws and regulations.
  - Developing new rules and regulations to help in the implementation of the current policy and addressing new health issues.
  - Strengthening mechanisms for implementation of the health laws and regulations.
- **Health service organization shall be systematized and rationalized by:**
  - Standardizing the human resources, physical facilities, and operational system of the health units of all levels.
  - Defining and instituting the catchment areas of health units and referral systems based on assessment of pertinent factors.
  - Regulating private healthcare and professional deployment by appropriate licensing.
- **Administration and management of the health system shall be strengthened and made more effective and efficient by:**
  - Restructuring and organizing at all levels in line with the present policy of decentralization and democratization of decision-making and management.
  - Combining departments and services, which are closely related and rationalizing the utilization of human and material resources.
  - Studying the possibility of designating undersecretaries to ensure continuity of service.
  - Creating management boards for national hospitals, institutions, and organizations.
  - Allowing health institutions to utilize their income to improve their services.
  - Ensuring placement of appropriately qualified and motivated personnel at all levels.
- **Financing the health services shall be through public, private, and international sources, and the following options shall be considered and evaluated:**
  - Raising taxes and revenues.
  - Formal contributions or insurance by public employees.
  - Legislative requirements of a contributory health fund for employees of the private sector.
  - Individual or group health insurance.
  - Voluntary contributions.

6.4. Domains of Government Role in Health Development

The duties of Ministries of Health involve spearheading health development by enhancing and executing key health system functions such as leadership and governance, healthcare financing, health service provision, and generating resources for health development. These efforts are aligned with other relevant ministries and departments.

6.4.1. Leadership and Governance

As expressed in their constitutions, ratified treaties, and attended conventions, governments are the custodians of social commitments and values like solidarity, social justice, and equity. The right to healthcare and education is enshrined in many international constitutions, as well as those of the Eastern Mediterranean Region. Governments have to guarantee that everyone has unhindered access to these services and to uphold the importance of health as a fundamental human right.

Health ministries are responsible for overseeing the development of health systems through governance functions. This includes analyzing and creating policies, regulating service delivery among partners, setting quality standards, and ensuring policies and strategies are implemented. To support these functions, health ministries rely on information systems, surveys, and health legislation aligned with national values. With the increasing complexity of health systems and changing demographics, the governance role is crucial. Health ministries evaluate system performance in terms of equity, quality, efficiency, and population satisfaction, using tools provided by the WHO for evidence-based decision-making.

The unique nature of health services, which makes them incapable of being solely generated and distributed by market forces, explains why government involvement in the sector is necessary. Research demonstrates that several factors, including the information asymmetry between patients and healthcare providers, the existence of public goods with positive externalities, moral hazard, adverse selection, and others, have contributed to the failure of market forces to operate in the health sector. Patients depend on medical professionals to make decisions about their health and treatment because they lack knowledge about their conditions. Patients should concentrate on the environmental and interpersonal aspects of clinical services, which they are most qualified to assess, rather than judging the suitability of doctors' decisions and actions. Several significant health services, sometimes known as public goods, including mass vaccination campaigns, environmental health initiatives, health promotion, and education campaigns, surveillance, and border control for communicable diseases, etc., are mostly supplied by governments because they are not profitable for private providers.

Overuse of health services, also known as "moral hazard," happens when patients, especially those with insurance, receive free services at the point of use. It also results from providers producing too many services at no cost to the patients. Such actions drive up healthcare costs and necessitate the implementation of cost-containment plans and initiatives, which are typically started by governments. Private insurers that refuse to accept elderly people, people with chronic illnesses, and other vulnerable populations that require more social protection are engaging in adverse selection. Typically, governments step in to make up for the market's unwillingness to guarantee that the most vulnerable groups are included. Additionally, governments play a significant role in creating pre-payment and insurance schemes, whether social, private, or a combination of both, due to the unpredictability of diseases and the possibility of impoverishment during illness.

6.4.2. Health Service Delivery

The delivery of healthcare services is ensured by nongovernmental organizations, public and private providers, and socialized healthcare financing. It is frequently the responsibility of the government to direct the advancement of general health through the creation of health policies and programs, the protection of vital public health services, and the control of health service delivery. Public goods like hospital care and promotional and preventive services are provided by governments as part of their healthcare services. Public hospitals continue to be the gold standard for healthcare quality standards, service costs, training of high-caliber medical professionals, and a variety of other aspects of health and medical research, even though the role of private hospitals in service delivery is expanding in these countries.

Health ministries are in charge of safeguarding public health and carry out this duty by putting in place the necessary surveillance systems and public health services, like mass vaccination campaigns and environmental and food safety and fortification programs. In light of growing globalization and its effects on shifting lifestyles, including eating habits and the sharp rise in international travel and communication technology, the provision of basic public health services is becoming more challenging.

Governments, through ministries of health, bear the responsibility of ensuring that necessary medications and vaccines, as well as supporting laboratory networks, are made available in order to fulfill their public health obligations and safeguard national health security. Several obstacles must be overcome for national immunization programs to have access to high-quality, reasonably priced vaccines. These obstacles include inadequate funding, unsuitable supply chains, and a dearth of strong national regulatory bodies to enforce safety and quality requirements. Governments must make strategic choices regarding national investment in fostering medical technology self-sufficiency and self-reliance, including medications and vaccines.

Clinical services are provided by governments at the primary, secondary, and tertiary levels of the health system. Communities, workplaces, and public institutions such as hospitals, health centers, and investigative networks offer these services. In most nations, special settings are used to provide health services to members of the armed forces, security personnel, and their dependents. In rural and isolated areas where there is a shortage of qualified private providers due to financial concerns, the government's involvement in service delivery helps to increase equity in access to healthcare. Governments that provide health services directly play a role in regulating the market in terms of both quantity and cost. Government-owned medical centers and hospitals serve as training grounds for future medical professionals and are frequently the best locations for studies on health, public health, and medicine. Government organizations have played a crucial role in the advancement of biomedical and health research by helping to plan, finance, uphold, and monitor research projects' effects on human health.

There is a growing focus among governments on balancing public and private involvement in health service delivery, due to the rise of privatization policies aiming to expand private services in welfare-oriented health systems. The late 20th century saw numerous waves of health policy and sector reforms aimed at enhancing health system efficiency and improving equity in healthcare access.

6.4.3. Human Resource Development

Governments are in charge of creating appropriate policies for human resource development that aim to meet the actual needs of the populace, secure a skills mix that is appropriate, improve equity in the distribution of human resources, manage them effectively, and monitor and evaluate the country's health workforce. This is because human resources are the primary inputs and assets in health systems. Governments create procedures for accrediting training facilities and establish national standards for the education of health professionals. The extent to which ministries of health, education, and other relevant departments collaborate intersectorally determines the policies and strategies that are appropriate for human resources development. Ineffective coordination between different stakeholders frequently results in redundant work and ineffective health workforce production.

6.4.3.1. Promotion of the Centrality of Health in Socioeconomic Development

Advocating for the centrality of health in overall social and economic development is a critical function of governments. Numerous studies, such as the Commission on Macroeconomics and Health report, have demonstrated the relationship between economic development and health and have come to the conclusion that, to fully utilize the significant synergies between development and health, intersectoral collaboration needs to be developed (Burda et al., 1993; Coase et al., 1960).

6.5. Economic Reasons for Government Intervention

The reasons behind government intervention in a market-based healthcare system are explained by two main alternative economic theories or viewpoints. These are the theories of government behavior regarding special interest groups and the public interest. The public interest theory holds that the government selects laws that improve equity and efficiency while also advancing the general interests of society, ensuring that each good and service is produced at the point where marginal social benefit equals marginal social cost for a given income distribution, resulting in an efficient allocation of resources. Market imperfections prevent markets from allocating resources effectively, such as monopolies or incomplete consumer information. In addition, market failure occurs when externalities like air pollution or public goods like national defense are at stake, or when distributive justice is an issue. When the government intervenes to rectify situations in which the market is unable to distribute resources or income fairly, the public interest is served. When the market breaks down, the government works to bring about efficiency and equity again by promoting competition, educating consumers, reducing negative externalities, or reallocating income within the community. As a result, the public interest model of government behavior anticipates that government policies, rules, and other initiatives will improve equity and efficiency.

The theory of special interest groups holds that the political arena can be compared to any private market for goods and services, where supply and demand determine the kinds and quantity of laws. Legislation is purchased by wealth-maximizing special interest groups, while politicians who prioritize winning votes are the ones who supply it. Under this model, incumbent politicians offer legislation that promises to redistribute wealth away from the general public and toward different special interest groups to increase their chances of being reelected. Politicians demand campaign contributions, political support, and votes in exchange. Professional lobbyists working on behalf of special interest groups bargain with legislators to determine the market-clearing costs and volume of various laws. Legislation about special interest groups evolves as the relative power of various interest groups changes. The amount of resources under control, the group's size, and the effectiveness with which the group converts resources into pressure are the factors that define power or political pressure. A successful politician maintains his or her position of power by fusing the legislative agendas of numerous special interest groups into a comprehensive budget that is then promoted in the political sphere. Special interest groups reap the benefits, but the general public bears a disproportionate share of the costs. For instance, the Automobile Workers Union, the American Dairy Association, and the National Education Association all profit from specific pieces of legislation that protect against imported cars, support milk prices, and increase the amount allotted to education. Each of these three groups can accept wealth transfers from the same politician in exchange for their combined contributions, votes, and political support. Politicians and special interest groups benefit from political exchanges, of course; otherwise, they wouldn't take place. Legislation enhancing wealth for special interest groups is passed while politicians hold or gain elected office.

But the political exchanges unintentionally worsen the lot of the general public. Because the personal cost of learning the true impact of legislation is high and the corresponding private benefit is low, people are generally rationally ignorant about the wealth implications of government activities. For example, suppose a certain piece of legislation redistributes $300 million a year away from the general public to a special interest group. Although this wealth transfer is a large amount of money in absolute terms, it is insignificant when expressed in per capita terms. In the United States, the cost of this wealth transfer is only about $1 per person. Raising the per capita cost of special interest group legislation to $100 increases the total wealth transfer to $30 billion. Yet even at a potential per-person savings of $100, few people are likely to become involved due to the money and time costs associated with political activity. To challenge special interest group legislation, a group or an individual must organize a legitimate counter-political movement, inform others, circulate a petition, and engage in lobbying. All these activities entail sizable personal time and money costs.

According to the special interest group model of government behavior, laws that transfer wealth are intended to "nickel and dime" the average individual consumer. Worse yet, the special interest groups are not receiving a dollar-for-dollar transfer of wealth from the general public. Scarce resources, including the politicians' time and professional lobbying, are involved in the political negotiations that result in the wealth transfer. Fewer resources are available for useful purposes as more are being redirected to political negotiations. Furthermore, any additional taxes levied on the general populace serve as a deterrent to people investing in production. Consequently, laws about special interest groups are typically linked to inefficiencies.

Public laws and regulations are therefore necessary because some special interest groups profit at the expense of the broader public, by the special interest group theory of government behavior. Because they have a concentrated interest in the same thing, members of a special interest group have significant collective power. However, consumers as a whole are typically dispersed, diverse, and helpless. Even when wealth transfers are known, organization costs usually prevent general consumers from acting.

Analyze whether various state regulations concerning AIDS-related health insurance underwriting practices are influenced by the pressure of special interest groups. They focus on state regulations prohibiting – (i) questions during the insurance application process about past HIV testing; (ii) insurers from requiring insurance applicants to submit to HIV antibody tests; (iii) questions on the application regarding sexual orientation; and (iv) the exclusion of any AIDS-related costs from the services covered by the health insurance contract.

The authors contend that private health insurance companies (because of decreased profits) and private insurance holders who have a low average risk of AIDS (because of higher premium costs) lose out on these insurance regulations. Both those at high risk of AIDS (lower premium costs) and private healthcare providers (larger profits from more generous private insurance coverage) benefit from this. The hypothesis that state regulations restricting AIDS-related health insurance underwriting practices are related to pressure from special interest groups is generally supported by the empirical findings of their regression analysis. In particular, states with high AIDS prevalence rates (as a proxy for the AIDS group) and weak insurance industries are more likely to have underwriting regulations.

There are two opposing theories concerning the economic justifications for government intervention in a market-based system: the public interest model and the special interest group model. In the actual world, governments probably get involved for both of these reasons. Sometimes the government steps in to address market failure and advance equity and efficiency. In other cases, policies implemented by the government improve the welfare of particular groups at the expense of society as a whole, leading to an inefficient use of resources and an uneven distribution of income. Determining the winners and losers and the implications for efficiency and equity for each piece of legislation would require a thorough cost-benefit analysis. It is crucial to keep in mind that because both the government and the market are fallible establishments, failure on both sides is possible. In other words, failure on both sides of the aisle can coexist. It is our responsibility as consumers and policymakers to research which institution can achieve which goal in a way that is more equitable and efficient.

6.5.1. Types of Government Intervention

Through the provision of public goods, the imposition of regulations, the enforcement of antitrust laws, the correction of externalities, the operation of public enterprises, and the sponsorship of redistribution programs, the government can modify the efficiency and equity of market performance. A government health officer's inspection of local restaurants' hygienic practices to safeguard the public's health serves as an example of a public good. To offset an externality, the government levies taxes on businesses' emissions to lower local levels of air and water pollution. In the medical field, a certificate of need (CON) law essentially limits entry into the hospital and nursing home markets, while the Sherman Antitrust Act of 1890 forbids independent physicians from discussing their pricing strategies to prevent price fixing and other monopolistic practices. An illustration of a government-run medical facility is a Veterans Administration hospital. Last but not least, public healthcare redistribution initiatives include the Medicare and Medicaid programs. Each of these government policies either directly or indirectly influences the allocation of medical resources and the distribution of medical care in the U.S. health economy.

6.5.1.1. Public Goods

Providing public goods is one of the government's authorized roles. A public good needs to meet two requirements. First, a public good can benefit multiple people at once, in contrast to a private good. In other words, a public good displays nonrivalry in consumption, allowing one individual to increase their use of it without reducing the amount that is available for others. Second, it is expensive to deny those who do not pay access to the advantages of a public good.

One excellent illustration of a public good is national defense. It is impossible to deny nonpayers the advantages of national defense since everyone benefits at the same time. Another example of a public good is the local public health department's preservation of the water quality in public swimming areas. The advantages of better water quality can be experienced concurrently by a large number of people (at least until the beaches become overcrowded). Furthermore, barring non-paying individuals from enjoying the advantages of better water quality at the neighborhood pond is expensive (unless the pond can be fenced off entirely). Government intervention is required because private enterprises are unwilling to produce and sell public goods due to the high cost of excluding nonpaying individuals. As a result, the private sector fails to provide public goods. The government collects the necessary funds through taxes and makes sure that public goods are produced in both the public and private sectors. Because medical services are so necessary for survival, some people mistakenly believe that they are public goods. Theoretically, however, the costs associated with denying nonpayers access to medical care are relatively minimal, and the advantages of medical services are virtually entirely internalized by the individual buyer. To put it plainly, potential patients may be refused access to medical services if they fail to pay the required amount at the door of the facility. Medical services are not public goods as a result.

6.5.1.2. Externalities

In a typical market transaction, the parties directly involved absorb all costs and benefits, leaving others not participating in the exchange unscathed. Think about a person who decides to visit the dentist after waking up one morning with a severe toothache. Following some examination, the dentist advises that the patient have the wisdom tooth extracted right away because it is the source of the issue. The $100 fee is paid at the desk, the task is completed expertly, and the (uninsured) patient gives their consent. The $100 charge, in a competitive market, covers both the dentist's marginal cost of providing the service and the marginal benefit the patient receives from being pain-free. You'll see that in this instance, the dentist and the individual customer are the only ones who internalize the costs and benefits of the market exchange. This transaction is efficient since it benefits both parties; if it hadn't happened, the transaction would not have happened. On occasion, parties other than the buyers and sellers are impacted by a market transaction. There is an externality in this scenario. An unpriced byproduct of production or consumption that has an impact on a third party not directly involved in the market transaction, either negatively or positively, is called an externality. The buyers and sellers do not fully internalize all of the transaction's costs and benefits when an externality occurs. As a result, there is usually under- or overproduction of the product from a societal standpoint as well as external costs and benefits.

6.5.1.3. Demand-Side Externalities

When the marginal social benefit of an item or service differs from the marginal private benefit, this is known as a demand-side externality. When there is a positive demand-side externality, the marginal benefit to society is higher than the marginal benefit to the individual; when there is a negative demand-side externality, the marginal benefit to society is lower. One modern example of a detrimental demand-side externality is cigarette smoking.

Cigarette smoking incurs external costs for nonsmokers in various ways. Firstly, collectively funded programs like health insurance, pensions, sick leave, disability insurance, and group life insurance are supported by taxes or premiums that do not distinguish smokers and nonsmokers. Because smokers have shorter life expectancies, they contribute less to these programs. Additionally, smokers generally have higher healthcare expenses than nonsmokers. Lastly, external costs are incurred when nonsmokers succumb prematurely to passive smoking and smoking-related fires. This means that nonsmokers end up subsidizing smokers and bearing unreciprocated costs in the private sector.

The impact of cigarette smoking on resource allocation is depicted in Figure 6.1. The marginal costs of using different inputs to produce and sell cigarettes are represented by the supply curve, S, which relates to both marginal private and social costs. Therefore, on the supply side of the market, it is assumed that all resource costs of production are internalized. The marginal private benefit (MPB) of cigarette smoking is likely to exceed the marginal social benefit (MSB), so we must account for this on the demand side. The marginal private benefit from smoking, or the private demand curve for cigarettes, is represented by the MPB curve in the figure. The MSB curve is lower than the MPB curve because it takes into account the extra costs imposed on society. The disparity between the two benefit curves is caused by the external costs.

We assume external costs per pack are the same at each level of cigarette consumption so that the two benefit curves are parallel. We also assume the marginal social benefit is positive at every level, although it might be negative if the external costs exceed the marginal private benefits of cigarette consumption. As an illustration, Manning estimates the external costs of cigarette smoking at approximately 15 cents per pack, exclusive of the costs due to passive smoking (2,400 deaths annually) and smoking-related fires (1,600 deaths annually). If we consider the value of lives lost from passive smoking and smoking-related fires, the total external costs increase to approximately 38 cents per pack.

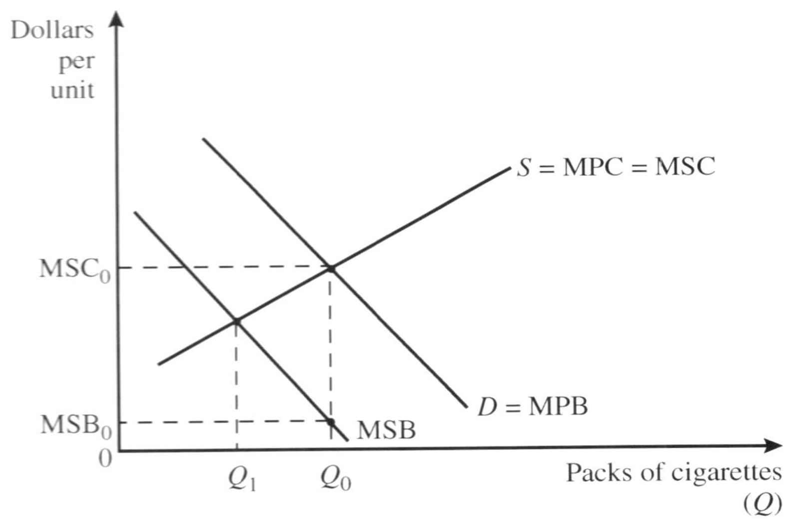

Figure 6.1. *External costs of cigarette smoking.*

Source: http://ndl.ethernet.edu.et/bitstream/123456789/90607/1/Health%20Economics%2C%205th%20Edition.pdf.

When choosing how many packs of cigarettes to buy, consumers only consider price, or their internal costs, in addition to their marginal private benefit. Thus, people buy Q_0 packs of cigarettes to maximize their utilities. From a societal standpoint, this level of cigarette consumption is inefficient because, at Q_0, the marginal social cost (MSC_0) of cigarettes surpasses the marginal social benefit (MSB_0); in other words, smoking cigarettes harms some nonsmokers, and smokers in the private market do not take these external costs into account. Cigarette production and consumption are excessive because both producers and consumers do not completely internalize the costs and benefits of their choices. In Q_1, where marginal social cost and marginal social benefit are equal, there is an efficient quantity of cigarettes. Some government intervention, like a tax on cigarettes, may be required to stop this harmful type of consumption activity because it is unlikely that producers and consumers will willingly change their production and consumption habits.

This example represents a negative consumption externality because others not directly involved are made worse off by the exchange. A positive consumption externality can also occur when a consumption activity generates external benefits. A vaccination to prevent an infectious disease, such as rabies, is an example of a positive consumption externality. Figure 6.2 illustrates the logic underlying this example.

On the horizontal axis of the figure, the number of dogs immunized against rabies is displayed. The marginal private benefit curve, or MPB, illustrates how important rabies vaccination is to dog owners. The MPB plus all external benefits are reflected in the marginal social benefit curve, or MSB. The monetary benefit that others receive when a dog receives rabies vaccination and stops the disease from spreading to people or other animals is one of the external benefits. The resource cost of administering the rabies vaccine is reflected in the supply curve, S.

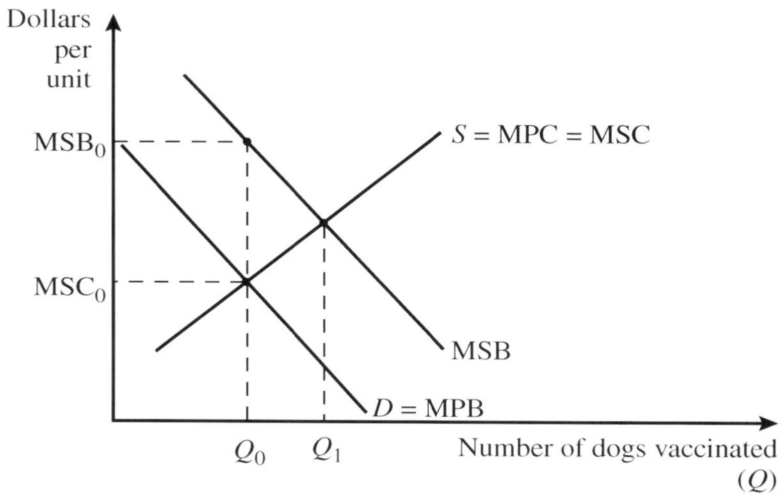

Figure 6.2. *External benefits of rabies vaccines.*

Source: http://ndl.ethernet.edu.et/bitstream/123456789/90607/1/Health%20Economics%2C%205th%20Edition.pdf.

In a free market, consumers weigh the price against the marginal private benefit of getting their dogs vaccinated against rabies. Because supply and demand intersect in a free market, Q_0 denotes the total number of vaccinations. However, take note that at Q_0, the rabies vaccine's marginal social benefit (MSB_0) exceeds its marginal social cost (MSC_0). When maximizing personal utility, some people place very little value on rabies vaccination because they do not take into account its external benefits, which leads to an inefficient outcome. Therefore, in a free market, there are insufficient rabies vaccinations from a societal standpoint. In Q_1, an effective number of immunizations take place. This suggests that some form of government intervention, like a mandate and a fine, might be required to guarantee an adequate number of rabies vaccinations. (For instance, obtaining a dog license is subject to fines in many states that require rabies vaccinations).

In conclusion, if the parties directly involved in the exchange do not fully internalize the social costs and benefits of a consumption activity, externalities may occur on the demand side of a market. From a societal standpoint, the good or service is likely to be under- or overproduced if the consumption activity results in external benefits or costs. As a result, government action might be required to address the market's inability to distribute resources to society effectively.

6.5.1.4. Supply-Side Externalities

As you are now aware, when one market participant's actions impact another without providing compensation, this is known as an externality, which results in an inefficient allocation of resources. Similar to demand-side externalities, supply-side externalities typically cause distortions in how resources are allocated in market economies. If a business places an unpaid expense on a third party during the production process, there is a negative supply-side externality going on. The marginal social cost and the marginal private cost of production diverge in this instance. The good is typically overproduced since the firm decides what to produce based on the private cost of production rather than the social cost. In a competitive market, this is what Figure 6.3 shows. D = MSB denotes the demand curve, or marginal social benefit curve, and S = MPC denotes the supply curve or the marginal private cost curve. The cost of producing each extra unit of output by the private sector is shown by the latter curve. The marginal social cost of production, or MSC curve, is higher than the marginal private cost of production (MPC curve) because it accounts for the additional per-unit costs incurred by the firm on behalf of others. The dollar amount of the costs imposed on society per unit is represented by the distance between the two cost curves. The price may be a reflection of increased health risks from things like toxic waste and air pollution, or it might be a reflection of longer travel times brought on by clogged roads.

To maximize profits, the good must be produced up to point Q_0, where the price is set so that the marginal private cost equals the marginal social benefit. However, at Q_0, the product's marginal social benefit is lower than the marginal social cost of production. From a social perspective, producing at the Q_1 level of output leads to efficient resource allocation as it maximizes the total social surplus and ensures that the marginal social cost of production equals the marginal social benefit. The market tends to overproduce the good, leading to inefficient resource allocation as it fails to internalize the firm's entire social cost of production.

Acid rain serves as a well-known example of a negative supply-side externality. The burning of fossil fuels releases sulfur and nitrogen oxides into the atmosphere, which, when combined with water, increase the acidity of water supplies. In regions like New England, acid rain has caused significant harm to marine life and wildlife. Estimating the cost of sulfur and nitrogen oxides is challenging due to the long-distance transport by wind currents. As a result, many emitters of these pollutants do not bear the full cost of production.

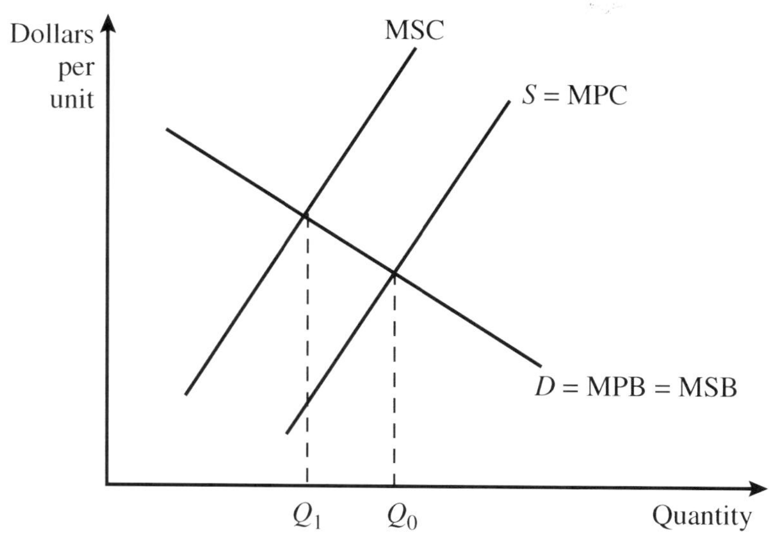

Figure 6.3. *Negative supply-side externality.*

Source: http://ndl.ethernet.edu.et/bitstream/123456789/90607/1/Health%20Economics%2C%205th%20Edition.pdf.

When businesses in one market (let's say A) give uncompensated benefits to businesses in another market (let's say B), this is known as a positive supply-side externality. The MSC curve in market A is below the MPC curve when the marginal social cost is less than the marginal private cost of production (*refer* Figure 6.4). The advantages enjoyed by the companies in market B are represented by the difference between the two curves. The companies in market A have no incentive to produce the optimal amount of output because they are not compensated. Q_0 is the output level that maximizes profits, but at this quantity, the MSB is greater than the MSC. The output should increase to Q_1 to maximize the overall social surplus. The businesses in market A do not produce to the point where the total social surplus is maximized because they are not compensated financially for the advantages other businesses enjoy.

One example of a positive supply-side externality is the international exchange of medical knowledge. Assume, for instance, that a major advancement in the treatment of cancer brought about by research funded by one nation results in a significant reduction in medical expenses. Without intellectual property rights, this advancement in medical knowledge will probably be documented in a medical journal and swiftly adopted at little or no cost by other nations. The entire benefit of the discovery is not paid to the national company that developed the treatment and incurred the research expenses. Because they wouldn't get a good return on their investment in research, private medical researchers in any given nation may be enticed to under-produce medical knowledge in the absence of government subsidies. According to economic theory, a supply-side externality makes it more difficult for the market to allocate resources effectively. This happens as a result of production decisions being made exclusively based on the firm's private production costs, not the social costs.

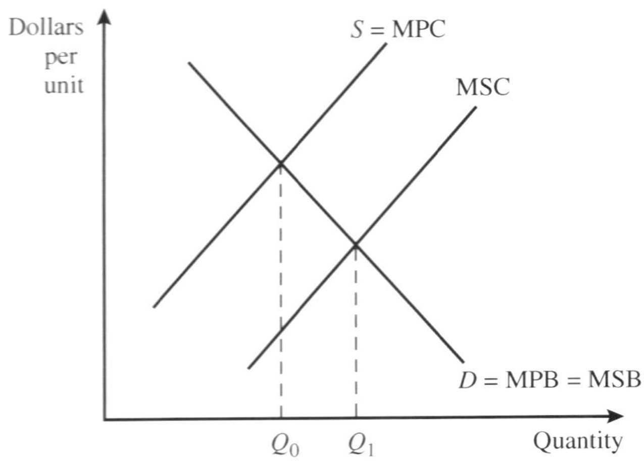

Figure 6.4. *Positive supply-side externality.*

Source: http://ndl.ethernet.edu.et/bitstream/123456789/90607/1/Health%20Economics%2C%20 5th%20Edition.pdf.

6.5.1.5. Taxes and Subsidies as Corrective Instruments

The government can modify economic incentives and correct the unbridled market's tendency to misallocate society's resources when externalities exist by enacting taxes and subsidies. To be more precise, taxes and subsidies can be used to change the cost of a good and deter excessive or insufficient consumption. Market players are compelled to think about the actual net social benefit of their decisions. For instance, by levying a tax, T, on cigarette manufacturers per unit, which is equivalent to the vertical distance between MPB and MSB in Q_1 in Figure 6.5, the government can promote an appropriate level of cigarette consumption. The market price of cigarettes rises to P_1 as a result of the per-unit tax, and cigarette consumption decreases to the level that is socially optimal (MSB = MSC). As after-tax revenues per unit, cigarette producers receive P_2, which is the difference between the market price of P_1 and the per-unit tax (or the vertical distance between the MPB and MSB).

Notice in this example that sellers and consumers share the burden of the cigarette tax. The consumers pay the portion P_1–P_0, and the sellers pay the portion P_0–P_2.

A lower profit margin or a transfer of costs back to input suppliers are the usual outcomes of the sellers' share of the tax burden. As we saw in our example, the cigarette tax may compel manufacturers to either reduce the prices they pay tobacco farmers or the wages they pay their staff. Depending on the relative strengths of supply and demand's price elasticities, producers or consumers will bear a larger portion of the cigarette tax. Producers typically bear a larger share of the tax burden when the price elasticity of demand (in absolute terms) surpasses the price elasticity of supply. When supply's price elasticity is higher than demand's, the consumer bears a comparatively larger share of the tax burden.

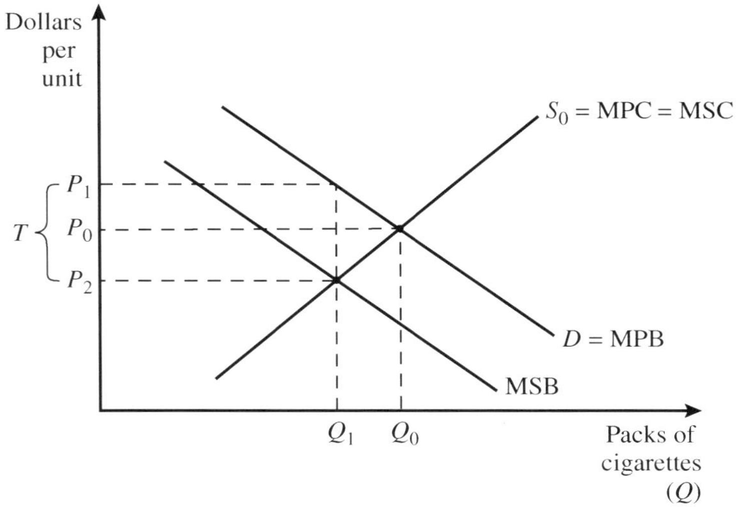

Figure 6.5. *A tax as a corrective instrument.*

Source: http://ndl.ethernet.edu.et/bitstream/123456789/90607/1/Health%20Economics%2C%205th%20Edition.pdf.

Taxing products for which demand is price inelastic gives governments an incentive to do so. This is because when demand is price inelastic, the quantity demanded decreases by a smaller percentage than the percentage increase in taxes. Therefore, when demand is price inelastic, the government's total tax revenue—which is the product of the tax per unit and quantity—increases. The fact that demand for alcohol and cigarettes is price inelastic makes "sin taxes" on these goods extremely popular politically. This provides the government with a reliable source of income. The idea is that socially detrimental behavior can be deterred by taxes or the threat of fines. Subsidies, on the other hand, can be used to support socially responsible endeavors that would otherwise go unappreciated in the market. Remember that when marginal social benefit surpasses marginal private benefit, underproduction, and under-consumption take place. A price-reducing subsidy encourages more consumers to participate in a socially beneficial activity.

6.5.1.6. Regulations

Another type of government interference is regulation that aims to regulate the cost, availability, or quality of a good or the introduction of new businesses into the market. The public interest theory states that the regulation is necessary because there is a market imperfection that would lead to an inefficient use of resources by society. For instance, inadequate customer data frequently serves as justification for quality standards imposed by the government. Another example is that if a large company can produce an output more cheaply than a large number of small companies, the government may grant the company monopoly status and regulate its price (that is, a natural monopoly, such as an electric utility or a local telephone company). It is difficult to forecast how government regulations will affect the medical markets. A multitude of factors, including market competitiveness, the cost structure each medical firm faces, the goals driving medical decision-makers, and the validity of the exclusion principle (i.e., externalities, third-party payers, or public good considerations), determine whether the government impedes or promotes efficiency and equity. The effect of a price ceiling in a monopoly and competitive market is discussed in the following section, assuming that consumers have health insurance, which is the most typical scenario in the medical market. The cost of a good or service is one thing that a third-party payer, like the government, may control. The government may control prices by setting a cap on prices or a level of reimbursement. Subsequently, the government establishes a maximum price for a good, and manufacturers are legally unable to charge consumers who fall under the ceiling a higher price. In a supply and demand model of a physician services market, Figure 6.6 illustrates the impact of a price ceiling.

The market demand, denoted as D in Figure 6.6, is the amount that numerous health insurers, acting on behalf of their customers or subscribers, are willing to pay for physician services. Remember that the market demand is theoretically determined by adding together the demands of each consumer while taking into account the insurance features that the consumer pays for, such as deductibles, copayments, and coinsurance. In essence, D is the total price that health insurance companies are willing to pay for various amounts of physician services, as well as the nominal demand for medical services at the market level. Supply, as we all know, is the range of quantities of medical services that doctors are willing to offer for sale at different prices. When the price is P_0 and the quantity is Q_0, the competitive market equilibrium is reached. Suppose that the government decides to cap a price ceiling at P_C in order to control costs.

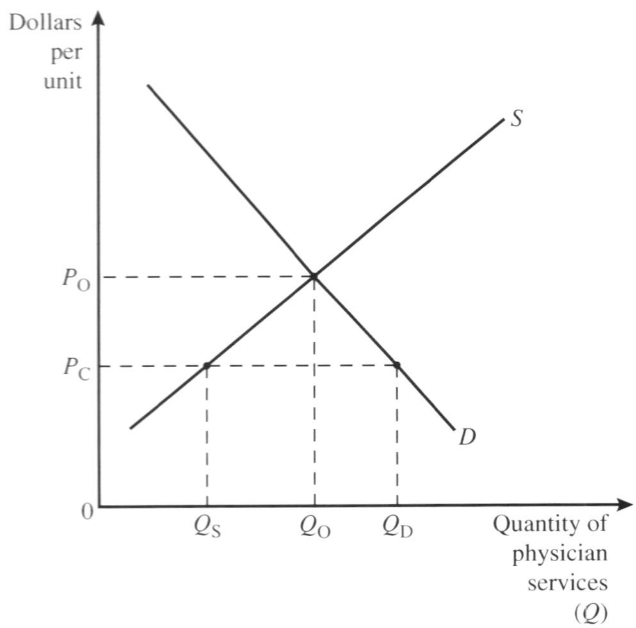

Figure 6.6. *Effect of a price ceiling in a competitive industry.*

Source: http://ndl.ethernet.edu.et/bitstream/123456789/90607/1/Health%20Economics%2C%20 5th%20Edition.pdf.

Because of the positively sloped supply curve, this lower price will incentivize doctors to supply fewer units to Q_S. The quantity demanded of physician services rises to Q_D, and the price ceiling incentivizes health insurers to purchase more of the now-cheaper service. Because of the price ceiling, there is a shortage of physician services in the market, as indicated by the difference between Q_D and Q_S.

Some unexpected consequences might happen in a price ceiling scenario where there is a shortage and the price mechanism is not used as a rationing tool. One possibility is that doctors will treat patients according to arrival time, even if some are more urgently sick than others. Doctors may also try to cut costs by decreasing the caliber of their visits. A longer wait time for an appointment or less time spent with doctors during the visit itself could result from the quality reduction. Furthermore, some dishonest doctors might take illicit side payments from affluent patients hoping to get ahead.

When there is a shortage of a medical service, political considerations may also influence how it is rationed. Politicians may decide that a person's age, illness, or the amount of money they donate to campaigns should determine how medical services are rationed. For instance, children's medical care is less rationed than adults in Great Britain, where price plays almost no role in rationing. The idea is that containing medical expenses is usually not a freebie. The previous model states that, in reasonable situations, cost containment may lead to shortages, longer wait times, non-price rationing, and lower-quality care. The trade-offs that society will inevitably face when implementing cost-containment measures must be carefully considered.

It should be noted that the medical firm's precise behavioral response is more complex than what has been shown thus far and is primarily dependent on the basis on which the price ceiling is implemented. In particular, medical professionals may respond to a reduced fee by modifying the number of patients, length of stay, or level of care. Hospitals might, for instance, respond to a lower per diem charge by increasing the number of patient days in order to obtain additional revenues and by lowering quality if they are paid based on a per diem price ceiling, which is the average revenue per patient-day. Increasing the number of new admissions or the average length of stay will increase the number of patient days. Hospitals can increase their profits by allowing patients to stay longer by using the money they make from the later days to subsidize the earlier, more expensive, and service-intensive days.

6.5.1.7. The Effect of a Price Ceiling in a Monopoly Market

We recently discovered that in a perfectly competitive market, a price cap may result in a shortage of medical care. We now turn our attention to the question of whether the result would differ if the price ceiling were implemented in a pure monopoly market setting. A hypothetical scenario in which a monopolist dominates the market for medical services is depicted in Figure 6.7. We still believe that there are a lot of health insurers and buyers in the market. Economic theory states that a monopolist/physician group charges P_0 and produces at Q_0 to maximize profits because MR=MC at that point. Physician services have a monopoly on the market, which causes quantity to fall and price to rise above levels of competition.

Assume for the moment that the government caps the cost of medical services at P_C. Either way, the price ceiling becomes the new fixed marginal revenue curve that the monopolist-provider must contend with over that range of the demand curve, thereby eliminating the incentive for the monopolist to restrict output by forbidding prices above the price ceiling of P_C. The physician organization delivers the quantity of services that buyers demand at the set price to maximize profits, provided that the price cap is higher than the marginal cost of production. The monopolist's Q_C amount of physician services is affected by the price ceiling, as shown in Figure 6.7. If the price ceiling were set at the intersection of S and D, then the monopolist provides physician services at a competitive level. But just like in a competitive environment, a shortage arises if the government sets the price ceiling below the level of competition. The price cap may also lead to the development of other detrimental effects like discrimination, long wait times, and a decline in quality. The exact response also depends on the base to which the price ceiling is applied (e.g., fee-for-service as assumed, per-diem, or per person).

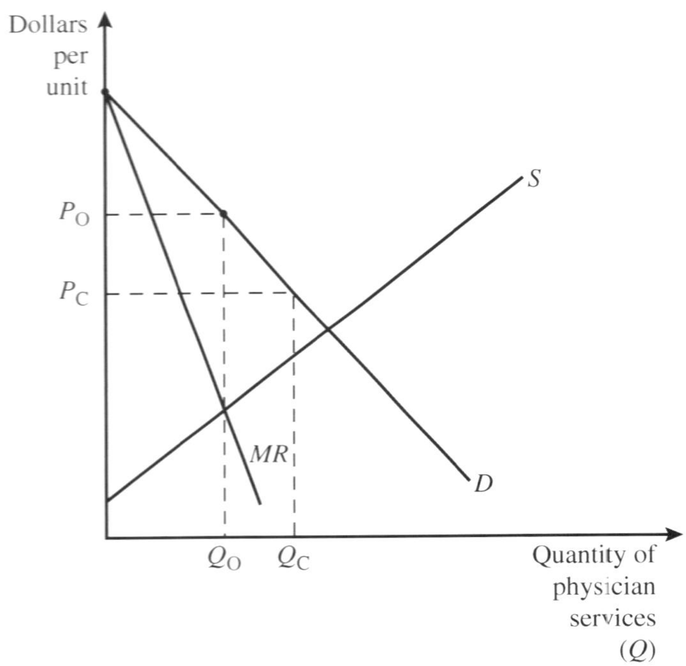

Figure 6.7. *Effect of a price ceiling in a monopoly industry.*

Source: http://ndl.ethernet.edu.et/bitstream/123456789/90607/1/Health%20Economics%2C%20 5th%20Edition.pdf.

6.5.1.8. The Efficiency Implication of a Price Ceiling

The impact of a price cap on the volume of services rendered is contingent upon the degree of competition present in the market. In a market with competition, setting a price cap causes a shortage of products and services. On the other hand, when a monopolist's profit incentive to limit output is eliminated, a well-crafted price ceiling in a monopoly market may lead to an increase in the amount of output supplied in the market. A more intricate query relates to how a price cap would affect efficiency. Remember that to be efficient, a good or service must be produced at the MSB = MSC point. A perfectly competitive market produces an efficient level of output, but a monopoly market in non-medical markets under typical conditions such as no externalities, utility-maximization, profit-maximization, and reasonably informed consumers paying the full price of the good.

However, upon closer inspection of Figures 6.6 and 6.7, we must acknowledge that, due to a certain amount of moral hazard, the market demand for physician services represents the nominal demand rather than the effective demand. The type of moral hazard determines the relationship between MSB and nominal demand. To illustrate our point, let's look at some extreme examples. Assume, on the one hand, that moral hazard is completely inefficient and that people utilize their insurance payout to pay for designer prescription sunglasses, additional hospital stays, or excessive medical visits. If so, the MSB is overstated by the nominal demand. Conversely, consider full efficient moral hazard as Nyman has described it. Then, because the insurance gives people access to life-improving medical care that they otherwise could not afford, the nominal demand is the same as the MSB.

6.5.1.9. Price Regulations

It is challenging to forecast how a price cap will affect an industry's performance. The extent of third-party involvement, the kind of moral hazard health insurance creates, the level of market competition, and the basis on which the price ceiling is implemented are just a few of the variables that determine its exact impact. Economists have learned from experience in other markets, like natural gas and housing, that price controls frequently result in unintended shortages of goods and can also have other unintended effects, like lower quality, longer wait times, and discrimination against certain groups, among other things. Price controls are occasionally used as a cost-containment strategy. If so, decision-makers need to understand that cutting costs could require a significant trade-off. But occasionally a price cap is implemented in order to make a certain good more accessible to more people. The irony is that imposing a price cap could cause a shortage, making the good or service less readily available but potentially more reasonably priced. This circumstance does not imply that people who cannot afford necessities should be disregarded. Rather, it appears to be more effective ways to provide equity based on this circumstance.

6.5.1.10. The Effects of Quality Regulations

When patients are irrationally ignorant, the government may also try to control the standard of medical care. As was already mentioned, variations in quality can be seen in the composition, methodology, and results of production. The structure of operation is usually the target of quality regulations, as procedural and outcome guidelines are more challenging to establish and implement. A public organization might, for instance, mandate a minimum staff-to-patient ratio or the professional licensing of medical personnel. The underlying premise in both situations is that improved structural quality encourages improved quality at the process and result phases.

Regulations focused on employee quality usually result in increased production costs, which lowers the availability of medical services in the market. The reason for the decrease in supply is that obtaining a professional license increases the cost of providing medical services and necessitates a larger human capital investment from the medical staff. The ramifications of a quality regulation, like professional licensing, are illustrated in Figure 6.8. The market wage and employment levels for medical employees are W_0 and N_0, respectively, and the initial supply and demand curves are

S_0 and D_0. Professional licensing lowers supply to S_1, raises the wage rate to W_1, and increases the cost of entering an occupation because it requires a greater investment of human capital. The compensating wage differential required to draw the marginal worker with the required professional license to the labor market is captured by the difference between W_1 and W_0.

The analysis raises two questions. First, does higher procedural and outcome quality follow from professional licensing? If not, the outcome might not justify the quality control strategy. Second, given that those in the labor group who are grandfathered in but do not have the necessary license benefit from the higher wage rate, was there a professional group behind the implementation of the professional licensing requirement? Analyzing the second question by drawing a comparison between a professional license and a trademark or brand name is an intriguing method. Customers may perceive all three of these gadgets as signs of quality assurance. Svorny specifically contends that the increased pay that comes with having a professional license provides financial motivation for the average medical worker to work effectively, meet patient needs, and produce a desired quantity and caliber of work. This is because opportunistic behavior, when discovered, results in job termination and causes the medical worker to receive a low or negative return on the original human capital investment. The quality assurance generated by the higher wage, in turn, raises the marginal value of the employee's services to the consumer. The higher quality assurance can be represented by a shift to the right of the demand curve from D_0 to D_1 in Figure 6.7.

With the increased focus on quality assurance, the wage rate rises to W_2, and employment increases from N_1 to N_2. Svorny suggests that this model can be used to determine if professional licensure requirements and other quality regulations benefit the public or if they only benefit specific interest groups, like established medical professionals. If the benefits of quality regulations outweigh the costs, as seen by a greater shift in the demand curve to the right compared to the supply curve to the left, overall employment should increase, indicating that society benefits from the regulation. However, if the supply curve shifts more to the left than the demand curve shifts to the right, it suggests that the quality regulations primarily benefit special interest groups.

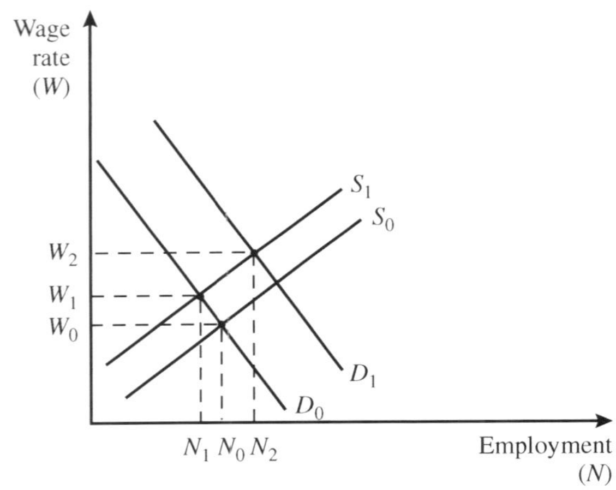

Figure 6.8. *Effect of professional licensure.*

Source: http://ndl.ethernet.edu.et/bitstream/123456789/90607/1/Health%20Economics%2C%205th%20Edition.pdf.

Svorny uses the data to investigate if the citizen requirements for medical licensure and basic science certification affected the per capita number of physicians in the 48 contiguous states of the US in 1965. She points out that to deter opportunistic behavior, both requirements may require a certain amount of human capital investment that raises wages and creates a future return. Svorny discovers an inverse relationship between the number of physicians and the existence of both requirements using multiple regression analysis. According to the theory, the regulatory process's special interest model is supported by an inverse relationship.

It is implied that instead of increasing the use of physician services, these quality regulations cause it to decrease. Because the license restrictions increased entry costs more than they increased consumer benefits from quality assurance, there is a lower consumption of physician services. Overall, the study discovered evidence in favor of the regulatory process's special interest group theory (Coase et al., 1960; Cromwell et al., 1976).

A Closer Look

Government Health Policy

Government health policy encompasses a range of strategies, regulations, and initiatives aimed at improving public health outcomes, ensuring access to healthcare services, and managing healthcare resources effectively. These policies are developed and implemented at various levels of government, including national, regional, and local.

At the national level, governments typically formulate health policies that address overarching public health challenges and priorities. These policies often focus on areas such as disease prevention, healthcare delivery systems, healthcare financing, and health promotion. For example, a government may implement policies to increase vaccination rates, improve access to primary care services, or regulate the pricing of pharmaceuticals.

National health policies also play a crucial role in shaping healthcare infrastructure and financing mechanisms. Governments may establish frameworks for healthcare delivery, such as public healthcare systems or private insurance markets, and allocate resources to support these systems. Additionally, they may implement taxation or insurance schemes to fund healthcare services and ensure financial protection for citizens against health-related expenses.

In addition to national policies, governments may develop regional or local health policies to address specific health needs and disparities within their jurisdictions. These policies may involve targeted interventions to address local health challenges, such as reducing rates of chronic diseases, addressing environmental health hazards, or improving access to healthcare services in underserved communities.

Government health policies are typically developed through a combination of legislative processes, stakeholder consultations, and evidence-based decision-making. Policymakers often collaborate with healthcare professionals, researchers, community organizations, and other stakeholders to identify priorities, design effective interventions, and assess the impact of policy initiatives.

Overall, government health policy plays a vital role in shaping the healthcare landscape, influencing health outcomes, and promoting the well-being of populations. By implementing strategic policies and initiatives, governments can address public health challenges, improve healthcare access and quality, and contribute to the overall health and prosperity of society.

Summary

- The poor lack access to basic health services and receive low-quality care. Government spending for health goes disproportionately to the affluent in the form of subsidies to sophisticated public tertiary care hospitals and to private hospitals.
- Public financing of an essential clinical package can be justified because the package creates positive spillover effects and reduces poverty. However, the case for government financing of discretionary clinical health services outside of the essential national package is far less compelling.
- The Health Policy of Ethiopia is based on the primary healthcare approach which has health education, education in personal and environmental hygiene, nutrition, immunization, and family planning as standard components.
- Ministries of health are responsible for leading health development through the implementation and improvement of main health system functions, including leadership and governance, healthcare financing, provision of health services, and generation of inputs for health development, including human resources for health and biomedical technology.
- While healthcare financing is socialized, delivery of healthcare services is secured by both public and private providers and nongovernmental organizations.
- Ministries of health are responsible for health protection and undertake that responsibility by implementing essential public health functions, including surveillance systems and provision of public goods such as programs for mass immunization, environmental protection, food fortification, food safety, etc.
- Government can alter the performance of markets in terms of efficiency and equity by providing public goods, levying taxes, correcting for externalities, imposing regulations, enforcing antitrust laws, operating public enterprises, and sponsoring redistribution programs.
- A demand-side externality occurs when the marginal social benefit diverges from the marginal private benefit associated with a good or service.
- Ensuring equitable access to healthcare services for all citizens, regardless of socioeconomic status or geographic location.
- Managing healthcare expenditures through budgeting, reimbursement policies, and cost containment measures.
- Implementing public health initiatives and disease prevention programs to promote population health and reduce the burden of illness.
- Engaging with stakeholders, including healthcare professionals, patients, and advocacy groups, to inform policy development and implementation and ensure accountability and transparency.

References

1. Aaron, H. J., & Schwartz, W. B. (1984). *The Painful Prescription: Rationing Hospital Care.* Washington, D.C.: The Brookings Institution.
2. Abel-Smith, B. (1969). *Value for Money in Health Services: A Comparative Study*. London.
3. Agency for Development and Coordination of International Relations. (2005). *The French Social Protection System*. Paris: ADECRI.
4. Becker, G. S. (1983). A theory of competition among pressure groups for political influence. *Quarterly Journal of Economics, 93*, 371–400.
5. Bryant, J. (1969). *Health and The Developing World*. London.
6. Burda, D. (1993). Flurry of merger plans has eyes focused on Iowa. *Modern Healthcare, 23*(15), 24.
7. Carrin, G. (1984). *Economic Evaluation of Health Care in Developing Countries*. London.
8. Cromwell, J. (1976). Hospital productivity trends in short-term general nonteaching hospitals. *Inquiry, 11*(3), 181–187.
9. Culyer, A. J. (1976). *Need and the National Health Service: Economic Social Choice*. Oxford.
10. Drummond, M. F., et al. (1993). *Methods for The Economic Evaluation of Health Care Programmes*. Oxford.
11. Green, A. (1996). *An Introduction to Health Planning in Developing Countries*. Oxford.
12. Health Evidence Network (HEN). (2006). What is the evidence on effectiveness of empowerment to improve health? Copenhagen: Regional Office for Europe.
13. Lynk, W. J. (1994). Tying and exclusive dealing: Jefferson Parish Hospital v. Hyde. In J. E. Kwoka, Jr., & L. J. White (Eds.), *The Antitrust Revolution* (2nd ed.). New York: HarperCollins.
14. Roemer, M. I. (1991). *National Health Systems of The World, Vol. 1: The Countries*. New York: Oxford University Press.
15. Scarpaci, J. L. (Ed.). (1989). *Health Services Privatization in Industrial Societies*. New Brunswick: Rutgers University Press.
16. World Health Organization. (1978). Declaration of Alma Ata. In *Primary health care: Report of the International Conference on Primary Health Care, Alma-Ata, USSR, 6–12 September 1978*. Geneva.
17. World Health Organization. (1990). *The Impact of Development Policies on Health*. Geneva.
18. World Health Organization. (2000). *The World Health Report 2000: Health Systems: Improving Performance*. Geneva.

Chapter

TECHNOLOGY TRANSFER IN HEALTHCARE

7

Contents

Introduction

The process of technology transfer involves the sharing of creative solutions developed in academic and research settings, with the goal of adapting and expanding these solutions to effectively meet local needs. Scaling up innovation is crucial to maximize the impact of these solutions and address a wide range of needs. Technology transfer plays a critical role in addressing global environmental and climate challenges by facilitating the implementation of innovative solutions that can reduce greenhouse gas emissions, improve energy efficiency, and promote sustainable development. In the healthcare sector, the transfer of medical technologies, pharmaceutical innovations, and healthcare management systems is essential for enhancing patient outcomes, improving the quality of care, and increasing the accessibility and affordability of healthcare services.

Orientation and Directional Terms:

Term	Definition	Illustration
Data analytics	The systematic use of data to obtain new insights and drive fact-based decision-making for patient care outcomes and clinical and operational improvements.	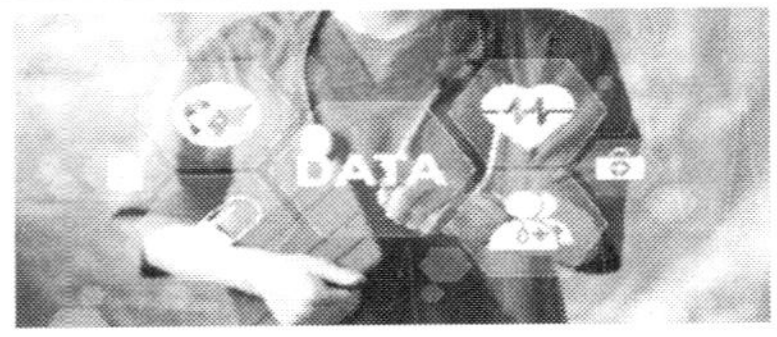
Electronic health record	EHRs offer a complete real-time record of a person's medical history that is easily accessible by health providers (and increasingly, by patients). In addition to being a comprehensive record of an individual's healthcare, the documentation inside EHRs supports the functions of billing, quality management, outcome reporting and public health disease surveillance and reporting. EHR is sometimes used interchangeably with EMR (electronic medical record).	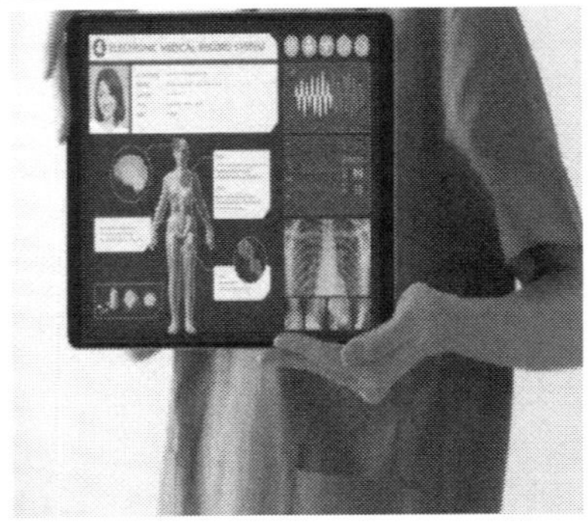
Big data	Big data, which has made an impact everywhere as computers have grown faster and more powerful, is becoming a major factor in healthcare. The three main characteristics of big data – volume, velocity, and variety – increasingly challenge healthcare organizations as EHRs, financial systems, and imaging systems spew out ever more data.	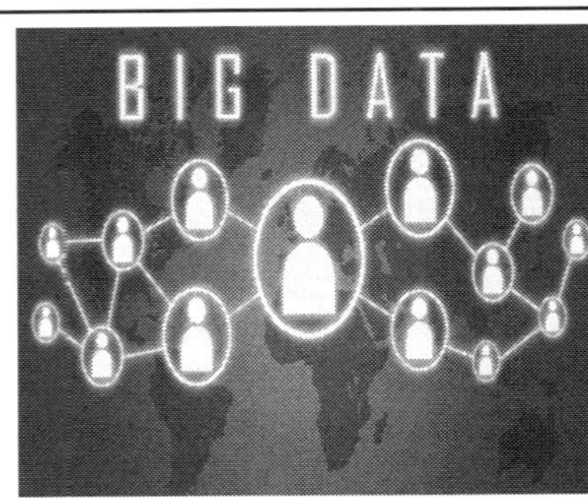
Health information exchange	Health information exchange, used as both a noun and a verb, focuses on utilizing technology to share healthcare information (including patient records). Health providers use HIE to deliver safer and more timely, efficient, and effective patient care; public health officials leverage larger data sets to analyze the health of patient populations.	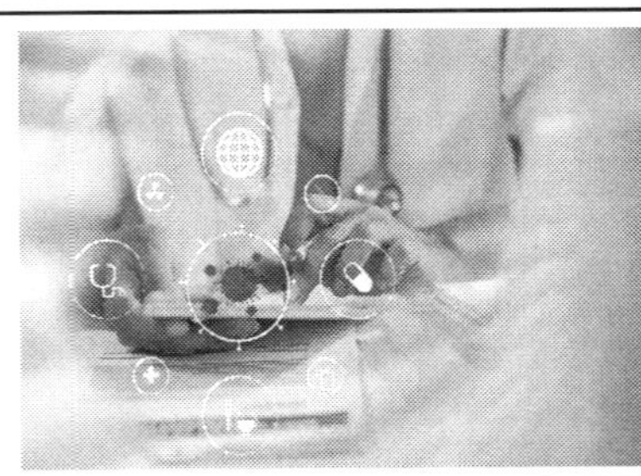
Remote patient monitoring	Remote patient monitoring uses digital technologies to collect medical and other forms of health data from individuals in one location and electronically transmit that information securely to healthcare providers in a different location for assessment and recommendations.	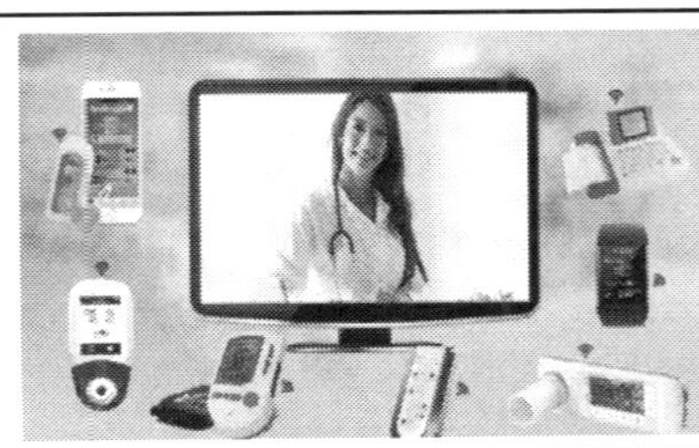

7.1. Developing Countries Need Up to Date Technologies

Despite 93% of preventable mortality occurring in developing countries, insufficient research funding is allocated to address health issues in these regions, resulting in a dangerous disparity in funding. Moreover, many modern laboratory technologies are not readily available in these countries. Both practical and ethical arguments support the training of scientists and healthcare professionals in developing countries in the use of modern laboratory and epidemiological skills. Given that pathogens can travel across the globe in a matter of days, enhancing capabilities in developing countries is crucial for preventing the global spread of infectious diseases. Furthermore, all countries, particularly those with high disease burdens, should have access to effective tools to manage infectious diseases as a fundamental principle.

7.1.1. Key Elements in Technology Transfer

By sharing biomedical technologies and engaging in collaborative research in developing countries, these are essential components of the technology transfer process. Along with technical considerations, the successful adoption of a new technology hinges on financial backing, governmental partnerships, efficient infrastructure, clear communication, cultural awareness, and environmental considerations. While these factors may be outside the researcher's immediate control, they can be addressed through well-structured research collaborations.

The 11 principles of research partnership:

1. Decide on objectives together;
2. Build mutual trust;
3. Share information and develop networks;
4. Share responsibility;
5. Create transparency;
6. Monitor and evaluate the collaboration;
7. Disseminate results;
8. Apply the results;
9. Share profits equitably;
10. Increase research capacity; and
11. Build on achievements.

By adapting equipment to local conditions, expensive technologies can become more affordable and accessible. For example, a blender can be transformed into a centrifuge or a record turntable into a lab shaker. Simplifying techniques, such as using water baths instead of a thermocycler for PCR amplification, can also reduce costs. Other strategies include streamlining protocols, like drying blood samples on filter paper, preparing reagents in-house, recycling, and repurposing outdated equipment. Breaking down the transfer process into smaller steps makes it easier to address and manage challenges (Figure 7.1).

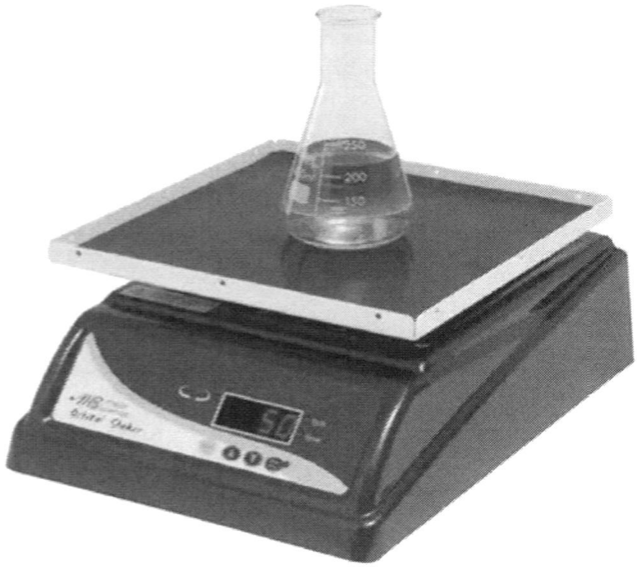

Figure 7.1. *Modifying equipment locally: The turntable of a record player becomes a lab shaker.*

Source: https://images.dutscher.com/reference/hd/022057B.webp

To ensure long-lasting knowledge transfer, the process must be built on a true partnership that values reciprocal exchange. It is crucial to have a fair, inclusive, and knowledge-driven approach where everyone is involved. In addition to simply teaching the technology, a deep understanding of its core principles must be shared for true independence to be realized. The recipients must take the lead in integrating any new concept or technology into their existing system.

Scientists in developing countries have created many innovations. For instance, in Nicaragua, they shortened a three-day ELISA test for dengue virus to just four hours while maintaining its effectiveness. In Cuba, they developed a micro-ELISA with a reaction volume of only 10 μl to reduce the amount of reagents needed.

The transfer of knowledge usually happens quickly in an intensive training workshop, but the implementation process is slow and needs ongoing support. The "donor" of technology must be available for scientific advice, technical help, resources, and materials to ensure success. Lack of proper follow-up is a common reason for failed technology transfer efforts. A dedicated contact person and a team committed to the project's success are essential for a successful outcome.

7.1.2. Examples of Technology Transfer Programs

There are two models for long-term partnerships and sustainable technology transfer; the first example focuses on technology transfer directly, while the second illustrates the circumstances surrounding successful technology transfer.

7.1.2.1. Sustainable Sciences Institute in San Francisco

To facilitate the proper transfer of laboratory and epidemiological techniques to developing nations, the non-profit Sustainable Sciences Institute was established in 1998. To better address infectious disease issues in their communities, it seeks to assist regional biomedical scientists in gaining access to resources such as funding, information, partners, training, tools, and supplies. With four primary program areas, the institute prioritizes long-term follow-up through material, financial, and technical support.

The integrated training program on site offers instruction in laboratory techniques, epidemiology, and scientific writing. Participants collaborate in inter-institutional teams focused on specific infectious diseases, receiving guidance from scientists from various countries in the region and the United States. The institute offers ongoing material and technical assistance to help ensure the success of projects developed during the workshops. The small grants program offers assistance to researchers who do not have access to other sources of funding. This initial funding can be used to generate scientific findings that are locally relevant and can be used as a basis for securing larger grants from other agencies. Applicants are encouraged to submit grants in their native language and can also send in preliminary proposals for feedback.

The networking and consulting program offers a database of health sciences experts who volunteer to provide consultations to researchers in developing countries. This program will soon be accessible online, allowing interested scientists to contact each other directly.

The material aid program makes it easier to send scientific equipment and supplies from labs in developed nations to researchers in developing nations.

7.1.3. Factors Affecting Technology Transfer

Various factors influence technology transfer, such as characteristics of the technology, the technology developer, users of the technology, organizations using the technology, attitudes, research policies, and regulatory and reimbursement policies. These categories are used for discussion purposes rather than to suggest distinct sets, as there is significant overlap and interrelationships among them. External factors like regulations and attitudes often impact internal factors like technology characteristics and user behaviors. Despite extensive research on these factors, there is still much to be understood about technology transfer.

The main goal of comprehending the variables influencing technology transfer is to apply that understanding to enhance transfer operations. But comprehending these elements and how they interact makes it easier to understand why public and private organizations' best efforts to influence technology transfer don't always succeed.

7.1.3.1. Characteristics of the Technology

The technology transfer process is influenced by the nature of the technology itself. Factors such as the stage of development, medical purpose, complexity, perceived effectiveness, initial test results, and potential marketability all play a role in determining how smoothly the transfer process will go.

7.1.3.2. Characteristics of the Technology Developer

The characteristics of an individual new technology developer can impact technology transfer, including personality, level of recognition, connections with other scientists, and understanding of the significance of the discovery. For instance, a little-known physician named Hammer first diagnosed coronary artery occlusion in 1878, but his findings went unnoticed until 34 years later when another scientist, Herrick, made the same discovery. Access to resources is crucial for both individual and organizational developers of technology. In the case of organizations, the size of a company can affect its capacity to innovate. Small companies are often at the forefront of technological advancements in the early stages, while larger companies tend to dominate as the field matures.

7.1.3.3. Characteristics of Individuals Using the Technology

There has been extensive research on how the individual characteristics of users impact technology transfer, with a focus on physicians. Key factors that influence technology transfer include the availability and accessibility of information on the technology, the individual's cosmopolitan or local mindset, level of education, prioritization of quality healthcare over economic efficiency, and willingness to explore new ideas.

7.1.3.4. Characteristics of Organizations (and Their Members)

The organizational structure and individual characteristics within an organization will impact technology transfer when using technology. Several sociological studies have been conducted on this topic, resulting in various theories with conflicting results. While it is not possible to resolve these conflicts here, it is important to acknowledge that the characteristics of the technology being adopted can also influence the organization's outcomes.

The size and resource base of an organization are significant factors that influence the likelihood of adopting innovations. However, these variables can be overshadowed by other factors such as organizational complexity, centralization of decision-making, and formalization of rules and behavior.

7.1.3.5. Attitudes

Attitudes play a crucial role in the technology transfer process at every stage. Positive attitudes can enhance the process, while negative attitudes can hinder it. The attitudes of individuals considering adopting or developing new technology are influenced by the attitudes of society, which can impact the decision-making process. For instance, if society had a negative view on technological interventions in childbirth, the adoption of electronic fetal monitoring may have been delayed. Currently, there is growing concern about technology due to increasing negative attitudes towards it. Although the exact impact of attitudes on technology transfer cannot be measured, their significance should not be underestimated.

7.1.3.6. Research Policies

Although basic research is not directly involved in technology transfer, different research policies can significantly impact the process. The distribution of research funds among various stages of technology transfer can affect the outcome. For example, dedicating more funds to basic research can lead to a greater knowledge base for technology development. Conversely, allocating funds to applied research can increase the number of technologies available for transfer. In this way, research policies play a crucial role in shaping the technology transfer process. The number of funds available for evaluation and demonstration will not necessarily affect the number of technologies transferred, it will affect the number of technologies that are transferred appropriately (i.e., those that are transferred after being shown to be efficacious, safe, cost-effective, etc.). Additionally, the criteria for determining research priorities, whether at an organizational level or within individual programs, will impact the technologies that are ultimately transferred.

Within an organization, research programs could place priority on filling gaps in knowledge in areas that:

- the diseases that most Americans fear (like cancer);
- are linked to a higher loss of "quality-adjusted life years;"
- have the highest financial impact on people or society but may not directly affect the greatest number of people (like renal dialysis);
- have the highest financial impact due to their direct impact on the greatest number of people; offer the most research opportunities;
- are currently trending politically or scientifically; or
- have the greatest impact due to a combination of high cost, high morbidity, and high mortality.

Projects within an organization's programs may be chosen based on scientific merit, potential clinical applications, political favor, cost, and the past achievements of the principal investigator. Additionally, the location where research takes place can impact technology transfer, with institutions closely connected to clinical practice likely to see new procedures adopted more widely compared to lesser-known clinics. For example, a prestigious medical school affiliated with a top-tier teaching hospital is more likely to facilitate the widespread adoption of innovative procedures.

7.1.3.7. Regulation and Reimbursement Policies

Government regulations and reimbursement decisions play a crucial role in ensuring that new technologies are effective, safe, and used correctly. Private industry relies on market-based criteria to determine which drugs and devices to develop, but government actions are necessary to address social and political concerns. These actions are primarily regulatory, focusing on the impact of technologies on health, safety, and the environment. Because these costs are widespread, government intervention is necessary to address them effectively. The government's role as a purchaser of technologies, particularly in healthcare, has led to the need to minimize reimbursement for ineffective technologies and determine which technologies are most appropriate. The regulatory process may slow the introduction of new technologies to the market and some may be filtered out. Reimbursement policies can also affect the speed of technology diffusion. Slowing the diffusion of new technologies can lead to more informed decisions before they are widely adopted.

The impact of regulatory and reimbursement policies on innovation and technology transfer not only depends on whether they hinder the process, but also on whether any unintended or undesirable consequences arise. Government support for research and development aims to speed up the process and steer it in certain directions. Regulations can influence the direction of innovation by affecting the competitive market, while reimbursement policies tend to impact the pace of innovation. Competition among medical care providers is typically not price-based, with incentives under current reimbursement policies prompting the adoption of diagnostic tools and therapies with perceived value, especially in hospitals. The majority of hospital care expenditures are covered by third-party payers. With technology costs having minimal impact on providers and patients due to health insurance arrangements, greater adoption of technology is likely to occur compared to scenarios with more price competition in reimbursement arrangements. In simplified terms, recent changes in regulations and reimbursement policies are moving towards a compromise between two extremes. Regulations are intended to slow innovation to a certain extent, especially during the diffusion phase, but adjustments are being made to ensure that innovation is not hindered more than necessary to meet regulatory goals. On the other hand, reimbursement policies are designed to promote the adoption of new medical technologies beyond what would occur in more competitive pricing systems, and reforms are focusing on limiting the adoption process.

The regulation aims to incorporate social considerations when evaluating the value of new technologies, so conclusions regarding the economic impact of regulatory requirements should be approached cautiously. It is expected that regulation will impact the innovation process, raising questions about whether the changes are intentional and if the benefits of regulation justify any resulting alterations to innovation. In terms of reimbursement policy, there is a need to introduce more price sensitivity in the adoption and use of new medical technologies. When combined with the regulatory framework, these adjustments could potentially allow socially worthy innovations to enter the market and enable competing new technologies to be assessed based on price. However, implementing a more price-sensitive approach to curb excessive demand may necessitate changes to the current medical technology innovation process. The key concern is whether such significant shifts in demand for new medical technologies could unintentionally impact innovation in negative ways.

7.2. Technology in Healthcare

The World Health Organization defines health technology as the "application of organized knowledge and skills in the form of devices, medicines, vaccines, procedures, and systems developed to improve quality of life and solve health problems." This covers information systems supported by computers and medications, tools, protocols, and organizational structures utilized in the healthcare sector. In the US, these technologies include both conventional and intentional social methods and means of patient treatment and care, as well as standardized physical objects.

7.2.1. Development

7.2.1.1. Pre-Digital Era

Patients suffered from defective and ineffective clinical systems, procedures, and circumstances in the pre-digital era. In the past, several medical errors were caused by underdeveloped health technologies. Adverse medication events and alarm fatigue are two instances of these medical errors. When numerous alarms are set off or activated frequently, particularly for insignificant events, employees may grow numb to the alerts. Alarm fatigue in healthcare personnel can cause them to disregard alarms that they consider unimportant, which can result in fatalities and hazardous circumstances. As technology advanced, a clever integration and physiological sense-making program was created, which assisted in lowering the number of false alarms.

Additionally, increased investments in health technologies resulted in a reduction in medical errors. Many healthcare organizations have replaced outdated paper records with electronic health records (EHR). Research indicates that this shift has significantly transformed the healthcare industry. Drug administration has become more efficient, healthcare providers have easier access to medical information, can offer improved treatments and quicker results, and have managed to save costs.

7.2.1.2. Improvement

The American Recovery and Reinvestment Act of 2009 included the HITECH Act, which Congress passed to encourage and expand the use of health information technology. The Health Information Technology for Economic and Clinical Health Act is referred to as HITECH. It granted the Department of Health and Human Services the power to encourage the use of health information technology to raise the standard and efficiency of healthcare. The act offered organizations monetary rewards or fines to encourage healthcare providers to enhance patient care. The act aimed to decrease health disparities by enhancing efficiency, quality, safety, and quality.

The HITECH Act's key component was the meaningful use requirement, mandating EHRs to enable electronic health information exchange and clinical data submission. The goal of HITECH is to ensure the secure sharing of electronic information among patients and clinicians, streamline healthcare provider operations, and minimize medical errors. The program was divided into three phases. Phase one aimed to enhance healthcare quality, safety, and efficiency. Phase two built upon phase one by concentrating on clinical processes and promoting meaningful EHR use. Lastly, phase three focused on leveraging Certified Electronic Health Record Technology (CEHRT) to enhance health outcomes.

Hospitals in the United States began using electronic records in 2014. The adoption rate increased from 10% to 70%. Healthcare providers that took part in the Medicare Promoting Interoperability Program were required to submit reports on the requirements of the Quality Payment Program starting in 2018. The initiative attempted to increase patient access to health information by putting a greater emphasis on interoperability.

7.2.1.3. Privacy of Health Data

Cell phones with location tracking, step tracking, and other features can be used as medical devices, and these phones and medical devices work in very similar ways. One study found that although people were willing to give their personal information to advance science, they were still apprehensive about who would access it. People are hesitant to divulge sensitive personal information by nature. The threat is increased by phones. Every year, the use of mobile devices grows in popularity. The possibility of an attacker obtaining unauthorized information is increased by the use of mobile devices as medical devices.

Healthcare is entering the digital age thanks to the Patient Protection and Affordable Care Act (ACA), commonly known as Obamacare, and health information technology. Nonetheless, it must be safeguarded in light of this development. Within the health industry, financial and health information that is now digital may become more vulnerable to cybercrime. Hackers manage to breach security despite numerous safeguards in place, so security updates are necessary to keep these breaches from happening.

7.2.1.4. Policy

Due to easier access and inadequate management, privacy violations were rising quickly along with the use of IT systems. As a result, privacy concerns have gained importance in the healthcare industry. When companies fail to protect the confidentiality of people's data, privacy breaches occur. There exist four categories of privacy breaches: unintentional disclosure by authorized personnel, purposeful disclosure by authorized personnel, loss or theft of privacy data, and cyberattacks. The high negative impact on individuals and organizations makes it even more imperative to protect the security and privacy of patient data. Credit card applications and other unethical actions can be made using stolen personal information. In addition, people must spend a lot of money to fix the problem. The disclosure of private health information may also have detrimental effects on a person's employment, relationships, or other spheres of their lives. The company may face financial penalties, legal action, lost business, and damaged reputation as a result of the privacy violation.

The Health Insurance Portability and Accountability Act was passed in 1996, and its acronym is HIPAA. The letter is U.S. Privacy and data security are the two main regulations outlined in healthcare legislation that govern the use of patient data. People's rights to privacy are safeguarded by the privacy rule, and precautions to preserve privacy are outlined in the security rule.

The three qualities of protected health information are confidentiality, availability, and integrity, as stated in the HIPAA Security Rule. Maintaining data confidentiality involves not allowing third parties or data loss to obtain access to protected health information. Availability gives authorized users access to the networks and systems at the precise moment and place when they are needed, like during natural disasters. In situations such as these, protected health information is typically printed out in paper copies or backed up on a different server for public access. Finally, integrity guarantees that patient data permanence is protected by not using erroneous information and improperly modified data as a result of a poorly designed system or process. Using data that has been erroneously or improperly altered may have detrimental or even deadly effects.

In addition, HIPAA-compliant health organizations developed technological, administrative, and physical security measures to help preserve patient privacy. Administrative protections often consist of workforce management and training, information access control, security staff, security management processes, and assessments of security policies and procedures. Security management processes are crucial examples of administrative safeguards that are essential for reducing risks and vulnerabilities in the system. Typically outlined as standard operating procedures in training manuals, these processes aim to educate individuals on the proper handling of protected health information.

Physical security measures include card swipes, lock and key, screen placement, private envelopes, and paper copy shredding. Physical safeguards include things like locks and keys. They may restrict who has actual access to a facility. Even though locks and keys are basic, they can stop people from stealing medical records. To open the lock, someone needs to have a real key.

Finally, transmission security, integrity controls, audit controls, and access control are examples of technical safeguards. One common illustration of a technological safety measure is the access control system. It permits authorized personnel to enter. Authorization and authentication are features of the technology. Authorization is the process of deciding whether a specific user is permitted to access specific data and carry out actions in a system, such as add and delete. Authentication is the identity verification that manages private information, such as username and password.

7.2.1.5. Assessment

The United States originally introduced the idea of health technology assessment (HTA) in 1967, in response to the growing need to address health technology's unintended and possible consequences, as well as its significant social role. The creation of the Congressional Office of Technology Assessment (OTA) in 1972–1973 further institutionalized it. HTA is characterized as a thorough type of policy research that looks at the risks, costs, and both short- and long-term effects of applying technology. Owing to its extensive reach, technology assessment necessitates the involvement of people beyond scientists and medical professionals, including managers and even consumers.

The Centers for Medicare and Medicaid Services (CMS) and the Veterans Administration, through its VA Technology Assessment Program (VATAP), are two American organizations that offer health technology assessments. These institutions use a variety of models, but they all center on whether the medical technology being provided is therapeutically relevant. According to a 2007 study, formal economic analyses were still not used in the assessments.

Apart from its advancement, evaluation in the health technology sector has been perceived as irregular and dispersed. Problems including identifying products that require development, affordability, and accessibility, among other things, have also surfaced. Some contend that these should be considered in the evaluation because health technology is never just a scientific endeavor but also a reflection of ideologies, values, and beliefs. Bioethics, also called the "fourth-generation" evaluation framework, is one of the mechanisms being proposed as a component of or a substitute for the existing TAs. Ethical HTA operates on two key dimensions. The first dimension focuses on integrating ethics into the methodological standards used for technology assessment. The second dimension pertains to the utilization of an ethical framework by researchers in their research and decision-making processes, ultimately shaping the information used in the industry.

7.2.1.6. In the Future

The United States is currently experiencing a significant change in the medical profession. There are numerous reasons for this shift, but the main one is the adoption and fusion of health technologies with healthcare. The electronic health record (EHR) has become widely used in recent years, and this has had a significant impact on healthcare. Future hospitals will be fewer, and as technology advances, more people will likely need to visit them for major medical procedures or life-threatening illnesses. Hospitals won't require nurse call buttons in the future. Rather, robots will administer the system, care for patients, and deliver medication. The electronic health record will also have a new appearance. Healthcare professionals will have real-time access to the notes through speech-to-text transcriptions.

To enhance the quality, information will be edited cooperatively by the patient care team. Furthermore, advances in natural language processing will aid in the extraction of keywords. In the future, patients' data will be stored on the cloud, where they can be accessed from any device or place by authorized providers, individuals, and patients. Big data analysis will advance continuously. As new data is received, machine learning and artificial intelligence will continue to advance and improve. Additionally, alerts will be smarter and more effective than they are now.

7.2.2. Medical Technology

Human-affecting diseases and medical conditions are treated with medical technology, or "medtech," which is a broad category of healthcare supplies. By reducing hospital stays and rehabilitation times, offering less invasive treatment options, and enabling earlier diagnosis, these technologies aim to enhance the quality of healthcare provided. Cost containment has also been a key focus of recent medical technology advancements. Biotech, medical devices, information technology, and healthcare services can all be considered forms of medical technology.

Medical technology has an impact on social and ethical issues. For instance, doctors don't have to read arbitrary patient reports when they can use technology to find objective information.

The medtech industry is growing due in large part to the consumerization of its products. Providers can reach a large audience at a low cost thanks to the widespread availability of smartphones and tablets; this trend is expected to continue as wearable technologies become more widely available. Over 30,000 investors have contributed US $11.7 billion to health tech companies since venture capital increased by 200% between 2010 and 2015.

7.2.2.1. Types of Technology

Smaller, portable devices like smartphones, tablets, laptops, digital ink, voice, and face recognition, and more have been made possible by advancements in medical technology. Innovations such as electronic health records (EHR), radio frequency identification (RFID), telemedicine, clinical decision support (CDS), mobile home healthcare, nanomedicine, genome-based personalized medicine, patient portals, health information exchange (HIE), Nationwide Health Information Network (NwHIN), nanomedicine, and cloud computing emerged with the use of this technology.

For a long time, medical research, patient reviews, and treatment analysis have relied on medical imaging and magnetic resonance imaging (MRI) as reliable medical technologies. The capabilities of medical imaging technology are expanding and producing better results as a result of advancements in imaging technologies, such as the use of faster and more data, higher resolution images, and specialized automation software. Patients will spend less time and money, as well as require fewer contrast agents, as imaging hardware and software advance.

Electromagnetic (EM) technology guidance systems, which are used in medical procedures and enable real-time visualization and navigation for the placement of medical devices inside the human body, represent a further advancement in healthcare. For instance, as the ENvue System illustrates, a feeding tube may be placed in the stomach or small intestine or a neuro-navigated catheter may be placed in the brain. An enhanced electromagnetic navigation system called ENvue is used to locate enteral feeding tubes. Using a field generator and multiple electromagnetic sensors, the system allows the display to be properly scaled to the patient's body contour. It also provides a real-time view of the feeding tube tip's location and direction, assisting medical staff in ensuring proper placement and preventing tube placement in the lungs.

Another significant advancement in healthcare is 3D printing. It can be utilized to create inert implants, prosthetic limbs, specialized splints, and parts for medical equipment. The ability to print replacement body parts that are customized is the ultimate goal of 3D printing. Further information on 3D printing in healthcare will be provided in the section that follows. Robotics and artificial intelligence are examples of new technology.

7.2.2.2. 3D Printing

3D printing is the process of automating the creation of specific objects using specialized equipment, materials, and software. Prosthetics, medical implants, new drug formulations, and the bio-printing of human tissues and organs are all experiencing rapid growth in this field. Businesses like Surgical Theater offer cutting-edge technology that can create 3D virtual representations of patients' brains for use in operating room practice. Medical companies can now create practice models for operations involving artificial tissue thanks to 3D printing.

Biomedicine benefits greatly from 3D printing technologies because the materials used in their creation enable fabrication with precise control over numerous design elements. The advantages of 3D printing also include more time savings, more effective designs, and reasonably priced customization. Since different drugs have different release times, 3D printing can precisely design pills to house multiple drugs. The pills can travel to the desired location and safely break down in the body thanks to technology. As a result, tablets can be made more conveniently and effectively. Instead of prescribing in the future, doctors may send patients a digital file with printing instructions.

Moreover, medical implants will benefit more from 3D printing. One instance is a surgical team that created a 3D-printed tracheal splint to help a patient breathe better. This illustration highlights the potential of 3D printing, which makes it simple for doctors to create new implant and instrument designs. All things considered, 3D printing will play a major role in medicine in the future since it can be utilized for surgical planning, artificial and prosthetic devices, medications, and medical implants.

7.2.2.3. Artificial Intelligence

Artificial intelligence (AI) systems are becoming larger and more capable, partly because big data is becoming more and more advanced. It is anticipated that technology will facilitate information accessibility in the healthcare industry and enhance treatment outcomes while cutting costs. The use of AI in healthcare generally results in more complex tasks being completed with greater quality and efficiency.

The possible lack of accuracy and privacy issues with the data collected are two risks associated with AI. Giving AI systems decision-making authority could also compromise accountability. Moreover, AI programs occasionally pick up undesirable behaviors from the data they use for training. For instance, since images of malignancies usually include a ruler to show the scale, an AI trained to detect skin diseases was found to have a strong tendency to classify images containing a ruler as cancerous.

AI has a multitude of benefits for the healthcare industry, including disease detection, chronic condition management, health service delivery, and drug discovery. It also can tackle critical health challenges by assisting with resource allocation in healthcare organizations and matching patients with suitable providers. Additionally, AI can enhance the healthcare experience by identifying patient anxieties through apps. In medical research, AI plays a crucial role in analyzing complex data patterns, aiding in drug discovery, and evaluating various studies. Moreover, in clinical care, AI helps with disease detection, data analysis, treatment recommendations, medical imaging, echocardiography, screening, and surgery. The groundbreaking capabilities of AlphaFold in predicting protein folding have also significantly accelerated medical research.

Medical virtual reality technology offers various surgical scenarios to doctors for practicing and preparation. It also gives medical students a chance to experience different procedures without the risk of errors. ORamaVR is a company at the forefront of using this technology to enhance medical education and training, ultimately improving patient outcomes, decreasing surgical errors and training time, and making medical education more accessible.

7.2.2.4. Robots

Modern robotics has advanced greatly and improved healthcare. Doctors can get assistance from robots for a range of tasks. Hospital robotics adoption is rising dramatically. There exist various approaches to enhance healthcare through the utilization of robots.

One type of robotic system that makes it possible for a surgeon to rotate and bend tissues more effectively and flexibly is the surgical robot. The system has a 3D magnification vision system that can precisely translate the surgeon's hand movements to perform surgery with fewer incisions. Cancer diagnosis and treatment are among the functions of other robotics systems. A large team of scientists started developing a next-generation robotic system to help surgeons replace bones in the knee and other joints. It will also be crucial for assistant robots to lessen the workload of regular medical staff. Simple and time-consuming tasks like carrying multiple racks of medications, lab specimens, or other delicate materials can be assisted by nurses.

Robotic pills are anticipated to lower the surgical future shortly. They can be relocated inside a patient and placed where needed. They can also perform biopsies, take pictures of the area, and unclog blocked arteries. In general, medical robots are a great help to doctors; however, it may take some time for a clinician to receive professional training in using medical robots and for the robots to react to their commands. As a result, numerous academics and new businesses are continuously striving to offer solutions for these problems.

7.2.2.5. Assistive Technologies

Assistive technologies are products specifically created to enhance accessibility for individuals with physical or cognitive challenges. Their primary goal is to enhance the quality of life through a wide range of solutions, ranging from simple low-tech tools to advanced technical devices. These technologies are divided into four main categories: visual impairment, hearing impairment, physical limitations, and cognitive limitations. The benefits of assistive technologies are numerous, including enabling individuals to care for themselves, work, study, access information more easily, improve independence and communication, and fully participate in community life.

7.2.2.6. Consumer-Driven Healthcare Software

Websites and apps that offer more details on the cost and quality of healthcare to assist patients in selecting their providers have proliferated as part of a broader trend toward consumer-driven healthcare.

As of 2017, Healthgrades, Vitals.com, and RateMDs.com had the most reviews among all websites, arranged in descending order. Although there were fewer medical reviews per doctor on Yelp, Google, and Facebook as of 2017, these platforms still host reviews with a lot of traffic. Online reviews can give rise to disputes involving defamation on the websites of medical professionals. Year 2018 saw the purchase of Vitals.com by WebMD, an Internet Brands company.

Hospital-Compare by CMS and hospitalsafetygrade.org by LeapFrog Group are two prominent examples of how patient safety organizations and government programs that have historically evaluated quality have made their data more accessible online.

Patient-oriented software may also help in other ways, including general education and appointments. It is now simpler to disclose legal disputes, such as complaints about medical licenses or malpractice lawsuits. Every state makes public license status and at least some disciplinary action available to the public; however, as of 2018, several states did not allow online access to this information. Customers can search for medical licenses in the medical licensing organizations' national database, DocInfo.org, which has some limited information. Consumers can look up medical licenses in a national database, DocInfo.org, maintained by the medical licensing organizations which contain limited details. Other tools include DocFinder at docfinder.docboard.org and certificationmatters.org from the American

Board of Medical Specialties. For instance, the Medical Board of California removes unfounded allegations from its website profiles, but these details can still be found by sending or picking up a copy of the request. There is a great deal of public debate surrounding the disclosure trend, especially about the National Practitioner Data Bank's opening. The first state to mandate a thorough disclosure of malpractice claims was Massachusetts in 1996.

7.2.2.7. Self-Monitoring

Individuals can now keep an eye on their health thanks to wearable computers, smartphones, and tablets. These devices are equipped with a multitude of applications that are intended to offer basic healthcare services and track an individual's health in order to identify any serious health issues. Fitbit, an activity tracker that is worn on the wrist, is one instance of this. People can track their heart rates, steps, miles traveled, floors climbed, active minutes, and even sleep patterns with wearable technology. Users can monitor and even help manage their health thanks to the gathered and analyzed data, especially when it comes to identifying health risk factors (Figure 7.2).

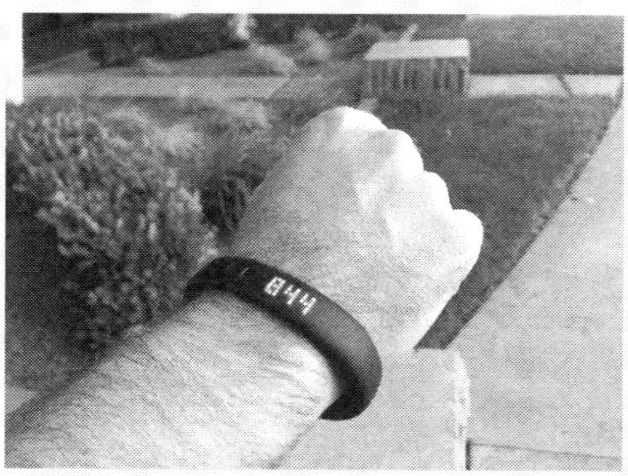

Figure 7.2. *The Nike+ FuelBand is one of the many kinds of wearable devices that people use as "quantified self" tools.*

Source: ByIntel Free Press, CC BY-SA 2.0, https://commons.wikimedia.org/w/index.php?curid=28115137.

Alternatively, there is the Internet, which functions as a clearinghouse of knowledge and professional material that allows users to "self-diagnose" in place of visiting a physician. For example, all it takes to identify an illness from the list of contents uploaded to the Internet is to list the symptoms as search parameters on Google, and the search engine will identify the illness based on those provided by expert/medical sources. The role of health professionals may eventually change as a result of these advancements from "gatekeeper to secondary care to facilitator of information interpretation and decision-making." In addition to Google's standard services in Search, other businesses, like WebMD, already provide specialized apps for symptom checking.

7.2.2.8. Technology Testing

Every medical device sold commercially has to abide by both international and US laws. The devices are tested for material properties, effects on the human body, mechanical aspects, and all parts, including those that come with other devices. The Medical Device User Fee and Modernization Act of 2002 introduced sponsor user fees for a faster review time with predetermined performance targets for review time, to expedite the FDA's approval process for medical technology. Additionally, the FDA approved 36 gadgets and applications in 2016 (Cordani et al., 2020; Garrett et al., 2006).

7.3. Technological Change

It's incredible to see how far technology has progressed in our world over the years. Regarding technology in healthcare, the same can be said. The healthcare revolution has improved the overall experience for patients and medical professionals, from increased operational efficiency to higher standards in patient care.

7.3.1. Promotion of Innovations

Among the numerous obstacles to fostering innovation in the healthcare sector is the industry's high level of regulation in the US. Because of this, entrepreneurs in this field need to be even more perceptive and imaginative in order to overcome obstacles and present fresh ideas. Adhering to regulations results in higher expenses and longer lead times, which hinders the release of novel solutions.

7.3.1.1. Successful Innovations Are Usable and Appealing

Innovations in healthcare that are successful must not only improve upon existing products or services, but also be aesthetically pleasing and easy to use. This implies that they have to be able to be commercialized, embraced by stakeholders as best practices, and modified for application in a healthcare environment. Asking themselves what their customers want, understanding their problem with stakeholders, and creating an adoption strategy are all steps that successful organizations take. They also promote a culture of innovation.

One excellent example of a successful innovation is DigiComp Kids, which was created in partnership with family partners and knowledgeable clinicians on the Complex Care Team. In order to build empathy for the circumstances and a sense of shared purpose, family members and clinicians discussed their struggles and victories throughout the project. Following the storytelling phase, team members gave case studies of potential medical remedies. They also provided instances of how the solutions had been successfully applied.

For innovators in healthcare, the Generative Co-Design Framework was made to be versatile and flexible. Because it enables end users to comprehend the difficulties present in the setting and context in which the innovations will be used, the co-design process is crucial. All too frequently, though, health innovations fall short of the expected gains.

7.3.1.2. Rigorous Evaluation of Influencing Variables

A lot of things need to be taken into account when encouraging innovation in the healthcare sector. These factors include the innovation's economics, the affordability of goods like outdoor seeds, complementary therapies, or services, and the existence of a market that is appropriate for the product. For instance, consumers have a significant influence on innovations in healthcare. They frequently become members of disease associations, advocate for more financing for healthcare, and put pressure on healthcare providers to offer innovative medications, tests, treatments, and equipment.

The value proposition of the new good or service should be taken into account in addition to the innovation's expenses. Although most innovations are intended to benefit society as a whole, they can have unexpected effects. It's critical to assess if the new offering will worsen existing disparities or have unanticipated consequences. Digital health technologies, for instance, have the potential to worsen already-existing health disparities and overlook the digital divide within the populace. Furthermore, conflicting inventions could lead to weariness and uncertainty, and a shift in healthcare services might raise medical expenses.

7.3.1.3. New Technologies

The healthcare sector is evolving thanks to new technologies, particularly in the areas of illness prevention and treatment. Healthcare professionals can detect and treat illnesses more successfully thanks to AI and digital health technologies. Additionally, the clinical experience of physicians and nurses is enhanced by these technologies. These technologies have produced advances in illness detection, prevention, and treatment during the last 10 years.

The delivery of care has also been affected by new technologies. In the past, the care team would frequently communicate via pagers. Providers can now more easily and successfully document clinical data thanks to new technologies. However, this kind of shift may hurt worker welfare and industry performance. Furthermore, new technologies have the potential to negatively impact worker voice and job quality if improperly implemented.

The healthcare system needs to be innovative in order to meet the challenges posed by the adoption of these new technologies and procedures. This is essential to getting better value. Novel approaches need to set themselves apart from pre-existing solutions. Regretfully, there is a lack of clarity in the healthcare industry as a result of the term innovation becoming overly generic.

The standard and security of care can be enhanced by new medical devices and technologies. Healthcare organizations should prioritize enhancing research and education in addition to patient satisfaction. Promoting innovative techniques and technologies requires proper education. Developing fresh approaches to patient care ought to be the aim of these innovations. It's also critical to acknowledge that data-driven methods for handling health data are still in their infancy. They also need to be impartial. This will make it easier to assess how much an innovation affects people. Nonetheless, intangible components of healthcare are indisputable and can only be evaluated through interpersonal communication.

7.3.2. Intellectual Property Rights

The use of digital technologies and data to improve health outcomes, boost the effectiveness of the healthcare system, and enable people to make decisions about their health and well-being is what the World Health Organization (WHO) refers to as digital health in its Digital Health Strategy (2020–2025). It also places a strong emphasis on the concepts of privacy, security, confidentiality, interoperability, scalability, replicability, and transparency.

Artificial intelligence (AI), wearable technology, telemedicine, electronic health records, health information systems, and mobile health (mHealth) apps are all part of the rapidly growing field of digital health. These innovations prevent fatalities. According to a recent study, the use of wearable AI—which includes gadgets like smartwatches with AI algorithms built in to monitor health in real-time—could prevent almost 4,00,000 deaths in Europe each year and save 200 billion euros in expenses. Furthermore, the industry is clearly profitable as seen by the over 100 unicorns in the digital health tech space worldwide.

In many regions of the world, the COVID-19 pandemic encouraged a greater uptake of digital health, expanding access to healthcare beyond conventional methods. Digital platforms helped limit the virus's spread and made contact tracing easier. The number of remote care services has increased, allowing patients to get critical medical advice and assistance from the comfort of their own homes.

The swift implementation of digital technologies, such as contact tracing software, presented prospects for mitigating health disparities. To facilitate scientific discovery and equitable distribution of the advantages resulting from scientific advancements and applications, knowledge transfer, IP collaboration, and sharing are essential for the successful implementation and accessibility of digital healthcare.

Digital health is supported by IP. In addition to making it simpler for users to take advantage of these developments, it offers protection for the creative ideas of scientists and business owners. IP guarantees that novel and ground-breaking digital health solutions can be developed and made broadly accessible to enhance healthcare outcomes for people, whether it is a cutting-edge software algorithm for remote patient monitoring or a mobile application that offers personalized fitness plans and health tracking features. IP contributes to the UN Sustainable Development Goals (SDG) of "good health and well-being" (SDG 3) and "industry, innovation, and infrastructure" (SDG 9) by safeguarding and advancing creativity and innovation in the field of digital health.

7.3.1.4. Patent, Trade Secrets, Copyright

Although patentable components like chemical, electrical, or mechanical parts are frequently found in digital health products, safeguarding technology-based components can be difficult because of their complex and intangible nature. The process of obtaining patent rights for data analysis methods can be lengthy in certain jurisdictions. As a result, innovators who wish to protect their digital health inventions may choose to have trade secrets protected. This strategy protects privacy and fits in well with the quick pace of technological advancement and the dynamic nature of digital health businesses. Additionally, in order to prevent unwanted use of these priceless assets, digital health software, databases, or documentation must be protected.

7.3.1.5. Other IPs That Protect Digital Health

In the field of digital health, other types of intellectual property are also important. For businesses to stand out in the marketplace, brand names and logos must be protected by trademarks. Businesses can gain a competitive advantage by using trade dress to preserve unique visual designs and design to protect distinctive product appearances.

7.3.1.6. Data Protection in Digital Health

The foundation of digital health is data. Patient data is regularly gathered and stored by digital healthcare products, and it can be sent to hospitals or healthcare providers. There are more threats to privacy and personal data protection. Under numerous IP laws, IP protection offers security for patient health data, including medical histories and results of diagnostic tests. In this regard, digital rights management technologies are a priceless resource.

7.3.1.7. WIPO's Role in Facilitating Discussions on Digital Technology and IP

To promote dialogue and information exchange about digital technology and intellectual property among Member States and other stakeholders, the World Intellectual Property Organization (WIPO) plays a crucial role. Its goal is to assist in making informed policy decisions and to offer useful tools and advice for navigating the intricate IP landscape in the rapidly evolving digital world. WIPO currently facilitates several open-ended discussions on subjects related to digital health. These include discussions about the implications of AI for IP policy, such as the IP and Frontier Technologies Conversation, which provides a forum for debating how frontier technologies affect all IP rights and fills in gaps in this quickly developing field.

7.3.1.8. Other Global Initiatives

0Initiatives to fully utilize the potential of digital health have been started by international organizations. The Global Initiative on AI for Health was recently launched by WIPO, the International Telecommunication Union (ITU), and the World Health Organization (WHO). Its objective is to guarantee that AI realizes its potential to assist in diagnosis and treatment, as well as provide more effective and inclusive healthcare services. ITU and WHO's "Be Healthy, Be Mobile" campaign uses mobile technology to enhance healthcare services, particularly in areas with limited resources. The Global Digital Health Partnership facilitates knowledge-sharing and interoperability efforts by bringing together governments, organizations, and experts in the field of digital health to advance global digital health standards and best practices.

7.4. Technological Diffusion

Throughout the COVID-19 pandemic, everyone has been curious about when things will return to "normal." This is a typical reaction of humans to trauma. But as 2020 keeps upsetting normalcy, we have to start considering whether we really should want things to go back to normal. The "normal" in the American health economy is deviant. In comparison to other industrialized nations, the United States had the highest percentage of healthcare in GDP (18%) in 2018. This percentage was higher than it has ever been.

7.4.1. Drivers of Innovation

Technological developments or social demands for change can spur innovation. The printing press, one of the most well-known and influential inventions in world history, resulted from the convergence of other technological advancements like the creation of manufactured paper and ink. There are three different kinds of innovations in healthcare:

- Firstly, innovations that enhance the patient experience are those that are focused on the needs of the end user. This can involve initiatives for price transparency, improved access to providers, or tools that promote collaborative decision-making.
- The second group consists of creative business plans. This broad category includes innovative insurance plans, risk-sharing programs focused on providers, direct primary care, and centers of excellence for specialized treatment of uncommon conditions.
- Technological innovation is the third type of innovation. Improved treatment plans, novel medications or medical equipment, or the application of artificial intelligence (AI) and machine learning to a growing corpus of medical data are some examples of technological innovation in the healthcare industry.

7.4.2. How Does Technological Innovation Spread?

Five characteristics of innovations determine how fast and far they are likely to spread. Within the framework of an intricate system like the U.S., none of these five elements—healthcare—is simple.

- According to the concept of relative advantage, an innovation cannot just be different from the element it would replace; it must be viewed as truly superior. Given the variety of frequently at-odds goals held by the various parties involved in the healthcare system, an innovation may be viewed as a relative advantage by some while being viewed as a relative disadvantage by others.

- The degree to which an innovation aligns with the tenets and values of the system in which it will be applied is referred to as compatibility. Even in cases where an innovation is beneficial, it must adhere to certain fundamental principles. We have preconceived conceptions about who should make decisions in the healthcare industry and how simple it should be to get care. If a solution puts one of these ideological pillars in danger, it might be hard to implement it.
- Complexity refers to the level of extensive training or new understanding needed to implement an innovation. This complexity can arise from challenges in understanding the need for innovation or from disruptions to existing systems and processes that require reengineering. In the intricate healthcare system, innovations typically impact multiple system components and cannot be made in isolation.
- Trialability is the ease with which an innovation can be tested to see if it is likely to produce the desired results. Trials of medical innovations require enormous amounts of work to be put into practice, ranging from expensive clinical trials of medications and treatments to demonstration projects testing novel payment schemes. These trials are expensive, time-consuming, and frequently hampered by ethical issues. Demonstrating improvements in cost or other outcomes may require very large samples and, occasionally, extended times.
- The degree to which an innovation's successes are apparent to others is referred to as observability. Particularly in the medical field, innovation can be expensive. It might be necessary to gather a critical mass of participants to lower that cost. To achieve this, potential adopters need to have easy access to information about innovations and their advantages. In a setting where results are hard to quantify and occasionally contradict amongst stakeholders, demonstrating innovative success can be a daunting task.

A 2006 case report identifies six key barriers to the adoption of new technology in healthcare:

i. Cost;
ii. Legality;
iii. Time;
iv. Fear;
v. Usefulness; and
vi. Complexity.

The tremendous advancements in medical technology over the past few decades demonstrate that there are solutions to these obstacles. The impact of venture capital has been a major driver of new technology in healthcare. It has been reported that over $4.05 billion in venture capital funds were allocated to digital health initiatives in just the third quarter of 2018. This funding may give stakeholders the much-needed push in the direction of adoption. The adoption of new technologies can also be aided by the power of regulatory agencies and Medicare's payment coverage.

Venture capital has significantly driven new healthcare technology. A new technology's ability to spread throughout society depends on caregivers' individual decisions to alter medical practice, even though funding and regulatory actions can have a significant impact on which innovations are most likely to succeed. This means that before a new technology's advantages can be felt, a certain number of early adopters must be attained. The use of electronic health record (EHR) systems in the medical field is one recent example. After a technology is widely used, its fixed costs are distributed among a greater number of users, potentially increasing the technology's benefits while lowering its cost. Numerous emerging technologies are on the verge of reaching the critical mass required to begin influencing the healthcare system as a whole.

7.4.3. The Diffusion of New Technology: Costs and Benefits to Healthcare

Technologies are praised for their ability to save lives, enhance health, and raise the standard of care. Simultaneously, technology is demonized as a primary cause of the ongoing rise in healthcare expenses. Organ transplants, diagnostic imaging devices, and new biotechnology products are examples of highly visible "big-ticket" items that draw a lot of attention and criticism.

This chapter is based on five facts about new medical technology. First, by enhancing health outcomes, new technologies do, on average, raise the standard of medical care. While this is true on average, it is not true for all technologies in all clinical settings. Second, new technologies don't improve health outcomes and are redundant or ineffective. The issue is that when new technologies are introduced, it can be difficult to distinguish between those that are effective and those that are not. Third, the overall cost of healthcare is increased by new technologies. Though the overall effect is to increase costs, some technologies may actually save costs by preventing costly health consequences or by replacing more expensive alternatives. Fourth, the incentives and rules incorporated into the US healthcare system cause an inappropriate spread of technologies, resulting in an excess of inefficient and expensively ineffective technologies as well as an under the diffusion of efficient and cost-effective technologies. The issue is exacerbated by patient demands, professional reward systems, reimbursement policies, and legal issues. The American public's insatiable appetite for new medical technology represents the fifth unavoidable truth about it. Our suppliers are generally pleased to comply when we ask for the newest and greatest products from them.

The issue is that medical expenses are still rising, making it more difficult for the public and private sectors to finance healthcare. The time when it will become impossible to give every American, regardless of cost, access to the best medical care possible is drawing near or may have already arrived in American society. The de facto solution has been to limit healthcare access for an increasing number of people—the uninsured—while upholding the myth that those who are fortunate enough to have coverage receive the best care available.

Pressure to drive up healthcare costs will only intensify during the 1990s. An expanding number of new technologies will demand a bigger portion of the country's resources. The "baby boomers," or the birth cohort born between 1945 and 1965, will enter an age range where the prevalence of chronic illness is expected to rise. Some sort of universal healthcare may be implemented. Each of these three factors will put difficult decisions in place, dispelling the fallacy that "best available technology for all." Medical technologies—especially those that are new—will have to defend their expenses in an environment where resource claims are conflicting.

Four facets of the cost-new medical technology relationship are covered in this chapter. We start by going over the data pertaining to how new technology affects the overall cost of healthcare. Second, we examine a normative model of the best possible diffusion of technologies, which is predicated on a cost-effectiveness analysis—that is, a technology's capacity to enhance health outcomes. Third, we look at how financial incentives impact new technology adoption in the U.S. and compare the priorities that emerge from the healthcare system to those that come from the normative cost-effectiveness model. We look at incentives for managed care organizations, hospitals, and physicians who charge by the service. Examples of incentives that promote the over-diffusion of cost-inefficient technologies and the under-diffusion of cost-effective ones are provided. In conclusion, we offer our thoughts on potential policy measures in the future that could lead to a more economical spread of technology.

7.4.3.1. New Technology Add to Healthcare Costs

Because health insurance lowers financial barriers for customers, it increases demand for technology and pushes service providers to charge more for a wider range of services. Nonetheless, it has proven difficult for researchers to quantify the exact amount that technology has increased costs. Determining what constitutes medical technology is one of the challenges. The word is often used in a broad sense to refer to medications, equipment, surgery, and organizational support systems that are used to provide medical care. It is nearly impossible to pinpoint the variations in cost that can be attributed to these items over any given time frame. The more significant inventions would be very hard to track down in terms of their overall economic impact, even if they could be named.

An additional warning is that the cost of purchasing a medication, a piece of equipment, or the payment made to a surgeon is sometimes mistaken for the economic impact of a technology. That is only one aspect of a technology's overall effect on healthcare costs; other effects may include induced costs and offsetting savings. A capital-embodied technology's total cost comprises both the capital cost and the operating costs necessary to put it into practice. Even the most capital-intensive technologies may have higher operating costs than expected due to the requirement for staff for supervision and operation, as well as for training, insurance, supplies, and space. In contrast, a novel medication or gadget might cost more to acquire but less to use than comparable options. A new technology may also have an impact on the use of other medical services. These outcomes make up a technology's "induced" costs and savings. A new imaging technology may make other diagnostic procedures unnecessary or increase the use of other tests to confirm a diagnosis that would not have otherwise occurred. A new diagnostic test may cause treatments that would not have been considered, or new technology may provide an alternative course of action, causing treatments to be avoided. Technologies and the processes they cause can have unintended consequences that call for additional testing and care, or they can prevent unintended consequences and side effects by enabling a safer clinical approach than would have been possible in the absence of the technology. Technology that prolongs life may necessitate longer stays in care, frequently in institutional settings and at high cost. Although few preventive technologies are cost-effective overall, they may save resources that would otherwise be needed for diagnosis and treatment. The way technology affects U.S. healthcare costs is by first calculating the effects of other, more noticeable sources, such as population growth according to age and price inflation. Technology is blamed for the portion of the rise in health costs that cannot be explained by these explanatory factors. Such research does not distinguish between the introduction of new technologies and the expanded applications of already-existing technologies. Some researchers have tried to track variations in the price of treating specific diseases over time. Others have examined the effects of significant technologies like computed tomography and intensive care units using case studies.

There are several issues with all three strategies. These methods are problematic for our discussion of the economics of new technology because they do not distinguish between the effects of new and existing technologies. Residual approaches typically fail to identify the exact cause of increases. Many studies link rising costs to rising "intensity per hospital admission," a finding that could be explained by non-technological variables like shifting disease severity or characteristics. Furthermore, these studies do not readily identify induced costs or indirect costs associated with the use of new technologies, such as the requirement for more qualified hospital technicians and nurses. While the case study and specific illness approaches do examine the effects of specific technologies, it is challenging to draw broad conclusions from them. This body of work does not try to link increases in costs to better health outcomes, in contrast to research on cost-effectiveness, which we shall return to.

According to empirical data from these kinds of studies, medical technology is responsible for between 10% and 40% of the long-term rise in healthcare costs. Between 1947 and 1967, the annual rate of increase in health expenditures was 8%, of which 0.6% was attributable to technology. Between 1962 and 1968, there was a 25% increase in hospital expenses per admission, which could be attributed to technological advancements. In more recent times, the "intensity per admission" was responsible for 21% of the increase in hospital costs between 1971 and 1981. The Healthcare Financing Administration (HCFA) estimated that, due to factors like changes in income level and demographics, "consumption per capita" and its intensity accounted for 35% of the variations in personal health expenditures between 1985 and 1986. Using a particular illness approach, changes in treatment that increased costs typically outweighed those that decreased costs between 1951 and 1971. The increase in ancillary services, like X-rays and laboratory testing, was the primary cause of cost increases.

The amount that each technology costs for healthcare is negligible. For instance, a 1979 study discovered that savings of 1% or 2% of the country's health expenditures would result from a 50% reduction in the annual operating costs of four costly technologies: renal dialysis, electronic fetal monitoring, coronary bypass surgery, and computed tomography. The use of intensive care units is one exception; Russell discovered that in 1974, this category accounted for roughly 10% of hospital expenses.

7.4.3.2. Optimal Diffusion of Technology: The Cost-Effectiveness Principle

To assess whether the degree of diffusion of specific technologies or technologies in general is appropriate, we need some standard or criterion. If new technologies raise healthcare costs, how much technology is appropriate? One such standard is predicated on the idea that the goal of medical technology is to enhance patient outcomes. Every time technology is used in a clinical setting, some of society's meager resources for healthcare are used, and hopefully, better health results result. Health improves more when society spends more on medical care. Furthermore, healthcare has diminishing returns; for every $1 billion spent, health improves more than it does for every $600 billion. More resources can be allocated to healthcare, which will improve health more, but at a higher incremental cost per unit of improved health.

This formulation of society's objectives leads to the cost-effectiveness criterion for resource allocation: a new technology should be adopted if it produces health outcomes at a lower cost per unit than existing technologies, or else it should not be adopted. The idea is that clinical procedures that are less expensive per unit of health benefit ought to take precedence over procedures that are more expensive per unit. Cost-effectiveness analysis is becoming more widely accepted in the medical community as a suitable standard for allocating resources, and it has been used extensively to support policy formation. One of the earliest examples of a cost-effectiveness analysis was one conducted on hemodialysis in end-stage renal disease. Cost-effectiveness analyses of new medical technologies are frequently helpful indicators of their potential role in healthcare. This study, which estimated a comparatively low annual cost of life extension, most likely had an impact on Congress's decision to fund Medicare's universal coverage. One study limitation that we will address is that the study only looked at the most advantageous target group, which is the relatively young and otherwise healthy people. It did not account for the possibility of expanding to older and sicker patients, for whom the cost-effectiveness ratio is significantly higher. The fact that adoption decisions are frequently made before complete cost or even satisfactory effectiveness data are available presents a barrier to the general application of cost-effectiveness analysis to new technologies.

Cost-effectiveness analyses have likely focused the greatest attention on the pharmaceutical industry. Cimetidine has been shown in analyses to be both cost-effective and to produce net savings when compared to standard treatment for peptic ulcer disease. When compared to conventional multiple-drug regimens, a study on the use of third-generation cephalosporins for hospital-acquired pneumonia also revealed cost savings, primarily due to lower costs associated with drug preparation and administration, monitoring, and side effects. Other medications have demonstrated incredibly favorable cost-effectiveness ratios in specific clinical applications, despite not being cost-saving. For instance, it has been demonstrated that the cost of life saved by beta-blockers after myocardial infarction ranges from $2,400 for patients at high risk of another infarction to, at most, $13,000 for those at low risk. Because quality-of-life effects are important for other drugs, quality-adjusted life years are used as a proxy for health outcomes. For instance, assessments of the effects of antihypertensive medications on longevity and quality of life are included in their cost-effectiveness analyses. Cost-effectiveness analysis has also been done on diagnostic technologies. Unfortunately, because it is challenging to link the use of individual diagnostic modalities to improvements in health, many significant imaging technologies, including magnetic resonance imaging (MRI), have not been the subject of formal cost-effectiveness analyses.

These and other instances highlight an important takeaway for studies on cost-effectiveness. In certain clinical scenarios, a technology that exhibits high cost-effectiveness may prove to be highly inefficient financially. Exercise tolerance testing is not a cost-effective screening test for asymptomatic individuals, but it is for those who have chest pain. Patients with left-main coronary artery disease can benefit financially from coronary bypass graft surgery, but those with single-vessel disease cannot. For patients without other risk factors, cholesterol-lowering medications are probably not cost-effective for the primary prevention of coronary heart disease. However, they may be cost-effective—or even cost-saving—for patients who already have coronary artery disease or who have multiple risk factors in addition to high serum cholesterol.

Early lessons from the story of end-stage renal disease indicate that even a life-saving technology that is clinically and financially effective will eventually spread into areas where it adds little to no value to health at significant additional expense. Employees will advance through the ranks until they reach their greatest degree of incompetence, according to the Peter Principle. The analogy for medical technology diffusion is that technology will spread until it is incorporated into medical applications that are not economically viable. This poses a problem for those who create, use, buy, and regulate new technologies: how to allow the adoption of new technologies that are cost-effective without letting them consume large amounts of resources for uses that are not cost-effective?

7.4.3.3. Effects of Reimbursement on the Use of New Technologies

Are the financial rewards in the U.S. healthcare sector encouraging the spread of cost-effective technologies? Whether a technology was cost-effective or not, the 1970s and early 1980s saw a rapid diffusion of new technologies thanks to fee-for-service physician practices, cost-based hospital reimbursement, and generous insurance plans. Relatively little thought was given to whether technologies were cost-effective because providers knew they would be paid for their services. Technologies were under pressure to be adopted within the system as long as they were thought to provide only slight advantages over current practices. In the 1970s, when healthcare costs were rising and policymakers started to address the issue, medical technology was identified as a major contributing factor. Whether technology was to blame for rising healthcare costs was the question posed in the title of a significant conference held in 1977. Payers started to doubt if the country's expenditure in cutting-edge healthcare was worthwhile. Articles promoting the application of cost-effectiveness analysis to direct resource distribution started to appear.

However, most observers realized that the real problem was not medical technology per se, but rather twisted incentives that shielded providers and patients from the true cost of care. Policymakers hoped that resources, including those for new technologies, would be allocated more economically by creating systems with more suitable incentives. There are now very different incentives for providers to adopt and use new technologies as a result of the extensive healthcare financing reforms implemented in this decade, such as the implementation of the Medicare Prospective Payment System (PPS) and the explosive expansion of managed care insurance plans. Although these systems create incentives for providers to be more frugal, they do not guarantee that cost-effective technologies will be adopted. Let's look at the incentives that three key players in the spread of technology currently have: doctors, managed care insurance plans (which include HMOs), and hospitals.

7.4.3.4. Hospitals

PPS has the potential to skew the adoption of new, affordable technologies in several ways. PPS encourages hospitals to concentrate on short-term costs and reimbursement levels because it sets fixed, predetermined payments per admission. However, from the perspective of society, the costs and health effects of a new technology are relevant for the patient's entire life. Hospitals are disinclined to offer new technologies that raise short-term expenses under PPS, even if those technologies save money or have significant long-term benefits. From a hospital's point of view, the measure of benefit associated with new technology is diagnosis-related group (DRG) payment levels, which may even surpass health effectiveness. Hospitals are also incentivized by PPS to move services to outpatient settings, even when doing so could be done more effectively on inpatients. Furthermore, because capital is still reimbursed based on cost, the system benefits capital-intensive technologies.

Of course, some opposing incentives work to encourage hospitals to adopt new technology. Hospitals compete with one another for doctors and patients by providing top-notch services that frequently rely on technological advancements. Technology use is often influenced by concerns about malpractice and the ethical obligation to provide each patient with the best care possible. Hospital doctors might support clinically useful technology regardless of its impact on profits, but they might also be just as indifferent to expenses as they are to income. As a result, there is frequent conflict between doctors' concerns about clinical effectiveness and meeting patient and professional demands and administrators' concerns about revenue and cost. To maximize health outcomes within financial constraints, neither party represents societal concerns.

Although they are unlikely to have much of an impact, two PPS provisions—the annual update factor and the recalibration of DRGs—mitigate the disincentives to use expensive new technologies. Hospital payments per patient are increased by the update factor, which raises the total amount of hospital reimbursement. It does not, however, impact incentives at the margin because the extra money isn't always designated to cover the cost of utilizing new technologies. Major time lags between the diffusion of new technologies and the annual readjustment of DRG weights limit the impact of the readjustment, which is meant to respond to the use of new technologies for specific diagnoses. These updates are not very effective at changing the system's inherent distortions toward underutilization because hospitals still bear the same DRG weight regardless of whether they use the technology or not.

Empirical evidence regarding the spread of new technologies under PPS is scarce. The number of community hospitals providing lithotripsy, open heart surgery, cardiac catheterization, and organ transplants has continued to grow in recent years, according to the Prospective Payment Assessment Commission. However, some evidence suggests that PPS has slowed the adoption of potentially cost-effective technologies. For instance, despite FDA approval and positive reviews from the Office of Health Technology Assessment and multiple medical associations, it has been reported that PPS has effectively stopped the spread of cochlear implants. The authors attribute the under diffusion to Medicare's choice to place patients with cochlear implants in a DRG whose reimbursement only pays a portion of the device's cost.

PPS, like all fixed-price systems, finds it difficult to adapt to shifts in resource usage that come with new technology. A few legislators have pushed for the creation of new or temporary DRGs as well as additional payments for significant new technologies like cochlear implants. Reimbursing technologies on an add-on payment basis, however, does not eliminate the other distortions from the cost-effective resource allocation mentioned above; rather, it reestablishes a cost basis for payment. Modeled after the Canadian system, global budgeting for hospitals is an alternative to prospective rate setting. Hospitals and other organizations are given a fixed budget under global budgeting, with the freedom to use it however they see fit. Global budgets reduce the incentive to concentrate on reimbursement levels because they do not link fixed payments to the use of specific technologies. They also frequently broaden the temporal context in which choices about the distribution of resources are made. They might therefore provide hospitals with more suitable incentives to devote limited funds to purchasing new technology. Global budgets, however, do not eliminate every distortion. For instance, the hospital's perspective is still restricted to inpatients. Furthermore, at least under the Canadian system, hospitals can get a yearly pass-through for justified cost increases, which lessens the incentive to be efficient. There is some evidence that new technologies spread more slowly in Canada than they do in the US, but it's unclear whether this is because of a more appropriate rate or because the most affordable technologies are embraced. Research indicates that, for instance, the US has eight times more MRI machines per person than Canada does, a difference that is unlikely to be explained by variations in disease or population. It is yet unknown which utilization rate—the American or Canadian—is more economical.

7.4.3.5. HMOs and Managed Care Plans

In terms of cost-effectiveness analysis, the viewpoints of health maintenance organizations (HMOs) and society are comparable in several significant ways. HMOs have an incentive to think about the long-term health and financial implications of decisions about new technologies because they are paid a set amount per enrollee. Furthermore, capitated plans offer hospital and ambulatory care for patients.

However, there are a few key differences between the societal perspective and the HMO perspective. An important distinction is that a large amount of enrollee turnover distorts the HMO perspective; in other words, an HMO is not a closed system as it might seem. The high disenrollment rate in many capitated plans could have significant effects on how inexpensively new technologies are adopted. From the perspective of society as a whole, technologies that raise short-term costs but reduce them over time may be cost-effective, but not for HMOs. It is reasonable to assume that an HMO's cost-effectiveness analysis of a new technology will discount expenses after the point of disenrollment, as well as potential health risks. Another distinction is that not all medical services, including stays in long-term care facilities, are covered by HMOs. Technology influencing these expenses (e.g., which averts stays in nursing homes) would not be regarded as highly by the HMO. Third, the majority of HMOs use financial incentives to incentivize doctors to limit utilization, which may have an impact on the uptake of new technologies. According to recent data, the type of HMO and certain financial incentives may have an impact on the frequency of outpatient visits and hospitalization rates. Similar to hospitals, there are opposing forces at play: the competition for doctors and patients, as well as worries about ethics and malpractice.

7.4.3.6. Incentives for Fee-for-Service Physicians

Physician reimbursement schemes that are currently in place have a significant impact on how affordable it is to implement new technologies. Fee-for-service doctors are incentivized to use new technologies beyond the point where marginal costs and benefits are equal because they are paid for the services they perform. Additionally, there is an inherent bias in the current reimbursement levels favoring procedure-based services. Reimbursement for technology-driven services is disproportionately higher than for more cognitive services, like clinical evaluation and management, according to a number of studies. Evaluation and management services are paid less than invasive, imaging, and laboratory services when it comes to resource costs. The system also has a bias towards inpatients. Research has indicated that services rendered to outpatients receive significantly less money than those rendered to inpatients.

The recent approval by Congress of a resource-based relative value scale (RBRVS) with a physician service expenditure ceiling will impact the adoption of new technologies in multiple ways. The goal of the new fee schedule is to give doctors a "level economic playing field" depending on the resources they use to deliver care. The goal is to make medical decisions income-neutral for the doctor, with clinical benefit as the foundation for resource allocation. However, maintaining the RBRVS current with resource costs to the doctor could cause temporary distortions that impact the adoption of new technologies.

7.4.3.7. Future Directions: How to Achieve Cost-Effective Diffusion of Medical Technology

While the average cost of new technologies does go up, in certain clinical settings, certain technologies may end up saving more money than they cost. The adoption of new technologies should be guided by cost-effectiveness, but other factors, like equity for the disadvantaged, must also be taken into account. Last but not least, the American healthcare management and reimbursement systems don't always encourage the use of the most economical combination of new and old technologies.

We offer some recommendations for the 1990s as we wrap up. First and foremost, new technologies need to be assessed as soon as feasible and then periodically reassessed. These assessments ought to take into account the effects on health and the economy. Although this nation hasn't yet established a reliable source of funding for these assessments, action must be taken to ensure a sufficient body of data on which to base policy decisions. Second, we need to align the incentives that consumers, providers, and insurers face with societal objectives and resource limitations. Medical professionals are already dedicated to enhancing health via efficient treatment, and organized medicine has acknowledged and embraced the difficulty of operating within financial constraints. Although it might not be without issues, a system built more on global, flexible budgets than on piecemeal regulations could be beneficial. Because HMOs do not fully bear the costs or realize the benefits of the technologies they use, care should be taken when applying the standard HMO model in this context. Therefore, managers should be financially accountable for both induced and external costs and savings in any decentralized global budgeting system. In such a setting, the role of information and guidelines for cost-effective care would be strengthened, and the body of research supporting the real-time provision of such information ought to be increased. Third, the existing Medicare PPS reimbursement system tends to maintain the status quo. New technologies that are more affordable than those that are not have a competitive advantage over the former. In this nation, we must promote innovation, level the playing field, and encourage—not inhibit—the replacement of clinical practices that are inefficient with those that are efficient in terms of cost. Ultimately, it is impossible to ignore the American public's voice. In addition to wanting cost containment, the public is open to new technologies if they can improve their health. Both goals might be achieved by implementing a system that incentivizes and encourages the use of affordable new technologies and healthcare.

7.4.4. The Future of Technological Adoption in the Healthcare Space

Shortly, the COVID-19 pandemic and developing medical technologies have both prepared patients to use new tools. The total amount of funding allocated to health innovation in the first half of 2020 was $9.1 billion, representing a nearly 19% increase over the $7.7 billion invested in the same period in 2019. Steven Krein and Unity Stoakes, co-founders of Start-up Health, note that, in contrast to previous years, there has been a significant uptick in the adoption of technologies in the last several weeks.

Wireless devices are used by digital companies such as Livongo and Proteus Digital to automatically read and report patient vitals and exceptions to clinicians. According to Zane Burke, CEO of Livongo, the pandemic has expedited the adoption of a more comprehensive virtual care delivery model, and remote monitoring will play a significant role in the individualized treatment of high-risk patients. Patients can receive warnings, early monitoring, and population surveillance, and they can be reached wherever they may be, at the exact moment when they need care most. Proteus Digital has created a pill that can be consumed that tracks patients' adherence to their prescription regimen. The use of virtual healthcare is spreading.

Numerous digital health companies are incorporating AI into their devices to improve decision-making and offer more individualized care management and patient guidance. This use of AI extends beyond merely detecting fraud and abuse or offering automated responses to implementing common questions or care management protocols. The trend of utilizing AI in this manner is expected to persist, with both patients and healthcare providers embracing these advancements.

Artificial Intelligence is an ideal tool for assisting with intricate modeling and sorting through data to choose variables for modeling the COVID-19 pandemic. While Stanford University and other pharmaceutical companies, like Editas, are developing a gene-editing technology called CRISPR that inhibits 90% of the coronaviruses, including COVID-19, Biopharma is investigating gene and cell therapies to help deal with HIV, COVID-19, and other viruses. The pandemic has caused some barriers to fall, and scientists worldwide are working together more closely as pharmaceutical companies work to find ways to combat the virus that causes COVID-19. Despite being in different stages of the development of antibodies, Eli Lilly, AstraZeneca, Roche's Genentech unit, Amgen, GlaxoSmithKline, and Lilly partner AbCellera all share information about their manufacturing facilities, capacity, raw materials, and other supplies required to produce successful monoclonal antibodies. The six companies are working together to secure manufacturing capacity so that, upon receiving regulatory approval, they can begin shipping their COVID-19-fighting treatments immediately.

Consequently, the use of diverse technologies by various stakeholders in the healthcare system cannot be reversed now that the genie has been let out of the bottle; the momentum will propel us ahead. The only thing left to determine is how many payers, providers, and members will adopt this new method of communication, education, and guidance about healthcare. As a result, we might witness a brief surge in the adoption of certain technologies and a marginally extended adoption curve for others. Rise in virtual healthcare, and the degree to which other technologies are adopted will differ depending on the population and, consequently, on the industry.

Younger generations live increasingly online lives, so it makes sense that they would shop for healthcare services online as well. Younger generations will demand more digital apps and increased transparency in their use. Additionally, this group will be more receptive to wearable technology and practical ways to obtain medical records and carry out online medical transactions.

Behavior change in older people will be driven by the necessity of maintaining social distancing and "business not as usual." Telehealth-enabled medical appointments for Medicare beneficiaries will proliferate, and as this pandemic has shown, both patients and providers are on board with it. A bill to permanently alter Medicare's telehealth provisions is being drafted, and the Centers for Medicare and Medicaid Services (CMS) is assessing whether the program's expanded telehealth policies should continue.

During the pandemic, third-party data management handled a greater volume of medical data; going forward, this increased portability may result in cost savings for health insurers and providers. Wearable technology that warns users when they are within six feet of other users, appointment reminder systems, and apps that share health information, offer advice, and notify users of possible infections are examples of third-party technologies that help with disease prevention and management. AI can be applied in even more ways in the future. During the pandemic, it was utilized for triage in emergency rooms.

The industry has taken several actions based on its predictions that new technologies will influence US healthcare in the future.

Regarding the prospects, some of the more sophisticated technologies like gene therapy and personalized medicine might have a longer timeline. We must consider the possibilities for the delivery of healthcare if the digital generations take the lead. Given that the majority of today's doctors were born and raised in the digital era, technology adoption may pick up speed. The Mayo Clinic is working with Google and has appointed a digital officer to move data to a secure Mayo cloud. This will protect data and enable cloud-based computing to create new knowledge and insights from the data. The medical community has made several decisions based on the industry's prediction that new technologies will influence American healthcare in the future.

7.4.5. Implications For Actuaries

What forces influence the adoption of technological innovation, and what do actuaries need to know about costs and diffusion of technology?

Providers tend to be risk-averse and resist implementing new technologies due to a certain amount of inertia. One can selectively overcome this inertia. Because they are busy people, providers won't alter their behavior unless compelled to do so by an outside force, such as a law or an emergency involving healthcare. Healthcare technologies have the potential to reduce costs, increase costs while improving quality, and in some cases, even improve both. In the long run, we might need to address funding mechanisms for these technologies with a combination of employers, payers, and providers.

Health plans and providers can monitor high-risk patients remotely and track adherence to treatment protocols, including medication compliance, with the help of big data and technology. Through better data coordination, technology use can enhance the experience for patients with average risk. Artificial Intelligence (AI) has the potential to amalgamate optimal clinical practices and insights, thereby facilitating their accessibility to physicians during treatment. It is simple to create and distribute wellness programs to patients in order to fulfill their individual needs. The demands of modern medicine seldom allow for many conversations about wellness with providers—perhaps only during the yearly physical. To expand the capabilities of providers and support them in patient care, payers, regulatory agencies, pandemics, consumer demand, and technologies like artificial intelligence (AI) can all contribute to the diffusion of technology. As is well known, some technologies gained prominence during the pandemic and will continue to do so; however, we should also anticipate further growth as a result of new "med tech" companies' increased investments in health technologies. As long as there is innovation in the healthcare industry, we should anticipate ongoing demands from consumers (Gondi et al., 2020; Herzlinger et al., 2006).

7.5. The Role of Technology in Healthcare: Advancements and Challenges

The way medical professionals diagnose, treat, and oversee patient care has been completely revolutionized by technology, which has completely changed the healthcare sector. Technological breakthroughs have improved healthcare in many ways, from telemedicine and artificial intelligence to electronic health records. But these developments also bring with them several new difficulties.

7.5.1. Advancements in Medical Diagnosis and Treatment

The possibilities for medical diagnosis and treatment have greatly improved thanks to technological advancements. Modern imaging methods, like CT and MRI scans, offer comprehensive views of the human body and help with precise diagnosis. Furthermore, robotic surgery systems allow for more precise minimally invasive procedures. Personalized medicine and targeted therapies are further products of the marriage of technology and pharmaceutical research.

7.5.2. Electronic Health Records (EHRs) and Data Management

The use of electronic health records has revolutionized the sharing, storing, and access of patient data. Electronic Health Records (EHRs) increase patient safety, improve provider-to-provider communication, and streamline workflows. When applied to electronic health records, data analytics and machine learning algorithms have the power to spot trends, forecast results, and encourage the use of evidence in decision-making. To guarantee the efficient use of EHR systems, interoperability, data privacy, and security issues must be resolved.

7.5.3. Telemedicine and Remote Patient Monitoring

In healthcare, telemedicine has shown to be a game-changer, particularly in remote locations or during emergencies. Geographical barriers are removed by allowing patients to consult with medical professionals through video calls. Wearable sensors and other remote patient monitoring devices make it possible to gather health data in real time and support proactive care management. In addition to increasing patient convenience and lowering healthcare costs, telemedicine also increases access to care.

7.5.4. Artificial Intelligence (AI) and Machine Learning

Healthcare stands to benefit greatly from AI and machine learning algorithms. Large-scale data analysis, pattern recognition, and insightful insights for disease management, treatment planning, and diagnosis are all possible with these technologies. Chatbots and virtual assistants driven by AI also help with patient education and engagement. To guarantee the safe and responsible application of AI in healthcare, however, issues with data quality, algorithm bias, and ethical issues need to be properly addressed.

7.5.5. Cybersecurity and Data Privacy

Concerns regarding data security and privacy have been brought up by the healthcare industry's growing reliance on technology. To safeguard confidential patient data from data breaches and cyberattacks, healthcare institutions need to make significant investments in cybersecurity measures. Maintaining patient privacy while allowing healthcare providers access to data is still a difficult task that needs constant attention.

7.5.6. Digital Divide and Technological Accessibility

Even though technology can lead to better healthcare outcomes, it is imperative to close the digital gap and guarantee that everyone has access to technology-based healthcare solutions. The impact and reach of these advancements may be restricted by disparities in affordability, technological literacy, and internet access. In order to guarantee that technology helps everyone, regardless of socioeconomic status or location, efforts should be made to close these gaps.

With its advancements in diagnosis, treatment, and patient care, technology has a significant influence on the healthcare industry. To optimize the advantages of technology in healthcare, however, issues with data management, cybersecurity, and equitable access need to be resolved. Healthcare providers can improve patient outcomes and improve healthcare delivery by adopting new technologies and offering more accessible, personalized, and efficient care.

7.6. Policy and Managerial Choice Points

Proactive government policy would support these actions. In most industries, active policy regarding technology adoption can be difficult; in the healthcare industry, this is less likely to be the case. As mentioned at the beginning, healthcare, in contrast to most other industries, has a moral responsibility that goes beyond straightforward economic considerations; the COVID-19 pandemic has only served to highlight this fact. It is hard to argue that it can or should operate in the same way as the competitive markets that form the basis of basic economic analysis because of a number of other sectoral peculiarities. Three stand out in particular.

First, as we've already mentioned, the majority of the projected job growth in the healthcare industry will be in positions that were, at least until COVID-19, seen as low status and low skill, positions that are typically held by women and people of color. Therefore, policy could encourage the adoption and application of new technologies in ways that raise the standard of these jobs as well as the productivity and pay of those who hold them. As a result, laws supporting high-road adoption strategies support labor market outcomes in addition to optimizing access, cost, and quality.

The second is the American healthcare system. It is almost entirely subsidized economically, primarily through preferential tax treatment. Anyone who sells a product would want the government to offer incentives for large purchases or for customers to be able to buy it before taxes. Since the majority of us are not able to afford this luxury, citizens and taxpayers have the right to demand that certain restrictions be placed on these market advantages granted by the government. For instance, policy might mandate that employers in the healthcare industry pay into a training fund for people who might otherwise be displaced by technology, or it might mandate the implementation of additional safeguards against worker organizing. In other words, it is only fair to insist that the government handouts be distributed widely if it is going to support an entire industry as it currently does. Benefits from employers to employees won't automatically trickle down, especially if there is no collective bargaining agreement in place.

Finally, the ability of employers to compete serves as justification for active healthcare policy. A country's healthcare system plays a vital role in its economic and social infrastructure from the standpoint of labor supply, encouraging a workforce that is robust physically and psychologically and capable of giving its all to both work and investments in its own human capital. Therefore, in addition to ensuring the steady and dependable flow of electricity, the government must also endeavor to keep the healthcare system thriving. In terms of the competitiveness of the national economy, requiring U.S. employers to compete while forcing them to buy employee health insurance in a struggling market places them at a significant competitive disadvantage compared to their foreign competitors. In light of this, policies that encourage the use of new technologies to raise the effectiveness and performance of the healthcare industry should be supported.

Here established the necessity of taking proactive steps to steer technological change in the industry and have identified three particular decision points for managers and policymakers:

- How willing are policymakers and managers to experiment?
- Which payment model—value-based care or fee-for-service—will they support?, e.g., practice and hospital administrators, be? and
- Which strategy—a work-centered strategy or a technology-centered strategy—will managers and policymakers choose for the adoption and implementation of technology?

Healthcare technologies will have the greatest and most widespread benefits when they are used to fulfill VBC, under the supervision of managers and policymakers who are willing to try new things, and by organizations that take a work-centered approach. The term "broad-based" is used to refer to all relevant parties, including front-line healthcare providers.

7.6.1. Leverage the Power of Payment Models

The divide between those funding healthcare and those delivering it creates a unique challenge not typically seen in studies of technological advancement. In most industries, companies adopt new technologies when the benefits outweigh the costs. However, in healthcare, providers' decisions are heavily influenced by the rules and structures that connect them to payers. This means that if a technology improves access, cost, and quality without directly benefiting the provider, it creates an economic externality.

The most prevalent example of this phenomenon concerns technologies that raise the standard of care provided. A particular hospital or doctor's office might be persuaded that a new machine or gadget yields results that are more accurate or dependable than those produced by outdated technology. However, the facility owners are not able to claim the additional benefits that come with using this technology under the traditional FFS model. That's why they won't buy it. This relationship explains why electronic health records (EHRs) were first adopted by health maintenance organizations (HMOs) and other integrated healthcare providers/payers like Kaiser Permanente and Health Partners. These technologies eventually affected the lives of transcriptionists and medical records technicians, among other occupations. It also clarifies the inclinations towards the adoption of more specialized, smaller-scale technologies.

Here is a great illustration of this. The hospital's chief financial officer clarified that tomosynthesis, or three-dimensional (3D) breast imaging, was a relatively new investment for the facility, even though it produced a sharper and more detailed digital image. When X-rays from different angles are combined, a process known as tomosynthesis is used instead of traditional 2D mammography to identify more cancers earlier and with fewer false positives. Regretfully, the machines are also significantly more expensive than those that are utilized for conventional mammography. This hospital, along with probably many others, would not be able to afford breast imaging because payer reimbursement is fixed at a single level regardless of how providers obtain the images.

On the other hand, if administrators find a piece of technology that can boost the number of procedures their hospital can perform each year or the efficiency with which it can perform a specific procedure, they may decide to invest in it. In this instance, it seems that technology can both lower costs and increase access; in fact, even the conventional FFS model would let the hospital keep the profits from the investment. As a result, there is less of a difference between the advantages this technology has for society and for individuals.

The use of semi-autonomous robots in hospitals is an example of this type of technological investment. Hospitals don't anticipate payers raising their rates just because food and linens are moved around the hospital by robots rather than by people. Instead, developers and administrators of service robots inform us that even with their expensive initial investment and ongoing maintenance costs, robots will prove to be more cost-effective than continuing to employ humans to perform these duties. If they are right, the hospital should benefit economically from the use of robots in this way as well as socially from a wider range of stakeholders—perhaps with the possible exception of those whose jobs are directly impacted by the deployment of robots, such as hospital orderlies. The decisions managers make regarding the treatment of potentially displaced workers during the implementation of new technologies will determine exactly how the deployment affects orderlies.

It is obvious that the division of labor between financing and delivery leads to market imperfections that hinder the industry's adoption of new technologies. Organizations investing in technologies that enhance quality should reap the benefits of improved quality, provided that society as a whole agrees that quality improvement is desirable. The system needs to compensate providers for being able to serve more patients if our goal is to increase access. They won't spend money on technologies until they've accomplished these objectives. Naturally, the third vertex of the Iron Triangle—cost reduction—applies the same principle.

It is up to policymakers to decide how to implement payment rules. They are able to recognize the institutional ability of Medicare and Medicaid to encourage the appropriate and appropriate use of technologies. One hospital administrator informed us that "private payers go where CMS goes." While it isn't always the case, private payers frequently take the Centers for Medicare and Medicaid

Services (CMS) as a model when determining which services to cover and at what cost. Bundled payments and accountable care organizations (ACOs) are two recent examples of value-based care's many forms. Therefore, private payers are likely to follow suit if Medicare and Medicaid adopt a more positive stance toward telehealth—as they did in their response to the pandemic—or new forms of care coordination and delivery that emphasize the importance of home care workers. Naturally, once researchers show how effective these high-road strategies are at optimizing across access, cost, and quality, the domino effect will happen faster.

Furthermore, accelerating the transition from fee-for-service payment models to value-based care models would hold providers accountable for the caliber of care they provide, placing an incentive to deliver high-caliber care—ideally, though debatably, without raising costs or limiting access. More people would then adopt technology as a result of this. As components of "value-based care" (VBC) are found in a growing number of health plans and health reform concepts, this trend is actually well underway. The goal of the ACA and Medicare's growing use of bundled payments is to incentivize providers to take an innovative approach to providing care that maximizes access, cost, and quality. This includes encouraging the formation of ACOs.

Long before VBC was introduced, private insurers realized that cost-conscious health plan participants, whether they were individuals or employers, tended to favor health maintenance organizations (HMOs) and other plans with cost-containment features. Therefore, policymakers can incentivize value in the system and then afford providers' independence toward achieving their goals, as opposed to paying providers based on the quantity of care they provide and then requiring them to adhere to strict treatment protocols. While some will embrace new technologies and others won't, their decisions will be based on their own in-depth understanding of whether or not new technologies will improve patient care. More precisely, by focusing more on VBC, policymakers support the uptake and application of new technologies in response to the four sectoral imperatives. The economies of scale and scope that result from organizational coordination and consolidation are undoubtedly valuable. In other words, if VBC is encouraged even more, businesses will be more inclined to use telepresence and digital technologies to optimize EHRs, which may eventually be enhanced or augmented with AI capabilities. They will also employ pick-and-delivery robots more frequently in hospital settings. On behalf of their patients, providers are also likely to take independent action to invest in telemedicine and telehealth as well as to create or acquire access to mobile health and medical apps, some of which may even use artificial intelligence. By doing this, they will be meeting the need to manage and prevent chronic illnesses on behalf of their patients in collaboration with them. Comparable arguments can be made for the other two sectoral imperatives, which are adapting to demographic trends and expanding access.

The shift from fee-for-service (FFS) to value-based care (VBC) has been gradual, primarily due to lobbying by those with vested interests in the FFS model. Therefore, why hasn't there been a tipping point already? The change in payment models was the main topic of discussion when it came to healthcare technology 10 years ago, according to investors and consultants. One venture capitalist in Austin, Texas said, "We were all thinking in big, systemic terms." Hope was abounding. Nearly nothing on the demonstration floor at the same conference this year was directly related to the switch from FFS to VBC, though it's possible that most of what was there was intended to support such a wide-ranging, sector-specific change.

7.6.2. Encourage Experimentation with Novel Uses of Technology

The slow emergence of HMOs in the 20th century and the creation and growth of ACOs in the 21st are arguably the best examples of policymakers' and managers' long-standing relative openness to experimentation in the healthcare sector. They now have to choose how adventurous they want to be in order to address the four sectoral imperatives.

Restrictive reimbursement policies limit provider organizations' ability to respond to the four imperatives by delaying the adoption of new technologies and reducing their flexibility in doing so. Telemedicine provides an example. For decades, medical professionals have been offering "low-tech" telemedicine, such as calling patients to inform them of test results or prescribing medication in response to their descriptions of symptoms. Nevertheless, prior to the modifications brought about by COVID-19, regulations forbade providers from billing for these services provided over the phone—and they still do, for the most part. In an attempt to divert low-acuity patients from ERs and doctor's offices, CMS and Congress temporarily loosened regulations governing telehealth provider reimbursements.

There are several reasons why policymakers are reluctant to relax regulations and why the current relaxation is only temporary. Many medical professionals worry that telemedicine will hurt their bottom line by forcing patients to see "virtualists" from home instead of PCPs in offices. Payers also fear that if telemedicine is covered, patients will "overconsume" the service and doctors and other providers will "overprovide," possibly trying to charge insurance companies for all the telephonic work they had been doing for free for so long.

CMS responded by gradually relaxing the regulations that prohibited Medicare reimbursement for telehealth services when early, pre-COVID-19 experience indicated that these worries were exaggerated. In certain situations, these benefits can now be used for online consultations, psychotherapy, and other medical or health services by senior and disabled residents who are dependent on government insurance. Even if there had not been a pandemic, we would have seen more providers utilizing telepresence and digital communications to boost access. It is unclear whether COVID-19's forced experimentation will result in long-lasting regulatory changes pertaining to telehealth.

Policymakers should not only address regulations that limit the use of new technologies, but they should also reconsider rules that restrict their full potential. For example, current rules require providers to be licensed in each state, making it difficult for entrepreneurs in telehealth to operate nationwide. This restriction became especially problematic during the COVID-19 pandemic when the need for telehealth services increased. While state-by-state licensing has its reasons, it is important to revisit these regulations in order to improve patient access and reduce costs.

Policymakers could encourage licensing boards to experiment with scope-of-practice rules that currently limit the effectiveness of new technologies, in addition to reconsidering the state-based licensing regime. For instance, as was previously mentioned, California has permitted the limited use of licensed practical/vocational nurses (LPNs/LVNs) in the home when they make use of point-of-care technologies, which essentially expand the scope of medical providers. Broadly speaking, technology has the potential to increase access and decrease costs by facilitating the transfer of responsibilities from registered nurses (RNs) to licensed practical nurses (LPNs) for patients with low acuity. To do this, though, would necessitate giving LPNs more power and permission to dispense a larger variety of low-risk medications. When these proof-of-concept studies show promise, policymakers should take them seriously and encourage licensing boards to expand their scope geographically and functionally.

A relaxing and potential harmonization of federal and state reimbursement regulations and scope of practice requirements might be more practical than the experimental easing of the medical licensing regime. While we shouldn't rush things, we should take into account how new technologies, in the hands of skilled users, can facilitate the assignment of tasks to those who are closer to the patient. In a similar vein, we ought to adopt a "blue sky" strategy when developing new healthcare jobs that leverage cutting-edge innovations, such as artificial intelligence (AI), and link them to patients in ways that benefit patients, payers, and providers without harming anybody.

Ideally, managers will allow experimentation within their own organizations, taking a cue from policymakers. In reality, when it comes to handling the politics of technological change, there is a very thin line dividing the responsibilities of managers and policymakers. Physicians' concerns about telemedicine are a sign of the larger political barriers that prevent the adoption of new technologies, many of which take place within organizations.

Digital technologies have the great advantage of decentralizing knowledge by providing providers at the point of care with the most recent information. But as research showed, RNs were never simply prevented from performing physician-level tasks by a "lack of information." Rather, specific policy-level scope-of-practice regulations define the kinds of tasks that each state's licensed roles are allowed to perform, under supervision or not. Employers typically set the restrictions for unlicensed positions; these are typically found in the collective bargaining agreement (if one exists) itself. Thus, in order to use technology to address the four sectoral imperatives, states need to amend their current laws to make room for new work arrangements that give front-line employees more authority. Similarly, managers and high-status providers—that is, doctors and surgeons—need to permit these modifications to occur at the point of care. Practice administrators, for instance, can accomplish this by showing individuals with high occupational status how new technological applications can eliminate tasks from their daily schedules that they likely view as low-value, time-consuming chores, freeing them up to take on more difficult and lucrative work for themselves.

Lastly, and in connection with this, home care offers an ideal environment for testing out new technologies to be applied to broader duties related to providing care. Speaking with union leaders reveals the barriers to the high-road application of technology that turns caregivers at home into on-site coordinators. Personal care and home health aides frequently feel uneasy utilizing new technology. Smartphones and tablets are unaffordable even for technically competent workers, and paying for a regular data plan will be particularly difficult given the wages of home care providers. As a result, in addition to investing in the required training, the home health agency hiring the aide would also need to buy the device and the app. Regretfully, the agency lacks both the incentive and the negotiating power to force additional public funding from the states under the current reimbursement model. This suggests that by moving work to less expensive, underutilized home care aides, there may have been a missed opportunity to lower overall costs and improve the quality of care. More importantly, it prohibits the application of technology to raise skill levels and pay in these positions, which many feel is the only way to draw more people into the home care industry.

7.6.3. Prioritize the Work, Not the Technology

Employees have both explicit and tacit knowledge of the care delivery process, so winning their cooperation would be essential to the project's success. Employers understand that, even if they are unsure of how to go about it, they should respect workers and value and utilize the information they provide. Consequently, no manager or employer offered to reduce headcount in order to defend their preference for technology. Instead, they focus on issues related to quality or cost, typically using language that is described as "enabling," outlining more productive, patient-centered ways that front-line healthcare workers could spend their time if new technologies were available to replace less-skilled, possibly even mind-numbing work. Nonetheless, the majority of employers adopt a technology-centered strategy by default, possibly unintentionally. Aside from the obvious tautology, this refers to managers or employers looking to use technology to handle any task that it can competently handle, based of course on the marginal benefits vs. marginal expenses. After shifting the tasks that can be reasonably transferred from labor to capital, human labor is still required for the remaining tasks. Refer to the alternate strategy as work-centered. Here, managers start by asking, "What are my people really good at?" and then look for the technology that best utilizes these skills, sometimes by taking on tasks that employees are not particularly good at or enjoy doing. These tech-advantaged jobs were usually those that needed a lot of strength or would put human labor in danger in the manufacturing sector in the past. As previously mentioned, in more recent times, we have come to define tech-advantaged tasks as those that, while still cognitive, can be easily proceduralized due to their mind-numbing repetition. It also includes jobs where employees must quickly process vast amounts of information; while they might not find these jobs monotonous in and of themselves, employees will probably be more prone to mistakes than with competing technologies. Lastly, humans are not particularly adept at remaining "on watch"—that is, keeping an eye on generally peaceful circumstances, waiting for something dubious or problematic to happen, and then reflexively reacting.

What skills do healthcare workers possess in particular? Since they are most likely to know the answer, employers ought to give workers a voice in the selection of new technologies. Workers can generally perform a wide range of inconsistent and frequently unpredictable tasks. A lot of these tasks call for discernment and a keen understanding of the nuances of the patient's emotions. Most importantly, primary healthcare providers provide patients with genuine empathy and emotional support. Managers who adopt a work-centered approach acknowledge these facts (Landi et al., 2020; Nunn et al., 2020).

A Closer Look

Implications for Future Spending on Healthcare

Future increases in healthcare costs will be the main factor influencing the country's long-term fiscal balance. If past trends of rising healthcare costs continue, the policies currently in place governing spending on Medicare and Medicaid will not be able to support these programs for many years to come. Simple modifications to the Medicare and Medicaid programs, like stricter eligibility requirements, higher cost sharing, or adjustments to provider payments, could partially reduce federal spending by shifting expenses from the federal government to private citizens. Such cost-shifting strategies, however, are unlikely to be sustainable in the long run, and slower cost growth in the healthcare industry as a whole will almost certainly need to be linked to limiting federal spending on healthcare while preserving widespread access to care under these programs.

Reducing the amount of current spending or slowing the rate of growth in spending are the two main outcomes of efforts to control healthcare costs. Creating long-term cost-control policies necessitates a clear separation between elements of the spending level and factors that propel spending growth because one sort of effect is easily confused for another. Cost pressures are lessened by one-time spending reductions, such as those attained by doing away with ineffective or wasteful procedures. Managed care organizations, for instance, have historically cut costs by reducing hospital admission rates, which removes ostensibly pointless or undervalued hospital stays. While this lowers costs, it has no effect on the factors—like technological advancements—that tend to drive up costs over time. If other factors affecting growth are not addressed, faster spending growth will resume once attainable savings have been exhausted. Reducing spending by focusing on waste requires ever-greater efficiencies.

Based on current estimates, the primary drivers of long-term spending growth are changes brought about by technology in clinical practice, an increase in the portion of funding from third-party payers (resulting in a decrease in the out-of-pocket portion of medical spending), rising income, and rising costs in the healthcare industry. Of these, cost sharing and technological advancement are arguably the most flexible in terms of policy. The healthcare system's adoption of new technologies will likely need to be addressed in any long-term strategy to control healthcare spending, since technological change is the biggest contributor.

If expensive new medical services were adopted more carefully than in the past and if the spread of currently expensive services was slowed, future increases in spending might be restrained. Despite the fact that using this strategy would result in fewer medical services being offered, data indicates that savings can be achieved without significantly sacrificing clinical value. The financial incentives that patients and providers currently face often encourage or at least facilitate the adoption of new, expensive medical services, and before these services become widely used in clinical practice, the additional clinical benefits are not always balanced against the additional costs. Older, less expensive alternatives may sometimes provide comparable results for patients; costly services that are well-established to be very effective in certain patient populations may occasionally be given to other patients for whom the benefits to clinical practice have not been thoroughly established.

To guarantee that future technologies and expensive services are used only when they provide clinical benefits greater than those of other, less expensive options, more data on the relative efficacy of alternative medical treatments may be helpful. Future spending levels could be lower than they otherwise would be if there was a stronger focus on the evidence-based delivery of healthcare (encouraged, for instance, by suitable financial incentives for providers and consumers). However, this could also lead to the more selective use of some expensive services. The findings of comparative effectiveness analyses would eventually need to influence medical treatment and lower healthcare costs by persuading physicians and patients to use fewer services or less intensive and costly services than are currently anticipated. In order to influence the incentives facing physicians and patients, enacting those changes would likely necessitate action from public and private insurers incorporating the results into their coverage and payment policies. Such measures could be contentious among patients and providers and are probably going to be challenging to execute.

Medicare's payment policies have not taken costs into account when determining which services are covered, and the program has only used a limited amount of comparative effectiveness data. However, if statutory changes allowed it, Medicare could use comparative effectiveness data to encourage higher-value care. Medicare might, for instance, base provider payments on the price of the most economical or successful course of care. The change in Medicare's payment policy would have the same practical effect as a decision about coverage if the payment was less than the cost of providing a more expensive service, which is likely what would happen if doctors and hospitals decided not to provide it. As an alternative, enrollees might have to foot the bill for more expensive but ineffective procedures (though this would have varying effects on patient incentives and care utilization depending on whether and how much they had supplemental insurance that covered all or part of Medicare's cost-sharing requirements).

Summary

- Factors affecting technology transfer can be placed into categories, including characteristics of the technology, characteristics of the technology developer, characteristics of individuals using the technology, characteristics of organizations (and their members) using the technology, attitudes, research policies, and regulation and reimbursement policies.
- Health technology is defined as the application of organized knowledge and skills in the form of devices, medicines, vaccines, procedures, and systems developed to solve a health problem and improve quality of lives.
- Medical technology, or "medtech," encompasses a wide range of healthcare products and is used to treat diseases and medical conditions affecting humans. Such technologies are intended to improve the quality of healthcare delivered through earlier diagnosis, less invasive treatment options, and reduction in hospital stays and rehabilitation times.
- Medical technology has evolved into smaller portable devices, for instance, smartphones, touchscreens, tablets, laptops, digital ink, voice and face recognition, and more.
- The scale and capabilities of artificial intelligence (AI) systems are growing rapidly, notably due to advances in big data. In healthcare, it is expected to provide easier accessibility of information and to improve treatments while reducing costs. The integration of AI in healthcare tends to improve the quality and efficiency of complex tasks.
- Modern robotics have made huge progress and contributions to healthcare. Robots can help doctors in performing a variety of tasks. Robotics adoption is increasing tremendously in hospitals.
- Successful innovations in healthcare are not just about making a product or service better; they must also be usable and appealing. This means that they must be able to be adopted by stakeholders as best practices, commercialized, and adapted for use in a health service setting.
- New technologies are driving the healthcare industry forward, especially in the prevention and treatment of diseases. With the use of AI and digital health solutions, healthcare providers are able to identify and treat diseases more effectively. In addition, these technologies improve the clinical experience of doctors and nurses. In the past decade, these technologies have led to breakthroughs in disease detection, prevention, and treatment.
- The scope of digital health is rapidly expanding, encompassing mobile health (mHealth) applications, wearable devices, telemedicine, electronic health records, health information systems, and artificial intelligence (AI). These technologies save lives.
- Innovations can be driven either by technological advancements or societal calls for action. One of the most well-known and impactful inventions in world history is the printing press, which arose from a confluence of other technological progress such as the development of manufactured paper and ink.
- Technology has transformed the healthcare industry, revolutionizing the way medical professionals diagnose, treat, and manage patient care. From electronic health records to telemedicine and artificial intelligence, advancements in technology have brought numerous benefits to healthcare.

References

1. Cordani, D. (2020,). Healthcare is on an unsustainable trajectory, requiring a renewed push for transformation. *Modern Healthcare*. Retrieved from: https://www.modernhealthcare.com (accessed on 1 July 2024).
2. Garrett, P., Brown, C. A., Hart-Hester, S., et al. (2006). Identifying barriers to the adoption of new technology in rural hospitals: A case report. *Perspectives in Health Information Management, 3,* 9.
3. Gondi, S., & Song, Z. (2019). The burgeoning role of venture capital in health care. *Health Affairs Blog*. Retrieved from: https://www.healthaffairs.org (accessed on 1 July 2024).
4. Herzlinger, R. E. (2006). Why innovation in health care is so hard. *Harvard Business Review, 84*(5), 58–66.
5. Kansteiner, F. (2020). AstraZeneca, Lilly, GSK and more will share COVID-19 antibody secrets to speed manufacturing scale-up. *FiercePharma.com*. Retrieved from: https://www.fiercepharma.com (accessed on 1 July 2024).
6. Landi, H. (2020). Investors double down on health technology as global funding reaches $9.1B in 2020. *Fierce Health Care*. Retrieved from: https://www.fiercehealthcare.com (accessed on 1 July 2024).
7. Nunn, R., Parsons, J., & Shambaugh, J. (2020). A dozen facts about the economics of the U.S. health-care system. *Brookings*. Retrieved from: https://www.brookings.edu (accessed on 1 July 2024).
8. Pennic, J. (2019). Mayo Clinic appoints Rita Khan as first-ever chief digital officer. *HIT Consultant*. Retrieved from: https://hitconsultant.net (accessed on 1 July 2024).
9. Rogers, E. (2003). *Diffusion of Innovations*. New York: Free Press.
10. Sawyer, B., & Cox, C. (2018). How does health spending in the U.S. compare to other countries? *Peterson-KFF Health System Tracker*. Retrieved from: https://www.healthsystemtracker.org (accessed on 1 July 2024).
11. Varma, S. (2020). Early impact of CMS expansion of Medicare telehealth during COVID-19. *Health Affairs Blog*. Retrieved from: https://www.healthaffairs.org (accessed on 1 July 2024).

Chapter 8

THEORY AND PRINCIPLES OF ECONOMIC EVALUATION

Contents

Introduction

To better understand and explain how people make decisions about their health and use of healthcare, health economics makes use of economic concepts and methodologies. It also offers a framework for considering the distribution of society's limited health resources to address the demand and need for healthcare services, prevention, and promotion of health. Health economics and economic evaluation are closely related fields. Economic evaluation produces evidence-based data to support and enhance the decision-making process when allocating healthcare resources, primarily through cost-effectiveness or cost-benefit analysis. Every decision pertaining to public health has resource implications, and it is crucial to take these into account. Economic evaluation and health economics are two significant areas. For those who want to work in the health field professionally, including healthcare workers, medical professionals, policy makers, and others, their theoretical viewpoints and empirical methodology are indispensable.

Orientation and Directional Terms:

Term	Definition	Illustration
Cost-utility analysis	An economic analysis in which the incremental cost of a program from a particular point of view is compared to the incremental health improvement expressed in the unit of quality adjusted life years (QALYs).	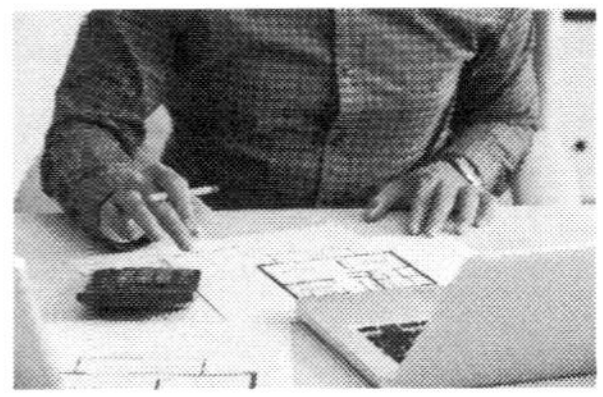
Probabilistic sensitivity analysis	Demonstrates the parameter uncertainty in a decision problem. The technique involves sampling parameters from their respective distributions (rather than simply using mean/median parameter values).	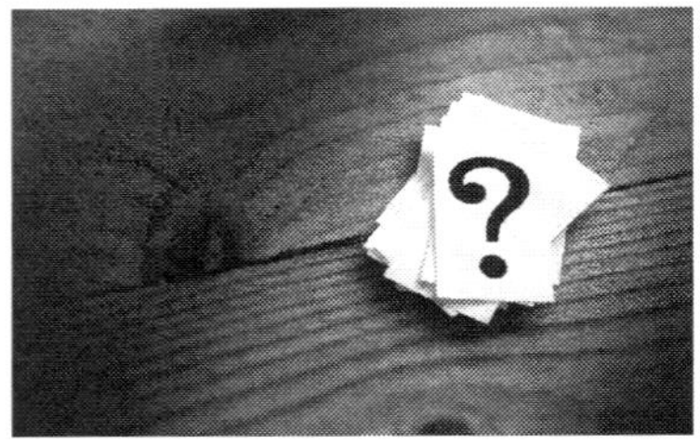
Incremental cost-utility ratio	Used to compare incremental cost and incremental utility to systematize the economic efficiency of medical interventions.	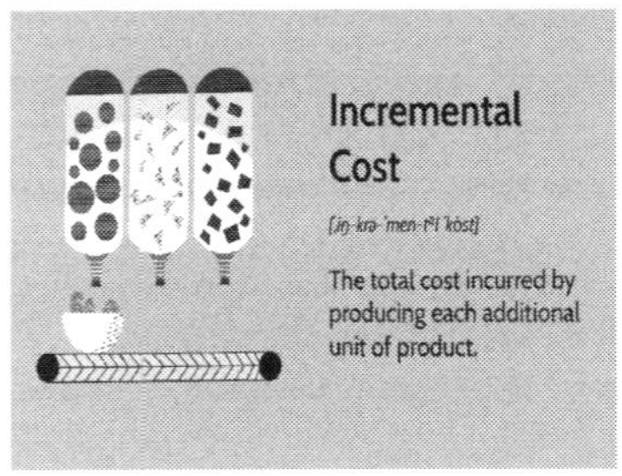
Public health intervention	Any effort or policy that attempts to improve mental and physical health on a population level.	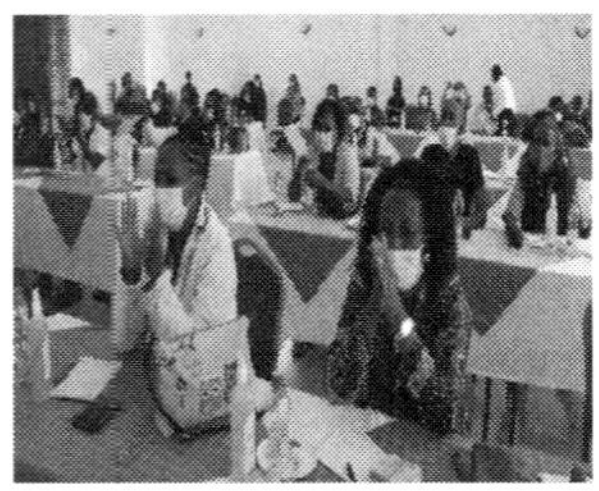
Gross domestic product	A monetary measure of the market value of all the final goods and services produced and rendered in a specific time period by a country or countries.	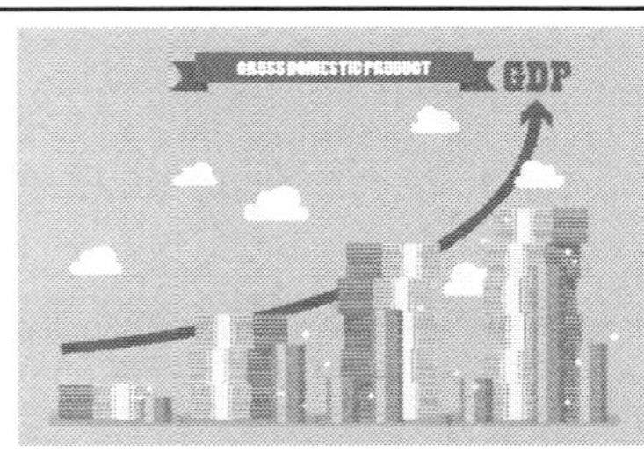

8.1. Health Economic Evaluation: Concept and Basic Principles

In order to help with decision-making, the multidisciplinary field of economic evaluation evaluates the costs and effects of healthcare interventions. It includes a number of techniques, each with a distinct focus and methodology, such as cost-effectiveness analysis (CEA), cost-utility analysis (CUA), and cost-benefit analysis (CBA). The costs and outcomes of alternative interventions are compared using CEA in natural units (e.g., life years gained or cases cured), offering insights into the relative effectiveness of various programs or treatments. Conversely, CUA builds upon CEA by assessing results using a common metric—such as quality-adjusted life years, or QALYs—those accounts for both the amount and quality of life gained. This makes it possible to compare various healthcare interventions, facilitating the allocation of resources in a way that prioritizes those that provide the greatest health gains for the least amount of money.

Concurrently, CBA considers a wider range of costs and benefits, including non-health-related elements like productivity increases or environmental effects, in addition to health outcomes. Health economic evaluation techniques assist stakeholders in balancing competing healthcare interventions while accounting for sustainability, equity, cost, and effectiveness. Economic evaluation helps to improve population health outcomes and the efficient use of resources by giving decision-makers evidence-based insights into the cost-effectiveness of healthcare interventions. However, methodological difficulties, data constraints, and ethical issues are some of the challenges that economic evaluation must overcome. Nonetheless, health economic evaluation continues to be a vital tool for directing policy and practice toward more effective, equitable, and sustainable healthcare delivery as healthcare systems work to optimize the allocation of limited resources to meet rising demands.

8.1.1. Cost-Benefit Analysis (CBA)

A methodical process for assessing how medical procedures, treatments, or health policies will affect the economy. By comparing the expenses and advantages of these interventions, it seeks to give decision-makers important information about how to allocate resources and set priorities in the healthcare industry. Fundamentally, a cost-benefit analysis of a given healthcare intervention or policy entails determining and measuring both of its costs and benefits. Costs include a broad range of elements, such as direct costs like prescription drugs, employee pay, and facility upkeep, as well as indirect costs like lost productivity and the opportunity costs of using resources in other ways. However, benefits could also include better patient outcomes, like lower rates of morbidity and death, better quality of life, and higher levels of productivity as a result of improving health. Although some aspects, like pain relief or emotional well-being, may be difficult to accurately quantify, these benefits are frequently evaluated in monetary terms. Following the identification and quantification of costs and benefits, the CBA compares them to see if the intervention or policy under consideration should be implemented because the benefits outweigh the costs. When an intervention's benefits outweigh its costs, it is considered economically efficient, meaning that resources are being used to maximize societal welfare. Decision-makers may need to reconsider the intervention's viability or look into other options if the costs exceed the benefits in order to more economically attain the intended results. The most significant benefit of CBA is that it gives decision-makers a methodical framework for comparing alternative healthcare options and determining which ones provide the best value for the money. CBA also helps to promote accountability and transparency in healthcare decision-making by clearly stating the trade-offs associated with resource allocation.

An economic analysis known as a cost-benefit analysis (CBA) expresses the costs and consequences in monetary terms. The treatment's financial benefit is expressed in the numerator, and the treatment's financial outlay is specified in the denominator. The role of CBA is to provide a monetary value to both incremental costs and outcomes, enabling a direct computation of the net cost of achieving a health outcome. One could consider a gain in life years to be the price of that life year's productive value to society. Techniques like willingness-to-pay, which measures how much people would be willing to pay for a quality-of-life benefit, are among the methods used to analyze improvements in quality of life (Table 8.1).

Table 8.1. *Summary of Various Types of Pharmacoeconomic Analyses*

Cost Minimization Analysis (CMA)	Cost Effectiveness Analysis (CEA)	Cost Utility Analysis (CUA)	Cost Benefit Analysis (CBA)
Compares the costs of two or more alternatives that produce equivalent health outcomes. No value is given to benefits; only costs, measured in monetary units, are compared.	Most common analysis used to decide between different treatments for the same condition. Measures cost per unit of effect. Costs measured in monetary units, benefits measured as outcome measures or in natural units (e.g., life-years gained, symptom-free days).	A type of CEA. Can compare treatments for different disorders, as the outcome measure is the same. Costs measured in monetary units, benefits measured as "utilities." Best known utility measure is the QALY.	Not often used in modern health economics. Both costs and consequences are measured in monetary units. Can use willingness-to-pay to value benefits. Any treatment with benefits greater than costs is considered "worthwhile."

Source: https://www.sciencedirect.com/topics/nursing-and-health-professions/cost-benefit-analysis#:~:text=Pharmacoeconomics%20in%20Healthcare&text=Cost%20benefit%20analysis%20(CBA)%20is,monetary%20investment%20for%20the%20treatment.

8.1.2. Cost-Effectiveness Analysis (CEA)

A quantitative technique used in healthcare to compare the costs and health outcomes of various interventions or treatments is called cost-effectiveness analysis, or CEA. It assesses the cost of achieving a specific health outcome, giving decision-makers important information about the relative efficacy of various healthcare strategies. Assessing the cost per unit of health outcome gained—typically expressed in natural units like life years gained, cases cured, or days without symptoms—is the main goal of CEA. Policymakers, healthcare providers, and other stakeholders can make well-informed decisions about resource allocation and prioritize interventions that offer the highest health gains per unit of cost by using comparative effectiveness analysis (CEA), which compares the costs and outcomes of various interventions. When evaluating healthcare interventions, CEA takes into account both the direct costs—such as medical bills, staff salaries, and equipment costs—as well as the indirect costs, such as lost productivity or patient travel expenses. Decision-makers can identify interventions that offer the best value for money by balancing these costs against the health benefits that the intervention generates.

It's important to note that CEA takes into account the trade-offs between costs and health outcomes in order to identify interventions that offer the most efficient use of resources, as opposed to prioritizing interventions only based on their cost. Nevertheless, there are a number of drawbacks to CEA, such as difficulties obtaining data, unpredictability in projecting future expenses and results, and the requirement to make assumptions regarding the efficacy of interventions. Furthermore, not all pertinent expenses and results—especially those that are hard to measure or commercialize—may be captured by CEA. In spite of these drawbacks, CEA continues to be a useful instrument for healthcare decision-making and resource allocation, assisting in making sure that scarce resources are used efficiently to enhance population health and attain the best possible health outcomes while staying within financial limits. Healthcare systems are under constant pressure to provide high-quality care while keeping costs down, and CEA is essential in directing practice and policy toward more cost-effective and sustainable healthcare delivery.

8.1.3. Opportunity Cost

The opportunity cost of resources is taken into account in economic evaluation. This entails determining what more could have been accomplished with the funds allocated to a specific project or set of policies. Decision-makers can rank projects that offer the most benefit over their alternatives by taking opportunity costs into account. Opportunity cost is a key idea in economics that describes the cost of choosing not to pursue the next best option when making a decision. Opportunity cost is an important factor to consider when allocating resources and making decisions in the healthcare industry, especially when funding, time, or staff are scarce. Healthcare organizations and policymakers naturally forfeit the chance to use those resources elsewhere when they decide to fund a specific intervention, program, or course of treatment. The opportunity cost is the sum of these missed opportunities. Let's say, for instance, that a hospital decides to set aside some cash for the purchase of new medical supplies. The potential alternative uses of that budget, like adding more employees, funding training courses, or improving other facilities, would be the opportunity cost of this choice. Decision-makers can evaluate the trade-offs associated with resource allocation and work to optimize the total benefit from their use by taking the opportunity cost into account.

Opportunity cost is a useful concept for resource allocation in the healthcare industry, since demand frequently outpaces supply. Decision-makers can identify interventions or programs that provide the best value for their money and most effectively improve health outcomes by comparing the costs and benefits of various options. Opportunity cost should be taken into account when allocating resources to prevent inefficiencies and missed opportunities to meet urgent healthcare needs. Furthermore, opportunity cost takes into account non-financial aspects like patient outcomes, expertise, and time in addition to monetary considerations. For example, the time that medical professionals spend on administrative duties may be considered an opportunity cost because it takes away from their ability to provide direct patient care. It is crucial to carefully consider alternative uses of resources because selecting one healthcare intervention over another may have an impact on patient outcomes and the standard of care.

8.1.4. Sensitivity Analysis

Uncertainty surrounds economic evaluations; costs, benefits, and other variables can change. Sensitivity analysis is the process of examining how changing important assumptions or inputs affects the results and tests how robust the results are. This aids in the understanding of the range of possible outcomes and the causes of uncertainty by decision-makers. Sensitivity analysis is a quantitative technique for evaluating, in the face of uncertainty, the robustness and dependability of a decision model's or economic evaluation's results. Sensitivity analysis is a useful technique for determining how changes in input parameters or assumptions affect study results, particularly in the healthcare industry where decisions frequently involve complex and uncertain factors. Sensitivity analysis's main objective is to investigate the range of possible outcomes under various scenarios or assumptions. This helps decision-makers determine which factors have the greatest impact on the outcomes and assess how stable their conclusions are. Sensitivity analysis helps stakeholders understand which factors contribute to variability in outcomes and offers insights into the degree of uncertainty surrounding a decision by methodically varying key input parameters, such as cost estimates, probabilities, or effectiveness measures.

Healthcare research uses a variety of sensitivity analysis techniques, such as probabilistic sensitivity analysis (PSA), multi-way sensitivity analysis, and one-way sensitivity analysis. By changing one input parameter at a time while keeping the others constant, one-way sensitivity analysis enables researchers to evaluate the influence of specific factors on the outcomes. This method is expanded upon by multi-way sensitivity analysis, which simultaneously modifies several input parameters to investigate correlations and interactions between variables. Contrarily, PSA entails repeatedly running the economic evaluation or decision model and selecting input parameter values from probability distributions that represent uncertainty on each run. Instead of producing a single point estimate, this probabilistic approach generates a distribution of potential outcomes and offers a more thorough assessment of uncertainty. Researchers and decision-makers can better grasp the limitations of their analyses and the reliability of their conclusions by using sensitivity analysis. Sensitivity analysis directs efforts to gather more information or hone modeling assumptions in order to increase the accuracy and dependability of results by highlighting important variables and areas of uncertainty. Sensitivity analysis also makes it easier to communicate results transparently, which helps stakeholders make better decisions and comprehend how uncertainty affects the outcomes that matter.

8.1.5. Incremental Analysis

Economic evaluation frequently contrasts an intervention's costs and benefits with a baseline or do-nothing scenario. To help decision-makers understand the added value of the intervention, this incremental approach focuses on the additional costs and benefits that can be attributed to it. By comparing the additional or incremental costs and benefits that a proposed change or alternative would generate in comparison to the status quo, incremental analysis, also known as marginal analysis, is a decision-making technique used to assess the costs and benefits of the change or alternative. Incremental analysis is frequently used in the healthcare industry to evaluate the effects of implementing new programs, treatments, or interventions in comparison to current procedures. Focusing on the additional costs and benefits connected with the suggested change rather than the overall costs and benefits is the fundamental tenet of incremental analysis. Decision-makers can more precisely evaluate the net impact of the suggested change and decide if it is a cost-effective use of resources by separating the incremental effects.

Incremental analysis is frequently utilized in cost-effectiveness assessments in the healthcare industry to compare the expenses and results of various interventions. An incremental cost-effectiveness analysis, for instance, can be performed by researchers to evaluate the health benefits and additional expenses associated with implementing a new medical treatment in comparison to standard care. Using this analysis, decision-makers can decide if the new treatment's added benefits outweigh its higher costs or if more affordable alternatives are available. Other healthcare decision contexts, such as resource allocation, program evaluation, and policy planning, can also benefit from the application of incremental analysis. For example, decision-makers may use incremental analysis to rank investments according to the additional health outcomes attained per unit of cost when dividing up scarce funds among competing healthcare programs. Incremental analysis has the benefit of drawing attention to the marginal impact of a proposed change, which aids in decision-making by enabling better resource allocation and priority setting. Incremental analysis offers a simple and straightforward framework for assessing the possible effects of alternative options and determining the most effective use of resources by solely taking into account the incremental costs and benefits.

That being said, it's critical to recognize the limitations of incremental analysis. It might, for instance, ignore interactions between interventions or larger systemic effects that could have an impact on the final results. Furthermore, the results and assumptions made about the costs and advantages of the suggested change are crucial to incremental analysis and can be prone to error or variability.

8.1.6. Intangible Costs and Benefits

It is not always possible to put costs and benefits into monetary terms. It may be necessary for economic evaluation to take into account intangible elements like social cohesiveness, environmental effects, and quality of life. Even though they can be difficult to quantify, these elements may be essential for fully understanding the effects of a project or policy. The term "intangible costs and benefits" refers to elements of healthcare interventions or choices that are hard to measure or put into monetary terms. Tangible costs and benefits can be quantified, but intangible costs and benefits are more difficult to quantify using conventional economic measures because they frequently reflect subjective experiences, psychological effects, or larger societal values. The experiences of patients, the standard of care, and general well-being are greatly influenced by intangible costs and benefits in the healthcare industry. Pain and suffering, psychological distress, or a lower quality of life as a result of a disease or treatment are examples of intangible costs. Due to a variety of subjective factors, including social support networks, cultural background, and personal preferences, these costs can differ significantly between people. For instance, side effects like nausea, exhaustion, and hair loss can cause a patient receiving chemotherapy to suffer greatly from significant emotional distress and a lowered quality of life. Decisions about healthcare should take these effects into account even though they might not have a direct financial cost because they can significantly affect the patient's general well-being.

Conversely, intangible benefits refer to advantageous consequences that are difficult to measure in monetary terms but are still significant to people or the community. These advantages could come from healthcare interventions that lead to increases in social connectedness, mental clarity, or patient satisfaction. For example, even if treatment does not prolong life or improve clinical outcomes, a patient receiving palliative care at the end of life may benefit significantly from the emotional support and symptom management offered by healthcare providers. Even though they are difficult to quantify, intangible costs and benefits are crucial factors to take into account when making decisions about healthcare. Ignoring these elements may result in a partial comprehension of the complete effects of medical interventions on patients, caregivers, and the community at large. It is necessary to give considerable thought to patient preferences, values, and priorities, as well as techniques for obtaining and appraising these factors, when incorporating intangible costs and benefits into decision-making processes. It is possible to integrate intangible costs and benefits into healthcare decision-making in a number of ways. The intangible elements that are most important to patients and caregivers can be found and prioritized with the use of qualitative research techniques like focus groups, interviews, and patient questionnaires. Furthermore, preference-based metrics like patient-reported outcome measures (PROMs) and quality of life assessments can offer insightful information about the individualized experiences and preferences of patients undergoing healthcare interventions.

8.1.7. Economic Evaluation of Health Interventions

The use of a health program, action, or technology to lessen or completely eradicate a health issue is known as a health intervention. Improving people's health and quality of life is the ultimate goal of health interventions. The dynamic, intricate, difficult, and demanding environment in which healthcare organizations function exists, nevertheless. Healthcare organizations consequently confront numerous difficulties with regard to efficacy, efficiency, quality, and equity. For health managers and policymakers, there are a number of obstacles to overcome due to the growing need for efficient and high-quality healthcare as well as growing costs and resource shortages. In order to guarantee that everyone has access to healthcare services, it is imperative that these services be provided effectively. Nevertheless, there aren't enough resources to meet everyone's needs. The objective of the economic evaluation is to ascertain, quantify, appraise, and contrast the expenses and outcomes of multiple substitute initiatives or programs. Economic evaluation plays a significant role in determining priorities and allocating limited resources in the healthcare sector, where policymakers must select between programs with varying effects due to resource constraints. Health policymakers are able to execute more successful health interventions with the aid of economic evaluation.

Cost-benefit analysis (CBA) and cost-effectiveness analysis (CEA) are the two broad categories into which economic evaluation studies are separated. It is preferable to start an economic evaluation of health interventions with a cost-benefit analysis. The advantages and disadvantages of an intervention are compared using the cost-benefit method. An intervention with a higher monetary value will be selected after the costs and outcomes of the health intervention are valued. It is advisable to implement a healthcare intervention that has a benefit-to-cost ratio exceeding one. Low-cost, high-benefit interventions that improve people's health and quality of life can be subjected to cost-effectiveness analysis. More affordable and efficient interventions are recommended. If it is not possible to monetize the intervention's results, the CEA may be employed. It establishes the worth of a health intervention by displaying the cost of the intervention in relation to the health outcomes. Clinical criteria are used to quantify the advantages of healthcare interventions in CEA. It is preferable to employ CEA when the primary objective of a health intervention is to lengthen people's lives. Cost-utility analysis (CUA), on the other hand, is preferable if the health intervention has an impact on the patient's quality of life. CUA considers both the quantity and quality of health outcomes. The Incremental Cost-Utility Ratio (ICUR) is the result of measuring health outcomes in CUA using the Quality Adjusted Life (QALYs) index. Ultimately, the decision regarding whether or not to approve the cost-effectiveness of a health intervention is made by comparing the ICUR with the consumers' willingness to pay service (threshold). Stated differently, a QALY's monetary value is determined by establishing the cost-effectiveness threshold. Funding should be allocated to interventions whose cost per QALY (ICER) is less than this limit since they are economical.

By maximizing resource allocation, rationing, and prioritization, as well as by enhancing equity and access, economic evaluations contribute to the effectiveness of the health system. In recent years, numerous studies on economic evaluation have been carried out. Some studies, though, have shortcomings. A few of these investigations lacked the necessary analytical techniques. Some of the limitations of economic evaluation studies include using the wrong perspective and evaluation method, excluding some significant costs, not disclosing the sources of data, and neglecting to perform sensitivity analysis on the findings. The results of these studies are therefore skewed and deceptive. As a result, our goal was to assess the economic evaluations of health interventions with a critical eye.

8.2. Economic Evaluations for Priority Setting and Resource Allocation

The demand for healthcare is only increasing, but there are clearly not enough resources to meet this demand. As a result, governments all over the world now prioritize getting the best value for their healthcare budgets, and economic factors are playing a bigger and bigger role in the design, administration, and assessment of health systems. Health economic analyses can assist in the best use of the limited resources available for healthcare by evaluating the value for money of health interventions. When debating whether to use a public budget to pay for healthcare services, decision-makers find it especially appealing to use health economic analyses to look into the cost-effectiveness of various health interventions. Over time, health economic analyses have played a more significant role in shaping health policy. Nevertheless, non-health economists may not always fully understand the underlying principles of the various forms of health economic analyses, and in low- and middle-income country (LMIC) settings where this field of research is less well-established, inappropriate types of analyses as well as inconsistent methodologies may be used to inform health policy decisions. This restricts these tools' ability to help guide policy choices that will maximize health benefits. While there is information and methodological guidance available for these health economic analyses, it is primarily in the form of training programs and textbooks that are usually behind a paywall and available only in high-income country settings. While many of the ideas are applicable to all contexts, there are some issues that are unique to LMICs (like the various kinds of data that are available, effectiveness metrics, and decision rules), and capacity in these environments is a persistent problem. There is currently a dearth of current, easily accessible open-access literature aimed at public health professionals in low- and middle-income countries (LMICs) who are crucial to the distribution of health resources.

This review offers a thorough, open, and cost-free introduction to economic evaluations. It is meant to serve as a resource for public health professionals, particularly those working in low- and middle-income countries (LMICs), where such resources are usually unavailable. In particular, we offer a current, thorough overview of the fundamental ideas guiding the most popular economic evaluation techniques—cost-effectiveness/cost-utility and cost-benefit analyses—that are employed to inform decisions about the distribution of resources in the global health sector (Table 8.2). We also highlight the main characteristics, variations, benefits, and drawbacks of these techniques. By doing this, we hope to improve general comprehension of the fundamental ideas underlying the various forms of economic evaluations frequently employed in the context of healthcare priority setting, with an emphasis on low- and middle-income countries. It is crucial to comprehend the fundamental ideas in this context since they could affect how each approach should be used and how health economic evidence should be interpreted to guide health policy. It is anticipated that this will aid in the understanding of the approaches and aid in the selection or differentiation of approaches for those performing such analyses as well as stakeholders who must interpret their output [such as a cost per disability-adjusted life-year (DALY) averted, cost per quality-adjusted life-year (QALY) gained, net monetary benefit, return on investment, and benefit-cost ratio]. It should be noted that this review is not disease-specific; rather, it concentrates on the broad application of these methodologies.

Table 8.2. *The Key Types of Full Economic Evaluations*

Type	Description
Cost-effectiveness analysis	Cost-effectiveness analysis is a form of comparative economic analysis that evaluates two or more policy alternatives in terms of their relative costs and outcomes, where the outcomes are measured in a single natural unit (e.g., life-years gained, disease case averted, etc.).
Cost-utility analysis	Cost-utility analysis (a specific type of cost-effectiveness analysis) is a form of comparative economic analysis that evaluates two or more policy alternatives in terms of their relative costs and outcomes, where the outcomes are expressed by a generic measure of health status that considers both the effect on mortality and morbidity (e.g., quality-adjusted life-years (QALYs) and disability-adjusted life-years (DALYs)).
Cost-benefit analysis	Cost-benefit analysis is a form of comparative economic analysis that evaluates two or more policy alternatives in terms of their relative costs and outcomes, where both the costs and outcomes are expressed in monetary terms. In principle, it should value the interventions relevant costs and outcomes based on the preferences of those affected (i.e., the individuals' willingness to pay).
Cost-minimization analysis	Cost-minimization analysis is a form of comparative economic analysis that compares the costs of two or more policy alternatives which are all assumed to have equivalent health effects.

Cost-consequence analysis	Cost-consequence analysis is a form of comparative economic analysis that evaluates two or more policy alternatives in terms of their relative costs and outcomes, where the outcomes are not summarized in a single measure, and multiple outcomes of interest are reported.

Source: https://www.frontiersin.org/journals/public-health/articles/10.3389/fpubh.2021.722927/full.

8.2.1. Health Economic Analyses Used for Evaluating Resource Allocation Decisions

Health economic analyses are conducted using a wide range of methodologies. Certain analyses solely look at the expenses associated with a condition or intervention (e.g., cost of illness studies) separately, whereas other analyses assess an intervention's costs as well as its effects. Knowing the distinctions between partial and complete economic evaluations is essential. Complete Economic Assessments in Comparison to Partial Evaluations: A particular kind of health economic analysis known as a full economic evaluation compares the expenses (resource utilization) and outcomes (impacts) of the health intervention(s) under consideration to a comparator, or other course of action (Figure 8.1). Full economic evaluations, therefore, even when examining a single health intervention or policy, formally evaluate at least two alternative courses of action. The comparator, which is also called the baseline scenario or counterfactual, is usually selected to mirror standard operating procedures or best practices in the context of the economic evaluation. For instance, the current cervical cancer screening program would be used as the comparator in an economic analysis of the introduction of the human papillomavirus vaccine in the United Kingdom. Even though a "do-nothing" or no intervention scenario may be used as the comparator in some circumstances, this is still a formal component of the analysis that must be acknowledged and the pertinent costs and consequences quantified.

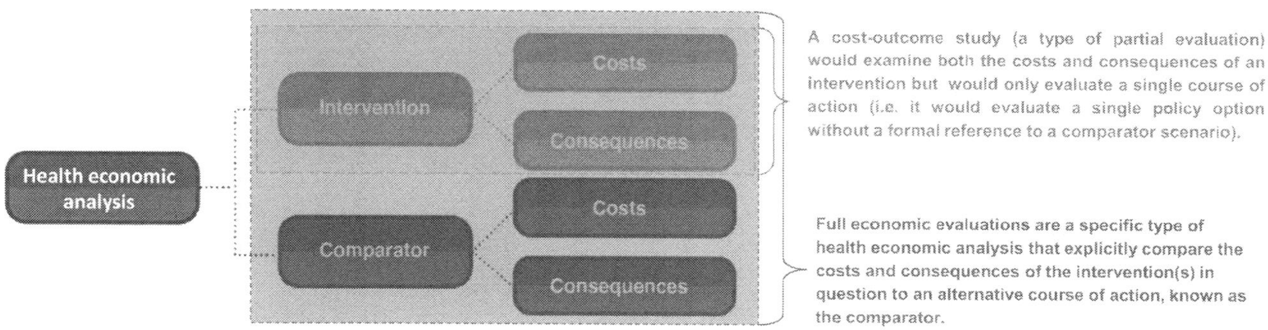

Figure 8.1. *The difference between full economic evaluations and cost-outcome partial evaluations.*

Source: https://www.ncbi.nlm.nih.gov/pmc/articles/PMC8424074/bin/fpubh-09-722927-g0001.jpg.

In contrast, partial evaluations (also referred to as partial economic evaluations) are studies that either:

1. Only examine the costs or consequences of an intervention independently, i.e., they do not look at both or relate the costs to the consequences. For example, a costing study would evaluate only the costs associated with an intervention (but not compare these to its consequences).

2. Examine both the costs and consequences of an intervention but only evaluate a single course of action (a cost-outcome study). By doing this, they are either explicitly or implicitly ignoring the comparator, which may overlook relevant costs/consequences and does not allow for comparisons to relevant alternative policy options for that setting. These analyses are therefore not a full economic evaluation—which has to formally compare the costs and consequences of the interventions in question to a comparator scenario (Figure 8.1).

While partial evaluations can yield valuable insights, they are insufficient in isolation to steer decision-making processes. This is because an intervention's financial worth cannot be determined solely by its cost or by the financial burden of a disease. It is critical to assess the costs and outcomes of the proposed intervention and compare it to a relevant alternative course of action or policy option (the comparator) in order to inform healthcare decision-making regarding resource allocation. Figure 8.2 emphasizes how crucial it is to take the comparator into consideration. In this hypothetical case, a partial evaluation would conclude that the use of the new treatment is encouraged because the monetary value of its health benefits exceeds its costs. Nevertheless, if a thorough economic evaluation were conducted using the current standard practice as the comparator and the new treatment as the treatment of choice, the analysis would reveal that the new treatment is more costly and less effective than the current standard practice, supporting the opposite policy recommendation (Figure 8.2).

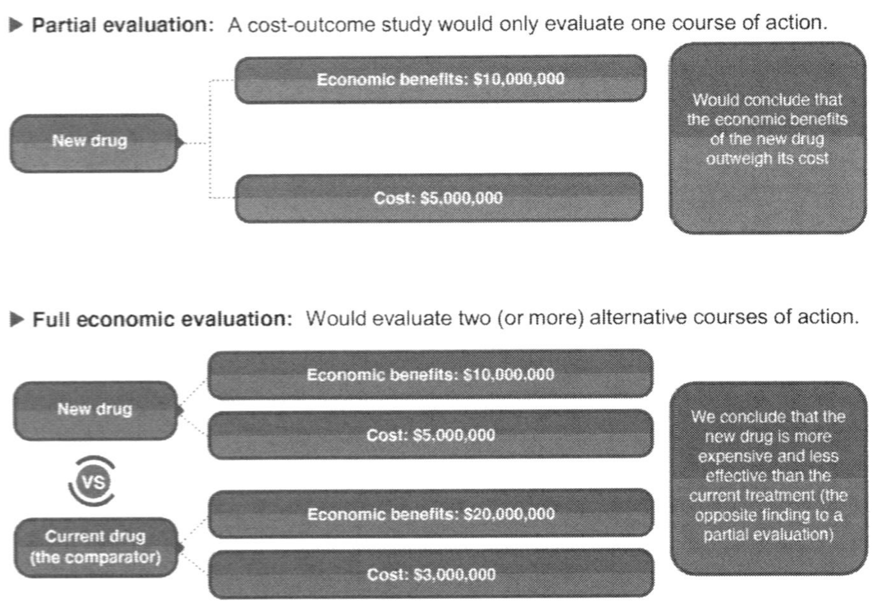

Figure 8.2. *A hypothetical comparison of the difference between a partial evaluation and full economic evaluation.*

Source: https://www.ncbi.nlm.nih.gov/pmc/articles/PMC8424074/bin/fpubh-09-722927-g0002.jpg.

This demonstrates how analyses can produce false conclusions if pertinent alternative policy options—like the standard of care—are disregarded. It should be noted that opinions in the literature differ on whether or not to call partial evaluations economic evaluations.

8.2.1.1. Different Types of Full Economic Evaluations

Health interventions are informed and evaluated by five primary types of full economic evaluations, as listed in Table 8.2. In this review, we concentrate on the most popular varieties, i.e., analyses of cost-effectiveness/cost-utility and cost-benefit. Cost-minimization analysis and cost-consequence analysis are two other forms of full economic evaluations. We won't go into greater detail about them in this review because they are less common and, in the case of cost-minimization analysis, only appropriate in specific situations. Similar principles serve as the foundation for these various economic assessments. Even though they might initially seem similar, their underlying methods and interpretations are different. How the result is expressed is a crucial distinction among the various forms of comprehensive economic evaluation (Table 8.2). The benefit or outcome of the health intervention in question is expressed in monetary terms using cost-benefit analyses. The health consequences of the health intervention are measured in a single natural unit (life-years gained, cases averted, or cases detected) in cost-effectiveness analyses, on the other hand, and in a generic measure of health status (DALYs and QALYs, a specific type of cost-effectiveness analysis) that takes into account the effects on both mortality and morbidity. The manner in which these various analyses evaluate the effectiveness of resource allocation varies as well (Table 8.3).

Table 8.3. *A Summary of How the Different Types of Analyses Consider the Efficiency of Resource Allocation and Examples of Their Use*

	Cost-Effectiveness Analyses	Cost-Utility Analyses	Cost-Benefit Analyses
How they consider the efficiency of resource allocation?	Cost-effectiveness analyses using disease or program specific metrics are often only concerned with how to use healthcare resources in a way that maximizes their output for the cost. As such, they are considering technical efficiency, identifying the option that provides the maximal healthcare for a given cost, or delivering a certain service at a minimal cos^{t}.1	Cost-utility analyses can consider the optimal allocation of healthcare resources (such as the mix of interventions) in a way that results in the maximum health gain for a given level of expenditure. In this way, it considers allocative efficiency within the health sector (i.e., it only deals with quasi-allocative assessments).	Cost-benefit analyses can be used to consider the optimal allocation of resources in its broadest sense because once the benefits have been converted into monetary terms, then the net economic benefit of different activities can be compared (including to those outside of the healthcare sector). It can therefore consider allocative efficiency across different sectors and across society.

Examples of when it is useful	Useful when a stakeholder is interested in a particular output metric and/or when you do not need to compare the outcome to other interventions/policy options. For example, comparing a range of different malaria interventions when investigating the cost per case averted.	Useful for informing health policy decisions when directly comparing different health interventions that fall within the same budget or benefit package (such as when considering the optimal allocation of a healthcare budget). For example, deciding if a new vaccine or treatment should be adopted within a national health benefit package.	Useful for cross-sectoral comparisons, such as looking at whether other government spending should be reallocated to the healthcare sector. Also useful when evaluating health policy/interventions where the health outcome metrics are not suitable (e.g., prenatal genetic screening for Down's syndrome), and in certain complex intervention contexts (such as interlinked packages of care, where maximizing health is not the only objective). For example, for considering non-pharmaceutical interventions for COVID-19 control in terms of both health and non-health outcomes.

Note: Cost-effectiveness analyses can be used to assess allocative efficiency within and potentially beyond the health sector for life-saving interventions when the outcomes are measured in terms of deaths averted or life-years gained, etc.

Source: https://www.frontiersin.org/journals/public-health/articles/10.3389/fpubh.2021.722927/full.

Disparities in the economic foundations underlie the variations in the way the outcome is expressed for economic evaluations. Traditionally, the foundation of cost-benefit analysis has been a welfarist approach, in which the health outcomes are assessed according to how much they contribute to the welfare of society as a whole, taking into account individual preferences and willingness to pay. On the other hand, cost-effectiveness and cost-utility analyses are grounded in an extra-welfarist approach, where the goal is customarily to maximize contributions to societal health, which is determined by adding up each person's health status. This review's focus on the most widely utilized kinds of comprehensive economic evaluations is one of its limitations. Health economic analysis is one of the frameworks or other approaches used in global health priority setting, in addition to comprehensive economic evaluations. Budget impact analysis, for instance, looks at the financial effects of implementing and spreading an intervention in a certain setting while taking affordability into account. Moreover, multicriteria decision analysis, or MCDA, can expand the scope of economic evaluation techniques to take acceptability, ethics, and equity into account. It also helps policymakers make decisions when there are two or more relevant criteria.

8.2.2. Factors of Cost-Benefit Analyses

A comparative study of the relative costs and results of two or more alternative courses of action, where the costs of an intervention and its subsequent outcomes are expressed in monetary terms, is known as a cost-benefit analysis (also known as benefit-cost analysis). It is also employed in other public sectors and has been dubbed the "gold standard" economic evaluation approach in the past. Because the net economic benefit of various activities can be compared (including to those outside the healthcare sector) once the benefits have been translated into monetary terms, cost-benefit analyses can be used to consider the optimal allocation of resources in the broadest sense. Thus, it can take into account allocative efficiency across various industries and throughout society (Table 8.3). Typically, cost-benefit analyses are summarized by calculating the intervention's net benefit, which is the monetized benefits less the costs incurred, or by calculating a benefit-cost ratio, which is the monetized benefits divided by the costs. However, additional outcome metrics, like the internal rate of return, can also be applied.

Traditionally, cost-benefit analysis adds up the costs and benefits of an intervention according to the preferences of the people who will be impacted. The welfarist approach serves as the theoretical basis for cost-benefit analyses in the healthcare industry. This is conceptually founded on three components. First, everyone is the best arbiter of their own welfare, or well-being. The second is that welfare metrics, which are based on the utility—or perceived value—that people derive from using healthcare products and services, are crucial for assessing health. The third is that the best course of action is one that maximizes social welfare; in other words, resource reallocation for an intervention is appropriate if it results in an increase in net benefits, or if gains could theoretically offset all costs and losses. Usually, "who" is winning or losing is not taken into consideration by the framework, and no real compensation is required. In well-functioning markets, the market can disclose social welfare according to people's preferences. However, because of shortcomings in the healthcare market, it is frequently necessary to elicit people's preferences through alternative means. In reality, a number of techniques are employed, such as willingness to pay and productivity gains valuation, to put the financial costs of the health effects into perspective. It is arguable how many analyses, when applied to healthcare decision making, fall within these original frameworks.

In cost-benefit analyses, an intervention is deemed optimal if its net benefit is positive or if its benefit-cost ratio is greater than one. In terms of boosting societal welfare, an intervention is judged justified if its monetized benefits outweigh its costs. Crucially, the main emphasis is not on saving money or cutting costs. Rather, based on estimates of willingness to pay, it usually represents the trade-offs people are willing to make between spending on the health intervention outcomes (like better health) and other goods and services. Formally speaking, a cost-benefit analysis should have a welfare economic basis, but the term is frequently used to refer to studies where the costs and outcomes are expressed in monetary terms. Other health economic analyses, such as return on investment and social return on investment analyses, quantify the financial benefit of a health intervention. When these formally assess an intervention's costs and outcomes in relation to a comparator or counterfactual scenario (i.e., examine two or more different options), they are a comprehensive economic assessment that shares many of the same benefits and drawbacks as a cost-benefit analysis. But these are only a partial evaluation (a cost-outcome study) when they only formally assess the costs and outcomes of one policy option and fail to adequately take into account the comparator or counterfactual scenario (Figure 8.1). Despite being frequently described as a continuation of cost-benefit analysis, these analyses lack precise definitions.

8.2.2.1. Cost-Benefit Analyses: Advantages

8.2.2.1.1. More Consistent with How Other Public Interventions Are Evaluated and Facilitate Cross-Sectoral Comparisons

The framework employed in cost-benefit analyses is more in line with the methods used to assess other public interventions and policies, not just those in the health sector, i.e., depending on the extent to which people are prepared to exchange the advantages. Because the net economic benefit of many different activities, including those outside the healthcare industry, can be compared once the benefits have been translated into monetary terms, cost-benefit analyses can therefore be used to consider the optimal allocation of resources in the broadest sense. A new health policy's "gain" to society, for instance, can be compared to spending money on infrastructure for transportation or education. This makes it easier to compare sectors to one another and enables analysis of the allocative efficiency of resources in various sectors and societies (Table 8.3). On the other hand, cost-utility analyses generally take into account only the healthcare sector's allocative efficiency of resources (Table 8.3).

8.2.2.2. Potential to Value a Wider Range of Benefits

This type of analysis can incorporate benefits and costs that fall outside of the healthcare sector. This can capture potential benefits of interventions missed by cost-effectiveness/cost-utility analyses.

8.2.2.3. Monetary Output Is Desirable to a Range of Stakeholders

The public, as well as decision-makers in the healthcare and non-healthcare sectors (like the ministry of finance and patient representatives), typically find value in a monetary output. Additionally, they can simultaneously take into account the opinions of multiple stakeholders regarding the impact by assigning "proxy" monetary values to all identified impacts that are important to the stakeholders. This makes it easier for stakeholders to be heard when allocating resources.

8.2.2.4. Cost-Benefit Analyses: Limitations and Areas of Debate

8.2.2.4.1. Methodological Difficulties Regarding Placing a Monetary Value on Health Benefits and Variations Between Studies

There isn't a widely accepted gold standard technique for valuing interventions' positive effects on health in terms of money. Consequently, even if the financial outcomes are the same, the methodologies used can vary significantly, making it tough to compare different studies. When comparing cost-benefit analyses of vaccinations, it's evident that using different methods to value health benefits can lead to very diverse results. It's crucial to compare different health economic analyses that influence resource allocation, considering the variety of approaches used and their quality. Moreover, different approaches could introduce biases in the findings of health economic analyses and consequently impact the health policies and decision-making they support. We believe that studies become less useful in guiding resource allocation within the global health context when they are too varied. A reference case for cost-benefit analysis has recently been established, aiming to bring much-needed consistency to this field.

8.2.2.5. Difficulties Capturing Non-Fatal Health Outcomes

In LMICs in particular, willingness-to-pay estimates are less common for non-fatal health outcomes. As a result, averted cost or averted cost-of-illness estimates are frequently used in this field of research as a proxy to measure the financial benefits of non-fatal health outcomes of health interventions (i.e., they consider the productivity losses and avoided direct costs related to a disease or treatment). The quality of these cost/illness studies varies, though. Because of this, evaluating interventions whose primary health benefits are unrelated to prevented excess mortality becomes more difficult when using a cost-benefit analysis. Furthermore, even though this is a practical response to the available data, one could argue that it deviates from the welfarist approach that underpins cost-benefit analyses. An additional technique is to assign a monetary value to QALYs gained or DALYs avoided by applying a willingness-to-pay threshold. Even though this is being used more frequently, some contend that these conversions are incredibly arbitrary and lack any theoretical foundation.

8.2.2.6. Potential Misinterpretation and Difficulties Regarding the Practical Interpretation

The findings of these research studies could be easily misinterpreted. In particular, these studies often aim to estimate social welfare measures or potential economic advantages rather than actual financial gains. Therefore, the economic benefits presented are usually approximations that reflect the health benefits of a population in monetary terms, derived from estimated productivity increases or willingness to pay assessments. For instance, the human capital method values potential productivity gains rather than the actual gains, while the willingness to pay approach determines benefits based on individual preferences and their willingness to pay for health improvements. It is crucial for stakeholders to understand that these estimated economic benefits may not be tangible and should not be mistaken for actual monetary gains to society. For example, an intervention with an estimated benefit-cost ratio of 6.0 may wrongly be seen as generating six times the initial investment, similar to a financial investment, even though not all economic benefits may be realized. This does not undermine the value of cost-benefit analysis, but it emphasizes the need for caution in reporting and interpreting such studies. The main objective of these analyses is typically to evaluate whether an intervention is justified in terms of enhancing societal welfare and determining if the economic benefits outweigh the intervention's costs, not necessarily leading to financial savings.

Similarly, when a study shows that the economic advantages of an intervention are greater than the costs, it is seen as having a positive return on investment. However, this can be misleading to policymakers because the concept of return on investment for public health interventions is often mistakenly equated with cost-savings. For instance, a review found that the average return on investment for public health interventions was 14.3 to 1. Many people wrongly assumed that this meant that for every £1 spent, the public sector would save £14.30 in cash, suggesting a 1,430% return. But this interpretation is not accurate, as not all of the economic benefits calculated translate into fiscal savings.

Another drawback is the absence of a specific threshold for determining when the perceived costs of an intervention outweigh the benefits in a given situation. The decision to implement an intervention is based on whether the benefits exceed the costs (i.e., if the benefit-cost ratio is above one). Cost-benefit analyses often do not consider fixed budget constraints in certain sectors (e.g., health), which means they do not fully capture the trade-offs of allocating additional costs within these budgets and displacing other health interventions.

8.2.2.7. Equity and Distributional Concerns

Avoiding death or morbidity is valued economically in cost-benefit analyses. Nonetheless, there may be implicit equity and distributional issues with this, and many have contended that this will inherently favor health interventions that benefit wealthier populations over impoverished ones. All other things being equal, the value of the increased social welfare or productivity gains of averting disease in richer populations will be higher than in poorer populations within the same country/setting. For example, when aiming to quantify the economic benefits experienced by a group of patients. Furthermore, it would be easy to estimate that treating a condition in women would have less economic benefits than treating a condition in men because women typically earn lower salaries and carry a heavier burden of unpaid work. This suggests that interventions aimed at treating diseases in men are more valuable than those aimed at treating diseases in women. Assuming that everyone has the same value of time or life (regardless of gender, socioeconomic status, and employment) is one way to get around this problem. On the other hand, one could counter that doing so makes the estimated economic benefits less evident and more speculative. What do the estimated economic benefits actually correspond to if everyone uses the same value of time? Once more, the issue lies in the fact that the economic benefits that are being touted are frequently theoretical or approximations and may not always be immediately applicable to the society or economy in question. It is noteworthy that efforts have been undertaken to modify cost-benefit analyses in order to tackle the issues of equity and distribution. It remains to be seen, though, if these will find their way into cost-benefit analyses focused on policy in the field of global health.

8.2.3. Cost-Effectiveness and Cost-Utility Analyses

Cost-effectiveness and cost-utility analyses are among the most common forms of economic assessments applied to the healthcare industry. They are a comparison of the relative benefits and expenses of two or more different options. Analyses of cost-effectiveness quantify the effects of an intervention on health in terms of one natural unit, such as life years saved or cases averted. The inability to compare studies examining interventions aimed at different diseases or stages of care, however, limits the potential utility of this information for educating policymakers because the health consequences of each intervention will be expressed in different units. A particular type of cost-effectiveness called cost-utility analysis was created to address this. Cost-utility analyses use a broad measure of health status, such as DALYs and QALYs, to account for benefits on both lower morbidity and mortality as well as the health consequences. The cost-effectiveness estimates for various healthcare interventions can be directly compared to one another because these metrics can be applied to a broad range of diseases (e.g., comparing the cost-effectiveness of a malaria intervention to a tuberculosis intervention). The lines between cost-effectiveness and cost-utility analyses have become more hazy in practice; consequently, cost-effectiveness literature frequently includes both of these methods, and cost-utility analyses are frequently referred to as cost-effectiveness analyses. The extra-welfarist approach, on which the goal is customarily to maximize contributions to societal health—measured as the sum of individual health status—is the foundation for most cost-effectiveness/cost-utility analyses.

A cost-effectiveness/cost-utility analysis can show what happens when a new health intervention is compared to a comparator, as shown in Figure 8.3. Standardized cost-effectiveness thresholds—an explicit cost per unit of outcome below which an intervention is considered cost-effective—such as £20,000 per QALY gained—are frequently used as a decision rule to classify whether an intervention is cost-effective or not when the analysis is using a generic measure of health status (such as DALYs/QALYs within cost-utility analyses) (Figure 8.3).

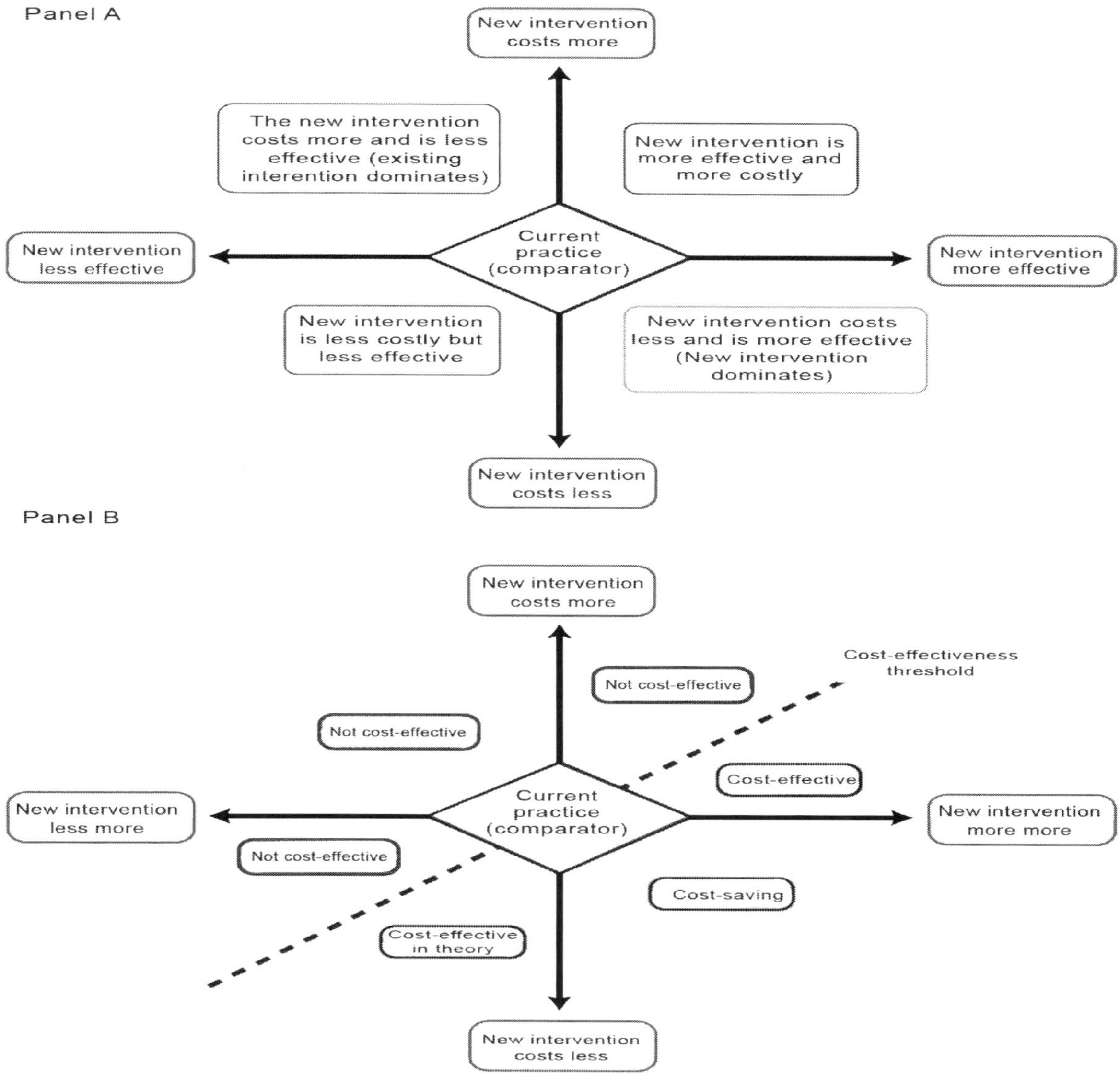

Figure 8.3. *A schematic of the cost-effectiveness plane. Panel A indicates the four different quadrants. Panel B illustrates the different decision rules in relation to a cost-effectiveness threshold within the different quadrants.*

Source: https://www.ncbi.nlm.nih.gov/pmc/articles/PMC8424074/bin/fpubh-09-722927-g0003.jpg.

Numerous techniques can be employed to ascertain these thresholds. Once this is completed, the analysis can take into account the healthcare sector's allocative efficiency of resources (Table 8.3), which is the distribution of healthcare resources so as to yield the greatest health benefit for a given amount of investment. In order to find the most effective option that is below the set cost-effectiveness threshold, the analysis looks at mutually exclusive policy options (such as various tuberculosis treatment options) incrementally (which is not necessarily the same as the option that has the lowest cost per unit of effect). On the other hand, it is uncommon to have a standardized cost-effectiveness threshold available to compare the results to when a cost-effectiveness analysis uses a disease- or program-specific outcome measure (like cases averted), and it is challenging to compare the results to those of other studies. In this situation, the analysis's main objective is frequently to determine which choice is the most cost-effective per unit of effect, i.e., determine which choice has the lowest cost-effectiveness ratio (e.g., lowest cost per averted case). Within this framework, analyses of cost-effectiveness based on disease- or program-specific metrics frequently focus solely on the most efficient use of healthcare resources in terms of cost, a concept known as technical efficiency (Table 8.3).

Ratios are commonly used to express the results of cost-effectiveness and cost-utility analyses (a cost per unit of effect). The results of cost-utility analyses can also be expressed monetarily (e.g., net monetary benefit). When a health metric has a net monetary benefit, the health outcomes are paid for according to a cost-effectiveness threshold that reflects society's assessment of the metric rather than an individual's willingness to pay for improved health. Because of this, even though it resembles a cost-benefit analysis, it employs a different decision rule and lacks the welfarist foundation.

8.2.3.1. Cost-Effectiveness and Cost-Utility Analyses: Advantages

8.2.3.1.1. Focus on Societal Valuation of Health

The framework of cost-effectiveness/cost-utility analyses is most appropriate if you acknowledge that, regardless of the amount people are willing to pay for it, health is a basic good whose value should be set by society (i.e., irrespective of their readiness to pay). This aligns more closely with the health rights theory that the World Health Organization (WHO) promotes. Furthermore, it circumvents the challenges associated with social welfare valuation that arise from market failure in the healthcare sector.

8.2.3.1.2. More Commonly Performed

Compared to cost-benefit analyses, cost-effectiveness/cost-utility analyses are performed and published more frequently. This facilitates decision-making by making it simpler for policymakers to compare various studies and interventions. Cost-utility analysis was created because cost-effectiveness analyses with disease- or intervention-specific metrics have trouble being comparable across various health programs and interventions and cannot be used to compare programs with different goals or outcomes.

8.2.3.1.3. Forgoing the Need to Monetize Health Benefits

The framework does not require assigning a monetary value to health gains. By foregoing this step, the analysis draws attention exclusively to health benefits and avoids the corresponding ethical and equity issues that can arise when monetizing them. However, it could be argued that some of these ethical and equity issues still arise when setting the cost-effectiveness threshold.

8.2.3.1.4. Guidelines for Reporting and Methodology

In the healthcare industry, there are more well-established standards and reference cases for carrying out and disclosing the outcomes of cost-effectiveness and cost-utility analyses. In certain contexts, national standards have also been established. It should be noted that methodological variation still exists between different cost-effectiveness/cost-utility analyses (such as the costs that are included, the perspective, and the assumed discount rate), especially for settings that lack standardized guidelines or reference cases, even though we would argue that the methodology used is more standardized than that of cost-benefit analyses.

8.2.3.2. Cost-Effectiveness and Cost-Utility Analyses: Limitations and Areas of Debate

8.2.3.2.1. Availability of Cost-Effectiveness Thresholds

To determine whether an intervention is cost-effective or not, a cost-effectiveness threshold is frequently employed as a decision rule. While some nations have set their own cost-effectiveness thresholds (89, 90), low- and lower-middle-income nations are less likely to do so. Interpreting the results of cost-effectiveness/cost-utility analyses can be more challenging in the absence of a predetermined threshold. Many have previously used the cost-effectiveness thresholds set by the Commission on Macroeconomics and Health, which are less than 3 and less than 1 times the nation's gross domestic product (GDP) per capita for an intervention to be considered cost-effective and highly cost-effective, respectively, in cases where no country-specific threshold had been established. But these days, a lot of people are criticizing them for being too high. According to the WHO, these thresholds were meant to serve as a general guideline for analyses conducted at the global or regional level rather than for specific investment decisions. They contend that as a result, these thresholds have not been applied in their intended manner. Regretfully, global health still makes use of these thresholds, which are one to three times GDP per capita. Even with guidelines in place, figuring out a nation's cost-effectiveness threshold is still a difficult task.

The health opportunity cost, or the amount of health that is anticipated to be lost if the resources in question are used for an intervention, can be estimated using the cost-effectiveness threshold, depending on how it is computed. When this is the case, the healthcare industry's financial constraints can be taken into consideration by the cost-effectiveness/cost-utility analysis. Nevertheless, in reality, the cost-effectiveness thresholds that are frequently applied in LMICs do not take this into account and are frequently just an expression of value made by a particular party (such as a government or international organization), without taking the limitations of the healthcare system into account.

8.2.3.3. The Generic Measures of Health Status (DALYs and QALYs) Have Limitations

Compared to merely gauging the impact of the intervention in terms of disease cases or deaths avoided, the use of DALYs or QALYs as outcomes within cost-utility analyses has been a noteworthy improvement, and these measures allow comparison across various diseases or interventions. These general indicators of health status do have certain drawbacks, though. These generic summary measures have a general limitation in that they might not be capturing all of the health benefits of an intervention and could be argued to be unduly reductionist and simplistic. Furthermore, in some circumstances—for example, when health outcome metrics are not the most appropriate—these metrics perform poorly. One could argue, for instance, that DALY/QALY metrics don't take into consideration the difficulties involved in examining the advantages of prenatal genetic screening and pregnancy termination for Down syndrome (such as the effect on caregivers).

8.2.3.4. Often Do Not Capture Non-Health Benefits and Limited Cross-Sector Comparisons

The goal of the cost-effectiveness/cost-utility analysis framework is to quantify the health gains that result from public health interventions. Cost-offsets and health savings (like avoided future medical expenses) resulting from an intervention can be added to and deducted from the intervention's total cost. However, many health initiatives also have a positive impact on other fields, such as education or the environment. There is variation in when and how broader benefits, both financial and non-financial, are included in cost-effectiveness/cost-utility analyses, even though they can all be monetarily valued and included when adopting a broad societal perspective. Consequently, the effects of public health interventions on other sectors are frequently left out of cost-effectiveness/cost-utility analyses, which often solely take into account the benefits to the health sector. This narrow viewpoint sometimes aligns with the mandate for the healthcare budget, which may be limited to the goal of improving health alone. Undervaluing the broader benefits of many health interventions may result from failing to account for these non-health benefits. This limitation is especially important when evaluating complex interventions (such as those with interconnected care packages), since their complexity may make it impossible for them to be evaluated using one of the current systems, and their primary goal may not be to maximize health.

Interestingly, the decision at hand might not only affect the health sector but also trade-offs between the goals of society and other sectors. Potential cross-sector comparisons are limited when non-monetary metrics are used. That is, it is difficult to directly compare the estimated value of funding a health intervention (based on the cost per QALY gained or DALY averted) to funding for purposes other than health, like education. Because of this, it becomes more challenging to use this kind of analysis to support the reallocation of other government spending to the health sector (like changing tax laws), and it becomes more challenging for decision-makers to evaluate the cost-benefit of funding a wide range of potential initiatives, including those from non-health sectors. When compared to cost-benefit analyses, cost-effectiveness/cost-utility analyses typically have less room to take resource allocation and efficiency into account (Table 8.3). It is becoming more widely acknowledged that people are concerned about more than just maximizing health gains when making healthcare decisions. This is because DALYs and QALYs may not fully account for all relevant outcomes when comparing various interventions. As a result, it is becoming increasingly important to report not just DALYs and QALYs but also other metrics and outcomes.

8.2.3.5. Variation in the Inclusion of Productivity Costs and Potential Double-Counting of Effects

The kinds of productivity costs that are taken into account when calculating cost-effectiveness ratios vary (Figure 8.4). From a societal perspective, it is generally agreed upon that productivity costs related to patients' productivity losses resulting from accessing an intervention should be included; however, there is disagreement over those related to productivity gains resulting from prevented morbidity/mortality (Figure 8.4) since the fact that it is arguable that the QALY/DALY effectiveness measure includes these benefits. Because of this, it is possible to double-count the effectiveness of the health intervention if these productivity gains are included in the cost component of the equation (Figure 8.4). Some have disputed this suggestion, claiming that the QALY measure fails to account for these productivity gains. Different guidelines apply to the inclusion of these productivity gains.

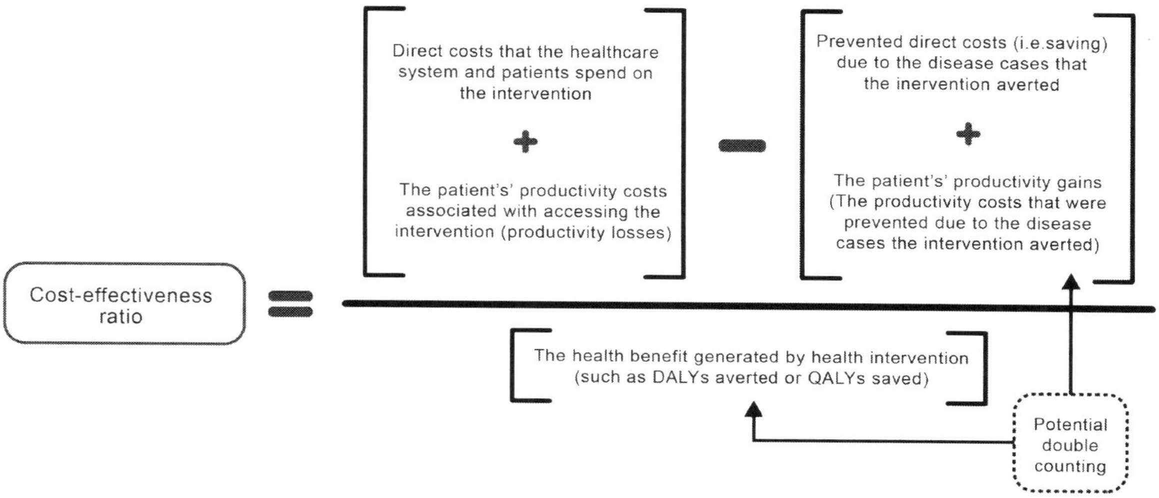

Figure 8.4. *Schematic surrounding the inclusion of productivity costs within cost-effectiveness ratios.*

Source: https://www.ncbi.nlm.nih.gov/pmc/articles/PMC8424074/bin/fpubh-09-722927-g0005.jpg.

As previously highlighted, estimates of productivity costs are highly sensitive to the method used, and it is important to be aware of the potential variation in methodology when comparing studies. This variation could lead to potential biases in setting health policy, and further guidance is needed.

8.2.3.6. Equity

Note that cost-effectiveness/cost-utility analyses circumvent the need to monetize health benefits, but they are nevertheless linked to ethical and equity concerns (e.g., DALY/QALY metrics, cost-effectiveness threshold setting). For instance, information about who benefits and who loses from health interventions is rarely provided by cost-effectiveness/cost-utility analyses (i.e., are equity neutral), and as a result, despite the fact that it might be a societal goal, they do not prioritize enhancing health among the poorest. Recent initiatives, such as the creation of distributional cost-effectiveness analysis and extended cost-effectiveness analysis, have attempted to include equity as a quantitative component in cost-effectiveness/cost-utility analyses, which may help to partially address these limitations. Nonetheless, there is still work to be done in this area in terms of practical application to help guide resource allocation decisions in the field of global health (Chisholm et al., 2007; Simoens et al., 2009).

8.3. Cost-Benefit Analysis versus Cost-Effectiveness Analysis

When confined to a hospital, healthcare provider, government agency, or other healthcare institutional setting, the application of cost-effectiveness analysis (CEA) may prove beneficial in identifying the least expensive intervention that yields a particular outcome. This is particularly true if funding has been allocated for the least expensive interventions. However, in a social perspective—one in which all members of society are involved, including family members, outsiders, and taxpayers—and no budget has been set aside, a CEA is wholly inadequate for determining the interventions that should be funded, if any at all. Here, the more applicable economic evaluation technique is cost-benefit analysis (CBA). This chapter aims to elucidate the specific rationale and methods by which CBA—for a CBA text that exclusively concentrates on the healthcare industry—is the more appropriate assessment approach when assessing interventions from a societal lens. The evaluation of five novel interventions aimed at mitigating dementia symptoms will serve as the primary framework for this work. A lifetime supply of hearing aids, lifetime vision correction, Medicare eligibility (and the additional services it offers), years of education (a dropout prevention program), and avoiding nursing homes (because living in one exacerbates dementia symptoms) are the new dementia interventions involved. It is not that the medical literature was ignorant of these five interventions; rather, their recent thorough evaluation using CBA and their newfound indication of being financially beneficial are what made them "new."

A sizable nationwide panel dataset from the National Alzheimer's Coordinating Center (NACC) was used to estimate costs and benefits for the five dementia interventions we will be highlighting. Alzheimer's disease is the most common type of dementia in the US. We cover all categories of dementia in our NACC data, which was utilized to perform the economic evaluation calculations reported in this chapter. However, some of the data used for the CBA evaluations will also be recast into CEA terms in order to fully transparently illustrate the difference between using CEA and CBA. The following is the paper's outline. To begin, we conceptualize CEA as a classical economic evaluation technique that considers mutually exclusive interventions both with and without a budget constraint. Next, we proceed to the cost-utility analysis (CUA), a broader variant of CEA. Although CUA can be thought of as CEA, it can also be transformed into a CBA with just one extension. This brings us to the proper analysis of CBA, which, in contrast to CEA, can be used to evaluate the social merit of any healthcare intervention. Some of the background information and broader issues regarding CEA and dementia interventions are provided in the discussion section. We wrap up with a summary and recommendations.

8.3.1. Examination of Cost-Effectiveness Analysis

8.3.1.1. Cost-Effectiveness Analysis with a Budget Constraint

Determining the effect unit for each intervention that needs to be costed is the first step in a CEA. The outcome of the five new dementia interventions was a decrease in dementia symptoms as determined by the Clinical Dementia Rating (CDR) scale, also developed by Washington University and referred to as the CDR® Dementia Staging Instrument. The CDR is a widely used dementia severity measure that is primarily based on a neurological exam and informant reporting. A clinician gave each NACC participant a CDR during each visit. The CDR consists of six domains: home and hobbies, memory, orientation, judgment and problem-solving, community affairs, and personal care. A questionable response receives a score of 0.5, and each domain is evaluated on a 0 to 3 interval (none, mild, moderate, and severe). With a range of 0 to 18, the CDR-SB, also known as the CDR sum of boxes, represents the total score obtained from all six domains. It is critical to realize that utilizing dementia symptoms as the outcome bases cognitive impairment not on the medical definition of dementia, which is based on brain pathology (e.g., fibers and plaques for Alzheimer's disease), but rather on the behavioral definition of dementia, which is defined as interfering with daily activities. Although therapies to modify brain pathology do not yet exist, there are interventions to lessen the symptoms of dementia. Any intervention must have resources allocated and costs to have an impact. In CEA, the costs are typically solely associated with the organization providing the funding; these are referred to as the private costs. Even though the CBA costs of the new dementia interventions were more extensive, we will assume for the sake of simplicity that the CBA costs were pertinent to the CEA (we will loosen this assumption when we address externalities and shift the analysis to social CBA).

For each intervention, the cost-effectiveness ratios are obtained by dividing these cost estimates by the outcome effects. The CEA then ranks every intervention in order of lowest to highest ratio. The five new dementia interventions are ranked according to CEA criteria in Table 8.4. According to this ranking of the five interventions, staying out of a nursing home would be deemed the least cost-effective intervention, and education would be the most cost-effective.

Table 8.4. *Cost-Effectiveness of Various Dementia Interventions*

Intervention	Effect: Reduction in Dementia Symptoms	Costs per Person	Cost-Effectiveness Ratio
Education	0.3459	USD 1,400	USD 4,047
Corrective lenses	0.1858	USD 765	USD 4,117
Medicare eligibility	0.9182	USD 6,540	USD 7,123
Hearing aids	0.7251	USD 8,498	USD 11,719
Avoiding nursing homes	3.2367	USD 54,545 *	USD 16,892

* The benefit and cost figures for nursing homes were in population terms. To convert them into per-person terms, one needs to divide by 1.1 million, the approximate number of older adults in Medicaid-financed nursing homes. The total cost of living in nursing homes in the CBA (which was the difference between total benefits of USD 1.93 trillion and the benefits without the nursing home cost savings, which was USD 1.87 trillion) was equal to USD 0.06 trillion. Dividing this sum by 1.1 million produces a cost per person of USD 54,545.

Source: https://www.ncbi.nlm.nih.gov/pmc/articles/PMC10001534/pdf/ijerph-20-04638.pdf.

Regarding the question of which interventions—if any—would be funded in reality, it is necessary to identify the budgetary restrictions, which entails being aware of the funds that the government has available to allocate to the interventions. We will take three potential spending caps: $10,000, $20,000, or $70,000 per individual. The government would only authorize Medicare eligibility, education, and corrective lenses for a $10,000 budget because the total is $8,705. Hearing aids would be added for a budget of $20,000, bringing the total to $17,037. The largest effect, not even avoiding nursing homes, would be approved for a budget of $70,000 because the total cost with this intervention added would be $71,748. The decision-maker who decided how big the institution's budget would be was deciding which interventions were worthwhile for that institution and would, therefore, be implemented, based on the CEA method for the new dementia interventions. The primary flaw in the CEA is that this budgetary decision would be made without knowledge of the interventions that would be available, their costs, and their expected effects.

8.3.1.2. Cost-Effectiveness Analysis Without a Budget Constraint

The primary function of CEA as an intervention evaluation method, in the absence of a predetermined budget constraint, is to identify which dementia interventions can be disqualified from consideration and, consequently, not be funded. Interventions fall into two categories that can be removed. Any ineffective interventions fall into the first category. Consider the scenario where a nursing home is tasked with providing skilled nursing care to an elderly person. Table 8.4 tells the decision-maker that living in a nursing home increases dementia symptoms by 3.3267 points in the case of the interventions listed in the table if living in a nursing home is under consideration (that is, not avoiding residing in a nursing home). This intervention should not be considered as it would be counterproductive. In the process, one avoids the worsening symptoms of dementia and saves $54,545 in expenses. Avoiding a nursing home turns into a fruitful intervention that can be included in Table 8.4 because of this effect gain and the avoidance of incurred costs. An effect gain, or a cost savings from an intervention not on the list but involving a variation of the listed interventions, is the second category of interventions that can be eliminated. The ones on the list are not exclusive of one another because both corrective lenses and hearing aids are eligible. The listed interventions also need not be repeatable so that funding can only be allocated to the most economical intervention once. The new intervention, however, is mutually exclusive with the listed intervention since it cannot occur simultaneously if it is a variation of the listed intervention that is the subject of the evaluation. In this instance, the new intervention's fate is determined by comparing its cost-effectiveness to the specific listed intervention. As a result, for instance, one is now evaluating buying six hearing aids over one's lifetime as opposed to the five sets of hearing aids that the hearing aid intervention indicated in Table 8.4 required. More generally, for mutually exclusive interventions where the new intervention has both a different cost and effect than an existing intervention, the CEA must be determined based on the incremental cost-effectiveness ratios rather than the average cost-effectiveness ratios that we have been using. If this sixth set costs more than $8,498, but does not produce greater effects, then it can safely be eliminated as it is dominated by the existing listed intervention. As we just saw, when there is no financial restriction, CEA can help remove certain ineffective interventions, which are primarily variations of the interventions on the list. The decision-maker is still unsure, though, if any of the interventions indicated in Table 8.4 are worthy of funding due to CEA.

8.3.1.3. Cost-Utility Analysis as Cost-Effectiveness Analysis

A quality adjusted life year (QALY), which is the most common healthcare outcome, is the focus of Cost-Utility Analysis (CUA) according to CEA viewpoints. The product of the quality of any given life year (QoL) and the number of life-years affected (LY) yields a QALY. It is the most general effect to use in a CEA because, in theory, every healthcare intervention that can be thought of that has an effect must affect either the quantity or quality (or both) of a person's life. CBAs for three of the new interventions shown in Table 8.4 used data that could be expressed in QALY units. Together with the costs from Table 8.4, the three QALY effects are shown in Table 8.5, where they are combined to create the cost-utility ratio, or cost-effectiveness ratio in a CUA.

Table 8.5. *Cost-Utility Analysis of Various Dementia Interventions*

Intervention	Effect: Increase in QALYs	Costs per Person	Cost-Utility Ratio
Corrective lenses	0.1012 *	USD 765	USD 7,559
Hearing aids	0.6785 **	USD 8,498	USD 12,525
Avoiding nursing homes	3.4282	USD 54,545	USD 15,911

* The outcome measure for corrective lenses was in terms of mortality and the reduction was 0.0044. Multiplying this mortality reduction by a life expectancy of 23 years produces the equivalent QALY increase of 0.1012.

** The outcome measure for hearing aids was in terms of the quality of a life year and the reduction was 0.0295. Multiplying this quality of life increase by a life expectancy of 23 years produces the equivalent QALY increase of 0.6785.

Source: https://www.ncbi.nlm.nih.gov/pmc/articles/PMC10001534/pdf/ijerph-20-04637.pdf.

The alternative cost-effectiveness ratios in Table 8.5 are interesting because, when measured in terms of QALYs rather than dementia symptoms, the ratios are significantly higher. This supports the apparent finding that the particular effect measure a CEA ratio employs has a significant impact on the ratio. Thus, unless it takes the form of a CUA, the applicability of CEA is not universal. The fact that other interventions that aren't being evaluated have a significant impact on an intervention's likelihood of being approved is less evident. The Medicare and education interventions are absent from Table 8.5 because QALY data for these two interventions was not available. Table 8.5, which does not take into account these two interventions, shows that avoiding nursing homes was previously rejected, but it would now be approved if the budget was USD 70,000 (since the total cost of the three interventions would be USD 63,808). Assigning a budget before knowing which interventions will be assessed and funded, even when using CEA in the form of a CUA, is not a sensible economic evaluation technique. CUA league tables are frequently cited when using CUA for decision-making when no financial limit has been imposed. These tables list a variety of interventions that have been reported in the literature in order of lowest to highest cost per QALY. Then, using CUA to evaluate a specific intervention related to dementia in our case, these tables are compared with that intervention. An abridged league table is provided in Table 8.6.

Table 8.6. *Cost-Utility Analysis of Various Non-Dementia Interventions*

Intervention	Cost-Utility Ratio
Cholesterol testing and diet therapy	USD 480
Hip replacement	USD 2,545
Kidney transplant	USD 10,276
Home hemodialysis	USD 37,658
Erythropoietin treatment for anemia in dialysis patients	USD 1,18,616

Source: https://www.ncbi.nlm.nih.gov/pmc/articles/PMC10001534/pdf/ijerph-20-04637.pdf.

By comparing the cost-utility ratios found in Tables 8.5 and 8.6, we can determine that diet therapy and cholesterol testing were the most cost-effective of the three new dementia interventions. All three dementia interventions, however, proved to be more economical than erythropoietin treatment. It matters which league table intervention you are comparing. League tables must be standardized so that the cost-utility ratios are determined using the same metrics for cost, utility, and discount rate in order to be considered legitimate. However, standardization does not address the issue of determining which league table intervention should serve as the benchmark. Equally significant is the fact that, even in cases where the CUA league table identifies a benchmark intervention, it remains uncertain if the benchmark is beneficial. To determine whether funding the intervention is justified because it is more cost-effective than the benchmark, a CBA of the benchmark intervention must first be conducted.

8.3.2. Utilization of Cost-Benefit Analysis

An effect that has a monetary value is what is referred to as a benefit. It is therefore commensurate with the costs since it is expressed in monetary terms, which are nearly always measured in monetary terms (except in cases where costs and benefits are both expressed in non-monetary terms). As a result, it is now feasible to directly compare costs and benefits to determine which is higher. From an institutional standpoint, an intervention is valuable only if the benefits outweigh the costs, or if there is a positive difference known as the net benefits. Positive net benefits show that the intervention is socially beneficial if the costs and benefits are related to every member of society, i.e., they are social benefits and social costs.

8.3.2.1. Cost-Utility Analysis as Cost-Benefit Analysis

A QALY is the result in a CUA; consequently, a QALY is in each person's utility function. The total number of QALYs for all individuals from an intervention, or the social utility, is just the sum of each person's utility function. The QALY needs to have a value or be assigned a cost, to be classified as a benefit. The price in a CUA that aspires to be a CBA is considered constant and is set apart from the specifics of the intervention under review. The CUA constant price is a floor price that is typically established at the federal level. It is the lowest cost attributed to the QALYs required for the intervention to be deemed beneficial (primarily by others). The threshold price is frequently set at a multiple of the national income per capita.

It is critical to realize that the price of a quality-adjusted life (QALY) in a cost-benefit analysis (CBA) is essentially intended to represent the WTP for that QALY. This suggests that converting a CUA into a CBA based on a single threshold price has two major drawbacks. The first flaw is that a QALY is given a fixed price. This is problematic because diminishing marginal utility is the foundation upon which an economic demand curve is constructed. This suggests that as one consumes more QALYs, the price they are willing to pay for a QALY decreases. Since donepezil had a higher total of 1.6 QALYs than any of the other interventions, Johannesson's point applies to the interventions in Table 8.7. The 0.6 additional QALYs are valued at 0.6 of $50,000 rather than 0.6 of USD 1,50,000 as in Table 8.7 if one QALY is valued at $1,50,000 but the second QALY is only valued at USD 50,000. The net benefits would drop to $1,31,824 from $1,80,000 for the Donepezil Monotherapy, which is less than the Memantine Monotherapy benefits. If there is no longer a valid assumption of a constant price, priorities may change. The fact that the threshold price used by CUA as the cost of a QALY is not determined by an individual's WTP is another flaw in the system. It is not at all based on an individual's preferences to use national income as a benchmark for human capital justification. The human capital approach, which is used for valuation in CBA in the healthcare industry, assumes that the value of a life is the foregone output that society no longer receives because the person dies. In national income accounting, the value of this lost output is determined by the prices others place on the goods—not by the value that the person whose life is in jeopardy places on it.

Table 8.7. *Net Benefits of Various Dementia FDA-Approved Medicine Interventions*

Intervention	Benefits per Person [1]	Costs per Person	Net-Benefits per Person
Rivastigmine oral monotherapy	USD 1,31,400	USD 58,277	USD 73,123
Galantamine monotherapy	USD 1,44,150	USD 60,793	USD 83,357
Memantine monotherapy	USD 1,94,100	USD 48,728	USD 1,45,372
Donepezil monotherapy	USD 2,41,350	USD 48,176	USD 1,93,174

*The benefit figures in this column were constructed by taking the QALY estimates for each intervention and multiplying them by the threshold value of USD 1,50,000 per QALY.

Source: https://www.ncbi.nlm.nih.gov/pmc/articles/PMC10001534/pdf/ijerph-20-04637.pdf.

8.3.2.2. CBA Not Based on CUA

It is not necessary to compare the social value of either drug, memantine or donepezil monotherapy, to any other intervention to justify it. This is because both drugs are listed as mutually exclusive rivals in Table 8.7. This is the only requirement, and the net benefits are positive. This is the standard by which any CBA-based dementia intervention is judged to be socially beneficial. This implies that dementia symptoms do not need to be standardized in any way, unlike Tables 8.4 and 8.5, and that any kind of effect that is legitimate for an intervention can be used in a CBA. Anything that adds value to both society and the individual can have an effect.

The net benefits from the CBAs of the five new interventions are provided in the upper portion of Table 8.8. Table 8.8 is not limited to the three evaluations that appeared in Table 8.5 that relied on effects on QALYs (consisting of corrective lenses, hearing aids, and avoiding living in nursing homes), because the effects can be anything that the evaluator considers relevant. Education and Medicare eligibility have been added, and the effect to be assessed is shown in Table 8.4, which uses the independent living cost savings of lowering dementia symptoms as the effect. Different measures of effects would indeed require different approaches to affect pricing. The key takeaway, though, is that any intervention with positive net-benefits is valuable if the valuation method—which is based on individual preferences—is valid. This holds regardless of the existence of other viable alternatives, as long as they do not conflict with one another.

Table 8.8. *Net Benefits of Various Dementia Interventions*

Intervention	Benefits per Person	Costs per Person	Net-Benefits per Person
Education	$5,500	$1,400	$4,100
Corrective Lenses	$14,249	$765	$13,484
Medicare Eligibility	$9,338	$6,540	$2,798
Hearing Aids	$2,48,425	$8,498	$2,39,927
Avoiding Nursing Homes	$1,700,000	($54,545)	$1,754,545
Preventing Elder Abuse	$50,000	$7,500	$42,500
Cognitive Rehabilitation	$8,875	$942	$7,933

Source: https://www.ncbi.nlm.nih.gov/pmc/articles/PMC10001534/pdf/ijerph-20-04637.pdf.

The Value of a Statistical Life (VSL) literature served as the foundation for the pricing strategy for the interventions related to avoiding nursing homes, corrective lenses, and hearing aids. This approach takes into account individual preferences because workers are ready to exchange a certain likelihood of dying at work for annual pay increases that offset the additional risk. In statistical terms, a thousand times $5,000, or $5 million, is what a thousand times greater risk would be worth if someone is willing to accept $5,000 as payment for a one-in-a-thousand chance of dying. This essentially means that, for that $5 million total compensation, one should anticipate that, on average, one person would die out of a population of 1,000 workers who have a one in a thousand chance of dying. The education and Medicare eligibility interventions were priced according to the savings that resulted from lowering dementia symptoms and raising the likelihood of independent living. Caregivers do not have to stop spending time and money on the dementia patient once they can move into independent living. This holds for both the public and private sectors since lower Medicare costs can result from fewer cases of dementia. Two additional dementia interventions are included at the bottom of Table 8.8, which do not rely on the NACC data but show the breadth and depth of potential applications for dementia interventions. The first is a decrease in elder abuse. People take advantage of those who have dementia, which leads to elder abuse that is psychological, financial, and physical. Humans are willing to pay to stay away from this abuse. Depending on the kind of abuse, a benefit amount ranging from $40,000 to $50,000 was estimated using the willingness to prosecute as a gauge of this willingness to pay. One can lessen the severity of elder abuse by reducing the symptoms of dementia. The $7,500 cost associated with helping the abusers be prosecuted was deducted, leaving $42,500 as the net benefit of lessening the symptoms of dementia.

Cognitive rehabilitation was the second intervention that was added to Table 8.8's bottom section. The effects of a person's dementia symptoms can be lessened, particularly for the advantage of the person caring for the dementia patient, even when the condition's symptoms cannot be eliminated. With cognitive rehabilitation, in the form of the Tailored Activity Program (TAP), an occupational therapist visits the home of the caregiver to determine which behaviors related to dementia need to be changed. The caregiver is then trained to modify their behavior to spend less time "doing things" or "on duty" for the person with dementia. The benefits of the TAP were easy to calculate because the time saved by the caregiver can be valued monetarily using labor market valuations, such as the federal minimum wage rate. The estimated time-saving benefits amounted to $8,875. The estimated cost of the occupational therapist's time spent training the dementia patient and caregiver at the caregiver's home was $942. The net benefits, after deducting these expenses from the benefits, came out to $7,933. Table 8.8 serves as an example of the numerous dementia interventions that have already been tested with CBA and determined to be beneficial for society. Numerous techniques have been used to assign a value to the effect that the intervention's evaluator determined to be the most significant.

8.3.2.3. Social CBA

The CBA's outcome measure cannot be unique to the institutional healthcare setting for it to qualify as a social evaluation. The effects on every member of society must be included in the outcome measure. In a similar vein, when it comes to costs, all parties impacted by the intervention—including those who provide the funding—must have their costs added up. An externality is an unpriced consequence of one person's actions on another, and it is a pertinent economic concept in this context. An essential component of a social CBA should therefore be the pricing of the effects on others. The impact on third parties is included in the externality if the patient is regarded as the first party and the doctor or hospital providing the service is the second party. The person who goes with the patient to get the service is frequently considered the third party in the healthcare industry. The total cost includes not only the amount the healthcare provider charges but also the cost of transportation and the value of the companion's time. When a friend or family member feels satisfied with the patient's improved functioning, the full benefit extends beyond what the patient gains. In the context of the cognitive rehabilitation intervention mentioned in Table 8.8, this externality was priced explicitly. The TAP's ability to save caregiver time was what determined the intervention's net benefits.

The reduction in dementia symptoms that the new interventions produced for the patient was the effect in all of the CBAs, and this resulted in benefits in the form of either cost savings from increased independent living or the value of the QALYs. It is crucial to realize that when a dementia patient experiences fewer symptoms, the caregiver will also probably experience fewer symptoms of dementia. This is because spouses of dementia patients have a six-fold increased risk of developing dementia themselves compared to those whose spouses have not had dementia. Therefore, in addition to the direct benefits that the dementia patient receives, any decrease in symptoms experienced by the patient will result in additional external benefits. Consequently, it is necessary to interpret all of the net-benefit estimates for the new interventions in Table 8.8 as conservative underestimates of their true social value. The net benefits of all new dementia interventions must be increased by the cost savings from the caregivers' increased level of independence and the value of the QALYs they receive from the patient's decreased symptoms. The literature supports our conclusion that including externalities would probably increase the net benefits of dementia economic evaluations. For 33 of the 63 CUAs of Alzheimer interventions surveyed, it was possible to compare CEA ratios with and without externalities. When externalities were taken into account, 28 of them (85%) had CEA ratios that were either more favorable or cost-saving. The primary externalities associated with informal caregivers were increases in QALYs and cost savings in terms of time. Around 21 (64%) of the CUAs that did include externalities and were therefore converted into CBAs using a threshold price did not cross the threshold to result in a negative net benefit (the threshold prices used to value the QALYs were $50,000, $1,00,000, and $1,50,000) (Chang et al., 2017; Robinson et al., 2019).

A Closer Look

Patient-Reported Outcomes (PROs)

A health outcome that has been directly reported by the patient who experienced it is known as a patient-reported outcome (PRO). It is not the same as an outcome that has been reported by another person, like an outcome from a doctor, a nurse, and so on. In clinical trials and other clinical settings, PRO methods—such as questionnaires—are employed to gain a deeper understanding of the efficacy or effectiveness of a treatment. In today's health research setting, the use of digitized PROs, or electronic patient-reported outcomes (ePROs), is growing. The term PRO refers specifically to patient self-reporting, but it encompasses a wide range of possible measurements. PRO data can be gathered through patient interviews or self-administered questionnaires that the patient completes on their own. The latter, however, will only be considered a PRO if the interviewer is eliciting the patient's opinions and isn't using the answers to form an expert opinion or assessment regarding how a treatment is affecting the patient's condition. Therefore, patient perspectives—as opposed to clinical or other outcomes perspectives—are gathered through PROs. Gaining approval for a medication or course of treatment can benefit greatly from the patient-reported viewpoint. Patients have no reason to report their outcome data other than to give back to the community and assist the medical community in preventing needless suffering in other patients.

A well-crafted PRO questionnaire should evaluate one main attribute or, in cases where it covers several attributes, several scales that each focus on a different attribute. The terms "constructs" refer to these measurement features, and "instruments," "measures," "scales," or "tools" refer to the questionnaires used to gather them. PRO tools usually need to go through a rigorous validation and testing process. A unidimensional questionnaire measures only one construct. It is possible to create a single scale score by adding items (questions) to a unidimensional questionnaire. A questionnaire is not, however, always one-dimensional. This needs to be proven empirically (using confirmatory factor analysis or regression analysis, for instance). A multi-dimensional questionnaire assesses several constructs. A profile of scores is produced by means of a multi-dimensional questionnaire, in which each scale is scored and reported independently. While some may see this as akin to adding apples and oranges together, it is possible to create an overall (single summary) score from a multi-dimensional measure using factor analysis or preference-based methods. Questionnaires can be condition-targeted (created especially to measure those aspects of outcome that are of importance for a people with a particular medical condition) or generic (designed to be used in any disease population and cover a broad aspect of the construct measured).

The most commonly used PRO questionnaires assess one of the following constructs:

- Symptoms (impairments) and other aspects of well-being;
- Functioning (disability);
- Health status;
- General health perceptions;

- Quality of life (QoL);
- Health-related quality of life (HRQoL);
- Reports and ratings of healthcare.

Symptom measures can concentrate on a variety of impairments or a particular impairment, like pain or depression. Functioning measures evaluate daily living activities, personal care, and locomotor activities. Health-related quality of life instruments are multifaceted questionnaires that evaluate various aspects of impairments and/or disability and provide information about the overall health status of the patient. QoL, on the other hand, inquires about the patient's capacity to meet their needs as well as their emotional reaction to their limitations, going beyond impairment and disability.

Summary

- Health economics uses economic concepts and methods to understand and explain how people make decisions regarding their health behaviors and use of healthcare.
- Economic evaluation is a multidisciplinary field that assesses the costs and consequences of healthcare interventions to inform decision-making. It encompasses various methods, including cost-effectiveness analysis (CEA), cost-utility analysis (CUA), and cost-benefit analysis (CBA), each with its unique focus and approach.
- Cost-benefit analysis (CBA) is an economic analysis in which both the costs and consequences are expressed in monetary terms. The numerator states the monetary benefit gained from the treatment and the denominator defines the monetary investment for the treatment.
- Cost-effectiveness analysis (CEA) in healthcare is a quantitative method used to compare the costs and health outcomes of alternative interventions or treatments. It provides decision-makers with valuable insights into the relative efficiency of different healthcare strategies by evaluating how much it costs to achieve a particular health outcome.
- Opportunity cost is a fundamental concept in economics that refers to the value of the next best alternative forgone when a decision is made. In healthcare, opportunity cost plays a crucial role in resource allocation and decision-making, particularly in contexts where resources such as funding, time, or personnel are limited.
- Sensitivity analysis is a quantitative method used to assess the robustness and reliability of the results of a decision model or economic evaluation in the face of uncertainty.
- In healthcare, incremental analysis is often used in cost-effectiveness evaluations to compare the costs and outcomes of alternative interventions. For example, when considering the adoption of a new medical treatment, researchers may conduct an incremental cost-effectiveness analysis to compare the additional costs incurred and health benefits gained by using the new treatment compared to standard care.
- Health intervention is defined as the use of a health program, action, or technology to reduce or eliminate a health problem. The ultimate goal of health interventions is to improve the health and quality of life of people and patients.
- Healthcare demand is continuing to grow; however, the resources available for healthcare are explicitly limited. Consequently, ensuring the best value for money spent in healthcare has been placed high on the agenda for governments worldwide, with economic considerations gaining an increasingly prominent role when planning, managing, and evaluating health systems.
- A cost-benefit analysis (referred to as benefit-cost analysis) is a comparative analysis of the relative costs and outcomes of two or more alternative courses of action, where both the costs of an intervention and its resulting outcomes are expressed in monetary terms.

References

1. Briggs, A. H., & O'Brien, B. J. (2001). The death of cost-minimization analysis? *Health Economics, 10*, 179–184. https://doi.org/10.1002/hec.584.
2. Chang, A. Y., Horton, S., & Jamison, D. T. (2017). Benefit-cost analysis in disease control priorities. In D. T. Jamison, H. Gelband, S. Horton, P. Jha, R. Laxminarayan, C. N. Mock, & R. Nugent (Eds.), *Disease Control Priorities: Improving Health and Reducing Poverty* (3rd ed., Chapter 9). Washington, DC: The International Bank for Reconstruction and Development/The World Bank.
3. Chisholm, D., & Evans, B. D. (2007). Economic evaluation in health: Saving money or improving care? *Journal of Medical Economics, 10*, 325–337. https://doi.org/10.3111/13696990701605235.
4. Drummond, M. F., Sculpher, M. J., Claxton, K., Stoddart, G. L., & Torrance, G. W. (2015). *Methods for the Economic Evaluation of Health Care Programmes* (4th ed.). Oxford: Oxford University Press.
5. Eddama, O., & Coast, J. (2008). A systematic review of the use of economic evaluation in local decision-making. *Health Policy, 86*, 129–141. https://doi.org/10.1016/j.healthpol.2007.11.010.
6. Hayati, R., Bastani, P., Kabir, M. J., Kavosi, Z., & Sobhani, G. (2018). Scoping literature review on the basic health benefit package and its determinant criteria. *Global Health, 14*, 26. https://doi.org/10.1186/s12992-018-0345-x.
7. Luz, A., Santatiwongchai, B., Pattanaphesaj, J., & Teerawattananon, Y. (2018). Identifying priority technical and context-specific issues in improving the conduct, reporting and use of health economic evaluation in low- and middle-income countries. *Health Research Policy and Systems, 16*, 4. https://doi.org/10.1186/s12961-018-0280-6.
8. Pitt, C., Goodman, C., & Hanson, K. (2016). Economic evaluation in global perspective: A bibliometric analysis of the recent literature. *Health Economics, 25*(Suppl 1), 9–28. https://doi.org/10.1002/hec.3305.
9. Robinson, L. A., Hammitt, J. K., Jamison, D. T., & Walker, D. G. (2019). Conducting benefit-cost analysis in low- and middle-income countries: Introduction to the special issue. *Journal of Benefit-Cost Analysis, 10*, 1–14. https://doi.org/10.1017/bca.2019.4.
10. Sassi, F. (2006). Calculating QALYs, comparing QALY and DALY calculations. *Health Policy and Planning, 21*, 402–408. https://doi.org/10.1093/heapol/czl018.
11. Simoens, S. (2009). Health economic assessment: A methodological primer. *International Journal of Environmental Research and Public Health, 6*, 2950–2966. https://doi.org/10.3390/ijerph6122950.
12. Udeh, B. L. (2020). Economic evaluation studies. *CHEST, 158*(5, Suppl), S88–S96. https://doi.org/10.1016/j.chest.2020.03.008.
13. World Health Organization. (2019). *WHO Guide on Standardization of Economic Evaluations of Immunization Programs*. Retrieved from: https://www.who.int (accessed on 1 July 2024).
14. Zarnke, K. B., Levine, M. A., & O'Brien, B. J. (1997). Cost-benefit analyses in the health-care literature: Don't judge a study by its label. *Journal of Clinical Epidemiology, 50*, 813–822. https://doi.org/10.1016/S0895-4356(97)00064-4.

Chapter 9

HEALTH EFFICIENCY

Contents

Introduction

The term "human health efficiency" refers to a wide range of variables that affect how well the body functions overall. Humans function within a delicate balance of biological processes designed to maintain homeostasis, from the molecular to the systemic. This efficiency, which maximizes resource use and energy expenditure to support life, is evidence of the complexity of evolution's design. The marvel of human metabolism is the foundation of health efficiency. The word "metabolism," which refers to all chemical processes that occur within the body, controls how food is converted into energy, how tissues are made and repaired, and how waste is removed. The distribution, absorption, and processing of vital nutrients to their sites of greatest need are all facilitated by this complex dance of biochemical pathways. Human metabolism is remarkably precise in responding to the body's needs, from the slow-burning of fats for prolonged endurance to the breakdown of carbohydrates for rapid energy bursts.

In addition, the immune system uses a sophisticated network of cells, tissues, and organs to protect the body from infections. The immune system's capacity to identify and eliminate foreign invaders while differentiating them from the body's cells is a clear sign of health efficiency. The immune system not only fights infection but also gains knowledge and adapts for defense in the future through the generation of antibodies, immune cell activation, and memory of previous experiences. The efficient structural design of human anatomy and physiology is visible even outside of the microscopic realm. Every cell in the body receives oxygen and nutrients from the cardiovascular system, which is made up of the heart, blood vessels, and blood itself. It also eliminates waste products. The heart effectively circulates blood throughout the body with each beat, guaranteeing a steady supply of essential nutrients. Similar to this, the respiratory system effectively exchanges gases, allowing carbon dioxide to be expelled and oxygen to be delivered to tissues. This process is made possible by the regular rise and fall of the lungs.

The musculoskeletal system, which functions remarkably well to produce force and maintain posture, provides the framework for movement and support. Coordinated contraction and relaxation of muscle fibers maximize energy efficiency while permitting exact control over movement. In the meantime, bones offer security and stability. They continuously remodel to adapt to mechanical stress, maintaining structural integrity throughout a lifetime. Maintaining health efficiency is largely dependent on nutrition, which supplies the building blocks needed for development, maintenance, and regulation. Tissue integrity is preserved, immunological function is bolstered, and metabolic processes are fueled by a nutritious, well-balanced diet. The body gets the most out of the food it consumes when nutrients are absorbed and used efficiently, which promotes health and vitality.

The effectiveness of human health is evidence of the complex interactions between harmonious biological systems. The human body functions remarkably well to support life, from the microscopic domain of cellular metabolism to the macroscopic coordination of organ systems. By following a healthy diet, engaging in regular exercise, and receiving prompt medical attention, people can maximize their health and fully utilize their biological capabilities.

Orientation and Directional Terms:

Term	Definition	Illustration
Health system efficiency	Healthcare efficiency is a comparison of delivery system outputs, such as physician visits, relative value units, or health outcomes, with inputs like cost, time, or material.	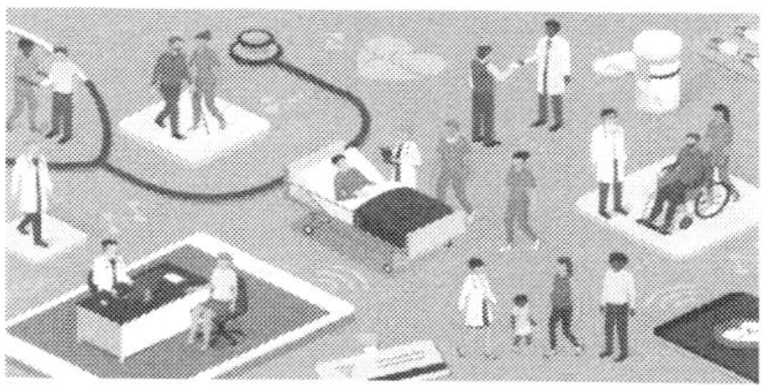
Healthcare	Healthcare is the improvement of health via the prevention, diagnosis, treatment, amelioration, or cure of disease, illness, injury, and other physical and mental impairments in people.	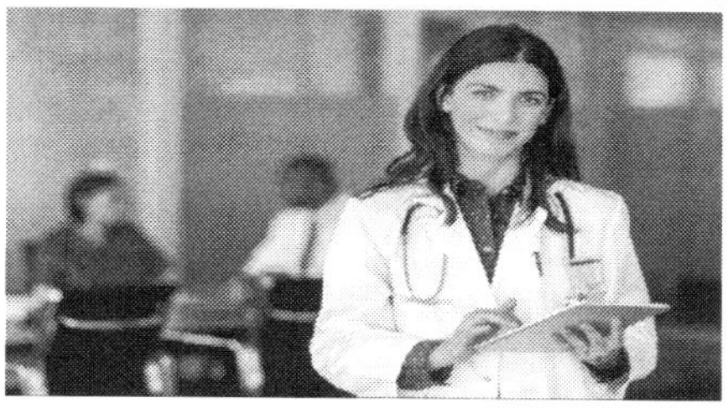
Electronic health record	An electronic health record (EHR) is the systematized collection of patient and population electronically stored health information in a digital format.	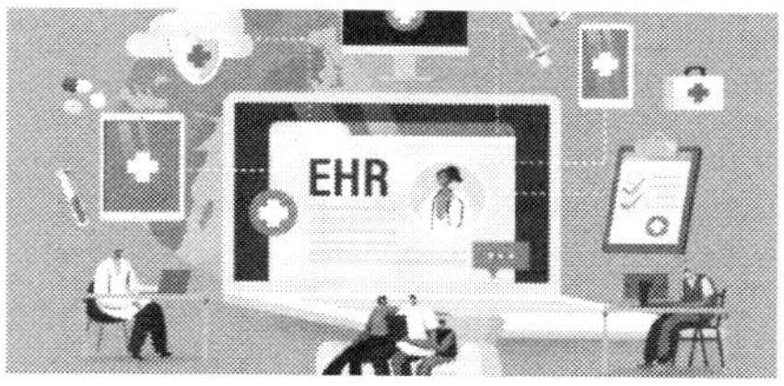
Clinical efficiency	Clinical efficiency is how well resources are used to meet needs or demands.	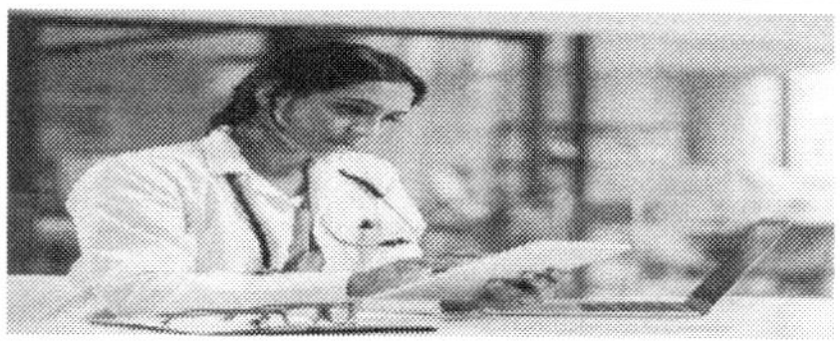

9.1. Concepts of Productivity and Efficiency

Two essential ideas that are vital to the prosperity of people, businesses, and economies are productivity and efficiency. Despite their frequent interchangeability, they stand for different but related aspects of output and performance. The rate at which goods and services are produced relative to the input of resources like labor, capital, and technology is known as productivity. It is a crucial factor in determining economic growth and prosperity because it quantifies the effectiveness of converting inputs into outputs. Put more simply, productivity is the amount of output produced per unit of input. For instance, the quantity of units produced per labor hour or dollar invested in capital can be used to calculate productivity in a manufacturing setting.

Contrastingly, efficiency is the capacity to produce a maximum amount of work with the least amount of resources or input. It entails streamlining activities, cutting waste, and optimizing processes to achieve objectives in the most efficient and resource-conserving way possible. Productivity and efficiency are closely related because raising efficiency frequently results in higher productivity. Through the reduction of inefficiencies, companies can optimize resource allocation, augment productivity, and ultimately strengthen their market competitiveness.

A combination of elements, such as organizational structure, management techniques, technology, and human capital, is needed to achieve high levels of productivity and efficiency. Technology is essential for increasing productivity because it can automate tasks, cut down on errors, and expedite procedures. The introduction of computer-aided design (CAD) software, for example, has transformed the manufacturing sector by enabling engineers to design products more rapidly and precisely, leading to higher productivity.

Enhancing productivity and efficiency also requires investing in human capital through skill development, training, and education. Employees who are motivated and well-trained are more likely to complete their work efficiently and make a positive impact on the success of the company. Furthermore, by encouraging staff members to find and apply process improvements, an innovative and continuous improvement culture can boost productivity.

Productivity and efficiency can also be significantly influenced by management techniques and organizational design. Streamlined decision-making procedures, efficient task delegation, and open lines of communication can all aid in removing obstacles and enhancing workflow. Performance measures and rewards can also encourage workers to work more productively and coordinate their efforts with company objectives. Although efficiency and productivity are crucial for the success of individual businesses, they also have wider effects on economies as a whole. Increased output, cheaper production costs, and improved living standards for the populace are all possible outcomes of higher productivity levels. Furthermore, increases in efficiency have the potential to boost innovation, accelerate economic growth, and raise competitiveness internationally. The fundamental ideas of productivity and efficiency support the competitiveness and performance of people, businesses, and economies. In the long run, entities can drive sustainable growth and prosperity by implementing effective management practices, investing in human capital, leveraging technology, and optimizing resource allocation to increase productivity and efficiency.

9.1.1. Improving Operational Efficiency in Healthcare

Healthcare is a complicated industry that is prone to administrative red tape and state intervention that can impede the adoption of new technologies, as well as rapid changes in medical practice as new treatments are developed. The transition from manual to digital healthcare processes must take patient safety into account in addition to system robustness and ability to adapt to changing data over time. Nonetheless, there can be significant advantages to process simplification and improvement while preserving the same standard of care, including lower costs and increased systemic efficiency.

Increasing patient satisfaction, health outcomes, cost-effectiveness, and healthcare efficiency are all dependent on it. Efficiency analyses show that between 20% and 40% of healthcare organizational resources are squandered, amounting to $760 to $935 billion in unnecessary medical expenses in the US alone. Your practice's care value, efficacy, and effectiveness can all be increased by cutting down on this unnecessary medical expense with a more capable medical staff and more efficient technology. We offer all-inclusive software to simplify the way healthcare services are run. You can handle everything with our end-to-end healthcare system, including electronic health records (EHRs), provider communication, appointment scheduling, and payment collection. For increasing productivity in your medical practice, whether it be in emergency medicine, sports medicine, dentistry, primary care, or any other area.

9.1.2. Why Efficiency in Healthcare Is Important?

Public health, organizational performance, and patient experience are all impacted by the effectiveness of the healthcare system.

Efficiency is important because it affects the following:

1. **Healthcare Expenditures:** Healthcare research on health economics shows that the healthcare industry wastes hundreds of billions yearly due to technical inefficiencies in service delivery and internal operations. These wasted funds could go toward necessary health affairs, like providing more affordable access to healthcare providers.
2. **Communication:** Modern patients see multiple doctors and specialists. For example, someone may seek out specialty healthcare workers for neurology-related problems. Because of this fragmentation, communication in an efficient health system has become necessary for providing consistent and accurate care.
3. **Patient Care:** The World Health Organization and U.S. National Guideline Clearinghouse consistently release new health services research and health policy guidelines surrounding optimal care techniques. These constant updates, combined with fragmented providers, make delivering successful patient care nearly impossible without an efficient system that can handle it. Improving healthcare system efficiency can help you stay on top of health records and best practices.

4. **Public Health Access:** Healthcare is not available, accessible, or affordable to all due to many factors relating to health economics. Economic research shows that poor organization-wide efficiency results in wasted resources, creating higher wait times and costs on the patient's end. Improved efficiency can reduce wasted spending, making healthcare more accessible and improving population health.

A comparison of the inputs, such as cost, time, or material, and the outputs of the delivery system, such as physician visits, relative value units, or health outcomes, is known as healthcare efficiency. Then, efficiency can be expressed as an output-to-input ratio or a comparison, using data envelopment analysis or stochastic frontier analysis, with optimal productivity. Examining latency times, the amount of time that passes between a care order and the completion of the task, and the accomplishment's stated value in relation to the estimated effort are some alternative methods. Outcome comparability is a challenge in developing a generalized efficiency measure. The assumption may be that hospital B is more efficient if, for instance, hospital A discharges 100 patients at an average cost of $8,000 while hospital B discharges 100 for $7,000. However, hospital B may be discharging patients with worse health, which will necessitate readmission and result in higher treatment costs.

9.1.3. Efficiency of Health Systems

As the variety of approaches isn't easy to compile and compare results from the literature on the effectiveness of health systems. This covers variations in methodology (qualitative and quantitative), as well as choices for models, exogenous variables, inputs, and outputs. For example, a sensitivity analysis of the World Health Organization's (WHO) initial efficiency analysis of 141 countries discovered that the model specification and definition of efficiency had an impact on the efficiency scores and country rankings. The main focus of qualitative papers was the opinions of stakeholders in the health system regarding the existence and causes of inefficiencies in the system. The degree of health system efficiency was reported using quantitative methods as an inefficiency score or as a proportion (with a range of 0–100). For instance, the most recent regional analysis of the effectiveness of the nation's health systems revealed that the mean efficiency for 45 African countries was 80% (range 31–100%), for 46 Asian countries it was 92% (range 81–91%), for 27 Latin American countries it was 93% (range 51–93%), and for 28 European countries it was 83% (range 54–94%). A mean efficiency of 93% (range 71–100%) was found in the most recent global analysis of the effectiveness of 140 country health systems. The regional means of this analysis were as follows: African countries (86%), Asian countries (95%), South American countries (95%), and European countries (96%). A health system that achieves a 100% efficiency score is considered highly efficient; on the other hand, a system that falls short of this threshold may still be able to improve its efficiency by increasing output or decreasing inputs.

9.1.4. Factors Affecting the Efficiency of Health Systems

9.1.4.1. Demographic Characteristics of the Population

It was discovered that several population/demographic factors influenced the technical efficiency of the health system. The density of the population was one of these. A high population density within a nation or sub-national unit (district, region, etc.) has been found in certain studies to be linked to higher levels of technical effectiveness. For example, a high population density in primary healthcare catchment areas improved the technical efficiency of regional health systems, according to a study on Chile's primary healthcare system. The technical efficiency of 46 Asian countries' health systems was examined, and it was discovered that those with populations of more than 200 per square kilometer were technically more efficient than those with populations of ≤100. Greater population densities improved the technical efficiency of regional health systems by lowering healthcare costs per capita and facilitating the organization and use of service infrastructure by health systems. They also reduced the distances to populations. Nonetheless, certain research findings indicated an inverse relationship between population density and the technical efficacy of the health system. Large populations, for example, were found to lower the technical efficiency of municipalities in a study of Finnish municipalities. The authors hypothesized that this could be due to other factors related to population size, such as quality differences, bureaucratic inefficiencies, or unmeasured outputs. According to a Kenyan study, population density and the technical effectiveness of the county health system were inversely correlated. It was hypothesized that this was probably because higher population densities were not accompanied by enough healthcare resources, which compromised health outcomes. The population's distribution between rural and urban areas was another aspect that was investigated. There is a consensus that technically less efficient regions are those with lower rates of urbanization. This was because reduced urbanization was linked to lower income levels and unemployment rates, both of which have an impact on healthcare utilization. The age distribution of the population was also examined; large percentages of very young people (children) or very old people decreased the technical efficiency of health systems because these vulnerable groups raised healthcare costs.

9.1.4.2. Socio-Economic Characteristics of the Population/ Social Determinants of Health

Numerous socioeconomic traits of the populace were looked at. According to certain research, the population's improved socioeconomic standing is positively correlated with the technical efficacy of the health system. For example, several studies discovered a correlation between higher per capita income and higher levels of technical health system efficiency in a nation or region. Nonetheless, certain research findings indicated an inverse relationship between per capita population income and the technical efficiency of the health system. This was assumed to be the case because health systems with higher per capita income catchment populations also tended to have higher rates of overprovision and higher overall healthcare costs.

It was discovered that the distribution of incomes also determined the technical efficiency of the health system, in addition to the average income levels in a nation. Low technical efficiency was linked to high-income inequality and poverty. Bekarogu and Heffley discovered that rising levels of poverty and income inequality had an impact on the health system's technical efficiency by lowering the system's overall level of outcomes. Employment status was a related socioeconomic factor; high unemployment rates were linked to lower technical efficiency of the health system.

Numerous studies have shown that having access to clean water and basic sanitation improves health systems' technical efficiency. This means that better sanitation leads to better health outcomes, which in turn improves the system's technical efficiency. For instance, the proportion of the population having access to sanitation services is linked to higher levels of technical efficiency, and the rate at which people have access to drinking water is linked to lower rates of water-related illnesses like cholera, fever, and malaria. Higher literacy rates have been linked to improved health systems' technical efficiency. For instance, the technical efficiency of the health system is higher in Asian nations with higher literacy rates. This is believed to be the case because educated individuals can convert health information and knowledge more readily.

9.1.4.3. Macro-Economic Characteristics

Mixed results were found regarding the impact of a nation's economic size on the technical efficiency of its health system. According to certain research, countries with higher GDP per capita also tend to deliver healthcare in a more technically efficient manner. This was believed to be the case because a wealthier nation may be able to invest more in the health sector and other areas that affect the social determinants of health, with better health and quality of life leading to better overall health outcomes. According to certain research, nations with developed road networks and easy access to electricity tend to have health systems that are more technically efficient. Other research, however, discovered a correlation between lower technical efficiency of health systems and higher GDP per capita. This was assumed to be caused by the rising relative costs of healthcare in wealthier nations due to overprovision.

9.1.4.4. Health and Wellbeing of the Population

The population's overall health and well-being had an impact on the health system's technical effectiveness. In general, the lower technical efficiency of the health system was linked to a higher prevalence of chronic disease. For example, Novignon & Lawanson discovered that HIV/AIDS hurts the technical efficiency of health systems in Africa and that a 10% increase in the percentage of individuals with chronic conditions would result in a 10% to 18% drop in the technical efficiency score of regional health systems in Canada. Moreover, health systems catering to populations with elevated levels of health risk factors, such as obesity, alcoholism, and smoking, are probably less efficient in terms of technology. As an illustration, a high alcohol intake raises inefficiency by hastening illness and death. High rates of chronic health-related risk factors had detrimental effects on the efficiency of the healthcare system by lowering health system outcomes and raising healthcare costs.

9.1.4.5. Health System Characteristics

It was discovered that several aspects of how health systems operate influence how efficient they are. First, there are multiple ways in which the financing of health systems has an impact on their efficiency. The efficiency of the health system was found to be adversely impacted by the fragmentation of financing arrangements, particularly the existence of multiple health insurance companies. The efficiency of the health system was also influenced by the amount spent on healthcare. The technical efficiency of health systems was positively correlated with total health expenditure as a percentage of GDP. This was believed to be because improving health outcomes required higher healthcare spending. However, some research indicates that when the health system is characterized by higher costs of care or unnecessary treatment, then higher levels of total health expenditure may be negatively correlated with efficiency. There is evidence that technical efficiency is also influenced by the funding source for the health sector. The technical efficiency of the health system was positively correlated with the portion of public funds allocated to healthcare. Moreover, higher population coverage through a prepayment health-financing mechanism (like health insurance) was linked to higher health system technical efficiency. According to a Chinese evaluation, provinces with a high percentage of out-of-pocket expenses had less technical efficiency. On the other hand, in contexts with sufficient population coverage and prepayment mechanisms, studies on the effectiveness of OECD (Organization for Economic Co-operation and Development) countries have found a positive correlation between out-of-pocket payments in the form of co-payments and health system efficiency. This occurred as a result of co-payments discouraging needless medical care. The efficiency of the health system was also impacted by public finance management arrangements. Increased efficiency can be attributed to factors including improved budget execution, money flowing directly to providers, prompt funding disbursements to local governments and healthcare facilities, budget flexibility, and resource autonomy for both.

The way that healthcare providers were compensated had an impact on the efficiency of the health system's purchasing function. For example, studies have found a positive correlation between health system efficiency and prospective payments like capitation, as opposed to fee-for-service payments, because the former disincentivizes unnecessary care and the latter gives purchasers greater cost control. The implementation of a zero-margin policy for drug sales in the public sector in the Democratic Republic of the Congo lessened the motivation for medical professionals to prescribe needless medications. The efficiency of the health system is also impacted by the layout and execution of benefit plans. By giving cost-effective health services top priority in their benefit packages, Chile, Mexico, and Uruguay have all increased the effectiveness of their healthcare systems.

It was also discovered that patients who interacted with healthcare providers had an impact on the effectiveness of health systems. Higher technical efficiency was linked to health systems where patients had a choice in healthcare providers. The implementation of gatekeeping by primary care providers, which necessitates a referral from a general practitioner for non-emergency access to a specialist, has improved the efficiency of the healthcare system by matching the level of specialization and cost of care with patient needs and lowering healthcare expenditures. However, in situations where primary care physicians had limited ability to coordinate patient care follow-up or where the health system's capacity to provide secondary care was limited, some studies found that gatekeeping could decrease the efficiency of the health system. Long wait times, a rise in the use of emergency rooms and hospital stays, and overall inefficiency were caused by the health system's inability to offer specialized care. Whether or not gatekeeping was combined with initiatives to raise the accessibility and caliber of secondary care services determined how beneficial gatekeeping was in improving the efficiency of the health system. Furthermore, it has been documented that price regulation and gatekeeping interact. It has been noted that gatekeeping, which encourages excessive specialization of healthcare professionals to obtain higher fees, may decrease efficiency when healthcare prices are regulated. To reduce their input costs as general practitioners, it also encourages them to refer patients to specialists for care that isn't necessary.

Strong controls over the operations of the health system, particularly those related to pricing, medication use, and the health workforce, have been linked to improved technical efficiency in the field of health governance. Pharmaceutical regulations that reinforced price control, authorized generic prescriptions, and enforced national essential drug lists enhanced the effectiveness of health systems in China and El Salvador. Efficiency gains in the health system were also linked to better coordination within the health sector, including the coordination of donor initiatives.

By matching and coordinating donor support with health sector priorities, and coordinating health sector planning, budgeting, and resource allocation to minimize waste and duplication, the Democratic Republic of the Congo and Zambia experienced improvements in the efficiency of their health systems. In addition to coordination within the health sector, multi-sectoral coordination and collaborations aimed at addressing social determinants of health were believed to enhance efficacy. According to certain research, national and sub-national health systems with more decentralized health functions have higher technical efficiency. An evaluation of the technical effectiveness of healthcare systems in a few middle-income nations revealed that decentralization improved technical effectiveness by enhancing care delivery in rural areas and improving health systems' responsiveness to community needs by increasing community involvement in healthcare decision-making. It has been discovered that efficient performance accountability and monitoring increase the effectiveness of Canada's health system. The effectiveness of the health system was also believed to be determined by leadership, management, and capacity. The technical efficiency of systems and the quality of governance are positively correlated, according to a study on the technical efficiency of 27 Latin American and Caribbean nations. The study's definition of governance quality was a multifaceted index that took into account factors like political stability, absence of violence or terrorism, rule of law, voice and accountability, and corruption control. Furthermore, evaluations of the technical effectiveness of the health systems in WHO member nations revealed a correlation between increased democratization and freedom and improved technical effectiveness of the health system. It has also been discovered that lower technical efficiency is linked to corruption.

Increased technical efficiency of health systems was correlated with the availability and distribution of hardware for health systems, such as infrastructure, equipment, and medical supplies. The ineffective combination of inputs caused by inadequate input availability had a detrimental effect on the effectiveness of the health system. An evaluation of the technical efficiency of health systems in Asian countries, for instance, indicated a positive correlation between technical efficiency and the density of hospital beds. An evaluation conducted in Canada discovered a correlation between the technical efficiency of national and subnational health systems and the unequal distribution of health workers. Inefficiency developed in Ethiopia as a result of an increase in primary healthcare facilities that was not accompanied by an increase in medical personnel. Health worker distribution and level had an impact on the effectiveness of the health system. Health systems at the national and local levels that lacked sufficient medical personnel performed less well. Inefficiencies in procurement were also found. This included procurement corruption, high procurement costs, supply chain issues resulting in stock-outs and delivery delays, and dispersed procurement of health commodities. Reduced health system efficiency was linked to higher pharmaceutical spending. This was believed to be a result of high pharmaceutical costs crowding out other healthcare inputs and decreasing the effectiveness of health resource utilization.

Reduced technical efficiency was linked to overprovision of health services, which includes extended hospital stays, high referral rates, high doctor consultation rates, high admission rates, and inappropriate drug use (such as antibiotic use), which is a component of care quality. For instance, the negative correlation between technical efficiency and admission rates suggested that using hospitalization services that require a lot of resources would be detrimental to the technical efficiency of the health system.

There is a correlation between higher health system efficiency and the arrangement of care to prioritize lower-level basic care primary healthcare. Provincial medical centers would become more technically efficient if a larger percentage of their services were provided in primary facilities. The efficiency of the health system was positively correlated with the percentage of basic and essential services in benefit packages. This was because basic and essential services were less expensive than advanced and costly care. Furthermore, it was predicted that health systems with a high proportion of primary care physicians—as opposed to specialists—would operate more effectively. It has been demonstrated that policy changes centered on increasing access to primary and community-based care and involving the community enhance the technical effectiveness of healthcare systems in OECD nations. Increased technical efficiency was linked to additional reforms aimed at improving the underprivileged and vulnerable access to healthcare and lowering access disparities.

9.1.5. The Impact of AI on Healthcare

Inspect immense amounts of patient info, including medical images, and electronic health records:

- Identify potential health issues with greater precision and speed than ever before.
- Provide a truly personalized approach to medicine.
- Tailor treatments as well as assist diagnosis and reduce the time before preventative healthcare interventions can be implemented.

This customized approach may also lead to better patient outcomes and lower costs for the patient and the healthcare provider. It also increases the possibility of successful treatments and shortens the time it takes to find a solution.

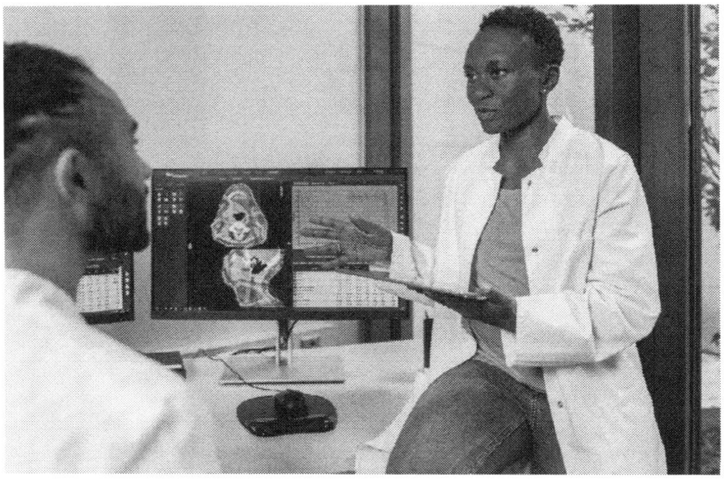

Source: https://assets-global.website-files.com/637e314d602973e4e6423677/647e03fc1c37abf7ac61beb5_644a2eb00dfd765053de69f6_Improving%20operational%20efficiency%20in%20healthcare.webp.

9.1.6. Utilizing Process Automation in AI

Through process automation, AI can also enhance administrative duties in the healthcare industry. Staff members have less time to concentrate on patient care because these procedures are frequently laborious and prone to human error. Healthcare providers can increase productivity, cut expenses, and improve patient care by simplifying administrative tasks.

While automation and artificial intelligence (AI) can improve the healthcare industry, patients' needs must always come first. This includes their treatment and health outcomes, as well as their health data and privacy rights. IT and operations leaders implementing new technology must be cognizant of these demands and find a workable solution to increase productivity.

9.1.7. Improving Operational Efficiency in Healthcare

Numerous crucial areas, scalable to larger healthcare organizations and provider groups as well as individual healthcare providers like hospitals, support improvements in the operational efficiency of the healthcare sector.

1. **Focus on Consistency:** First, addressing important processes establishes a solid foundation for subsequent change. To ensure meaningful progress, identify the critical points and bottlenecks in the critical processes that will have the greatest impact, concentrating on the issue's root cause rather than just its immediate effects. This is in contrast to a patchwork approach that addresses individual problems as and when they arise.
2. **Improve Processes, Not Just Working Conditions:** By concentrating on enhancing the way individuals work with processes rather than just personnel or workspace, it is possible to lessen the dependence on personnel management to produce outcomes using frequently outdated or patchwork-improved toolkits. By applying process mapping, operations managers can build an improvement model that tackles the essential operational aspects of a healthcare facility and involves employees in recognizing problems and formulating solutions.
3. **Get Organizational Buy-In:** People on the ground must accept any changes made to the process, and steps should be taken to ensure they receive ongoing training and support. Improvements in operational efficiency will be made possible by strong change management leadership and strategy. After all, without adequate employee onboarding and training, it is unrealistic to expect new processes and updated essential components to bring about change. This has an impact on the success of the new processes as well as any administration or treatments that the processes are meant to support.

   For operations managers, top-down training and communication are the only ways to achieve more effective process management. This strategy is also recommended by the NHS: "Organizational and system-wide multi-professional collaboration is necessary to improve value and efficiency." Only in an environment where team relationships are flourishing can organizations provide effective patient care given the resources at their disposal.

4. **Identify Barriers and Siloed Areas of Operations:** Creating a more cohesive healthcare system is essential to increasing effectiveness. When healthcare organizations operate in silos, the result is fragmented care, which produces inefficiencies and worse outcomes. The NHS has the chance to provide better value by adopting an integrated, more cooperative approach to the planning, designing, and delivering health services across local systems through the creation of integrated care systems (ICSs).

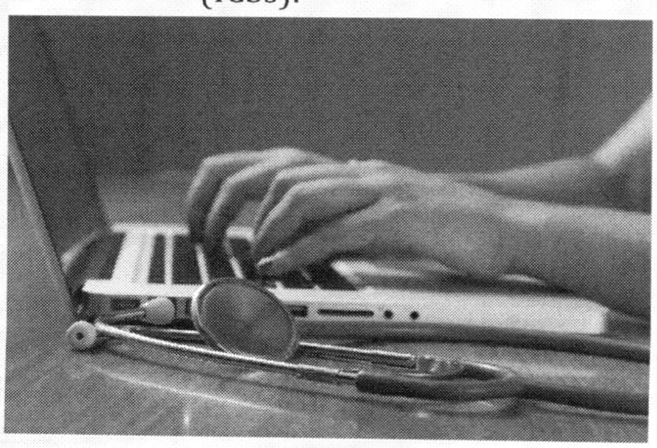

Source: https://assets-global.website-files.com/637e314d602973e4e6423677/647e04089bbc0f5feec91b78_644a2ebb121c527e152f585a_Improving%20operational%20efficiency%20in%20healthcare%20-%202.webp.

9.1.8. Orchestration in Healthcare

The largest lever for increasing operational efficiency is orchestration. Productivity can be increased by removing bottlenecks and emphasizing standardizing and streamlining procedures. The orchestration of care has been crucial for coordinating and creating positive change for IT and operations leaders in the healthcare industry. Data is used to identify problematic processes and develop new workflows that can be implemented across national (and international) health organizations.

Personalization is essential to well-executed care orchestration. This specifically means that well-orchestrated care must integrate disparate departments and procedures into a single, patient-centric continuum. This is more difficult than it seems because the patient's unique circumstances will inevitably cause that continuum to shift. Departments may be closely paired for particular patients at times, or if it is the appropriate course of action, they may be completely bypassed.

9.2. Data Envelopment Analysis: Introduction

In the field of health economics, Data Envelopment Analysis (DEA) is a commonly employed technique for assessing the relative effectiveness of healthcare providers, including clinics, hospitals, and healthcare systems. Researchers and decision-makers can evaluate how well these organizations use their resources to provide healthcare services and results thanks to this analytical technique. When used in conjunction with Introduction to Health Economics, DEA is a useful instrument for comprehending and enhancing healthcare delivery efficiency. The increasing need to make sure that resources are distributed effectively to maximize health outcomes while minimizing costs is a result of the global healthcare expenditure trend.

The idea behind DEA is to compare various inputs (e.g., personnel, equipment, and financial resources) to a variety of outputs (e.g., patient outcomes, and care quality) to assess each healthcare provider's effectiveness. Because DEA takes into account several performance dimensions at once, in contrast to traditional methods that concentrate on a single input-output ratio, it is especially well-suited for assessing complex healthcare systems. Researchers can examine many facets of healthcare delivery, including the efficacy of healthcare interventions, the influence of organizational structure on performance, and the efficiency of various healthcare facilities, by applying DEA to Introduction to Health Economics. The results of this analysis can help guide policy decisions that aim to improve the efficacy and efficiency of healthcare delivery by offering insightful information about areas that need improvement.

Additionally, DEA can help with benchmarking exercises so that medical professionals can find best practices by comparing their performance to that of their peers. To improve patient outcomes, healthcare organizations can maximize resource allocation and spearhead continuous improvement initiatives with the aid of this comparative analysis.

In Introduction to Health Economics, Data Envelopment Analysis provides a potent methodology for evaluating the effectiveness of healthcare delivery. DEA can help advance healthcare systems and promote better health outcomes for individuals and communities by assessing the performance of healthcare providers and identifying areas for improvement.

9.2.1. Data Envelopment Analysis: CCR Model

In health economics, Data Envelopment Analysis (DEA) is a potent mathematical tool used to assess the effectiveness of healthcare providers, including clinics, hospitals, and healthcare systems. The Charnes, Cooper, and Rhodes (CCR) Model, which evaluates the relative efficiency of decision-making units (DMUs) by comparing their inputs to outputs, is one of the most widely used DEA models. Researchers and policymakers can measure how well healthcare providers use resources to deliver services and meet goals when using the CCR model in the context of health economics. The basis of the model is the identification of the most effective DMUs, sometimes referred to as efficient units, which serve as benchmarks for other units.

The first step in the CCR model is to define a group of DMUs, each of which stands for a healthcare provider. These DMUs are distinguished by their outputs, which include patient outcomes, care quality, and rendered services, and their inputs, which include funds, personnel, and equipment. The objective is to ascertain each DMU's efficiency scores, which show how well they translate inputs into outputs in comparison to their peers.

The CCR model yields an efficiency score that runs from 0 to 1, where 1 denotes perfect efficiency—that is, the DMU uses all of its resources to produce outputs. Since they could produce more outputs with the same inputs or the same level of outputs with fewer inputs, DMUs with scores below 1 are regarded as inefficient. Researchers can identify inefficient healthcare providers and evaluate the factors influencing their inefficiency by using the CCR model in health economics.

This analysis can identify areas for process optimization, performance improvement, and resource reallocation, which will ultimately improve patient outcomes and the distribution of healthcare resources.

Additionally, benchmarking exercises are made possible by the CCR model, which lets healthcare providers assess how well they perform in comparison to their peers. Through the identification of best practices and the development of performance improvement strategies, this comparative analysis can help create a healthcare system that is more effective and competitive. In health economics, the CCR model of Data Envelopment Analysis is a useful tool for assessing the effectiveness of healthcare providers. Through performance quantification, inefficiency identification, and benchmarking facilitation, the CCR model optimizes resource allocation and enhances the provision of high-quality healthcare services to individuals and communities.

9.2.2. Data Envelopment Analysis: BCC Model

The Banker, Charnes, and Cooper (BCC) model is one prominent model offered by Data Envelopment Analysis (DEA) for evaluating the effectiveness of healthcare providers. The BCC model is a useful tool in health economics for comparing the relative effectiveness of healthcare organizations, systems, or facilities. Comparing the inputs and outputs of decision-making units (DMUs) in the context of healthcare is how the BCC model and other DEA models work. However, the BCC model stands out because it can handle efficiency analyses that are both output- and input-oriented.

The BCC model assesses how effectively healthcare providers use their input resources to generate a specific level of output in an input-oriented analysis. This viewpoint helps find ways to cut back on resource use without sacrificing quality or output. For instance, it can assist in determining whether a hospital is efficiently allocating its funds, personnel, and equipment to provide patients with high-quality medical care.

Conversely, an analysis that is output-oriented concentrates on the effectiveness with which healthcare providers produce outputs in relation to a specific level of inputs. This viewpoint is helpful in assessing how well healthcare delivery uses the resources at its disposal to achieve desired results. For example, it can evaluate whether a clinic is working within financial constraints while optimizing patient outcomes, satisfaction, or public health indicators. With its dual orientations of input and output, the BCC model offers a thorough evaluation of efficiency in healthcare economics. This adaptability enables scholars and decision-makers to customize their analyses to particular objectives, concerns, and situations.

Moreover, benchmarking exercises are made possible by the BCC model, which lets healthcare providers assess how well they perform in terms of efficiency in comparison to peers or best-practice standards. Within the healthcare industry, this comparative analysis can be used to pinpoint areas that need improvement, best practices, and chances for cooperation or knowledge exchange. In human health economics, the BCC model of data envelope analysis is a flexible instrument for assessing healthcare providers' effectiveness. Through the integration of input-oriented and output-oriented viewpoints and the facilitation of benchmarking exercises, the BCC model aids in resource allocation optimization and the provision of top-notch healthcare services to communities and individuals.

9.2.3. Introduction to DEAP Software

A useful technique in health economics for assessing the relative effectiveness of healthcare providers is the Data Envelopment Analysis (DEA). The Data Envelopment Analysis Program, or DEAP for short, is a software application made expressly to make DEA analysis easier. DEAP, which was created by Tim Coelli and associates, provides a user-friendly interface for efficiency analysis and has grown to be a popular tool in health economics research.

Researchers and policymakers can evaluate the effectiveness of healthcare providers, including clinics, hospitals, and healthcare systems, using the comprehensive platform that DEAP offers. Users can enter data on inputs (e.g., personnel and equipment) as well as results (e.g., patient outcomes and care quality) for a number of the healthcare industry's decision-making units (DMUs). DEAP's versatility in handling various DEA model types, such as input- and output-oriented models and models with variable returns to scale (VRS) or constant returns to scale (CRS), is one of its primary features. Because of its adaptability, users can customize the analysis to fit particular research questions or policy goals.

DEAP provides users with insights into different facets of healthcare provider performance by offering a range of efficiency measures, including technical efficiency, scale efficiency, and overall efficiency. Additionally, the software produces comprehensive efficiency reports that make interpretation and decision-making easier. These reports include efficiency scores, rankings, and graphical representations. Support for sensitivity analysis, which enables users to evaluate how resilient efficiency results are to modifications in input and output data or model specifications, is another noteworthy aspect of DEAP. This capability improves the validity and reliability of DEA findings and offers insightful information about the variables influencing healthcare providers' varying levels of efficiency. Additionally, DEAP has sophisticated functions for statistical inference, hypothesis testing, and model validation, making it a complete tool for carrying out thorough efficiency analysis in health economics research. The program comes with a wealth of online resources, tutorials, and documentation to help both new and seasoned users learn how to use it. A flexible and easy-to-use software program for performing Data Envelopment Analysis in health economics is called DEAP. To evaluate and enhance the effectiveness of healthcare delivery and ultimately improve health outcomes for people and communities, DEAP offers a variety of features for input data management, model specification, efficiency analysis, and result interpretation.

9.2.4. Application of DEA in Healthcare Using DEAP

The Data Envelopment Analysis Program, or DEAP, is a crucial tool for these kinds of analyses. Data Envelopment Analysis (DEA) is a valuable methodology that is widely used in the healthcare industry to evaluate the effectiveness of healthcare providers. By comparing the input-output relationships of hospitals, clinics, healthcare systems, and other healthcare entities, DEAP helps researchers, policymakers, and administrators assess how well these entities are performing. The evaluation of healthcare providers' efficiency is one of the main uses of DEA in the healthcare industry with DEAP. DEAP creates efficiency scores for each provider based on data inputs about a variety of inputs, including staff, equipment, and financial resources, and outputs, including patient outcomes, care quality, and services rendered. These ratings show how well healthcare professionals use their resources to achieve the intended results. Healthcare providers can also compare their efficiency scores to their peers or best-practice standards through benchmarking exercises made possible by DEAP. This comparative analysis can point out areas that need work and direct initiatives to raise standards of care and performance in the healthcare industry.

Additionally, resource allocation optimization is facilitated by DEA in healthcare when DEAP is used. DEA assists administrators and legislators in the healthcare industry in better allocating resources to enhance overall efficiency by spotting inefficient resource allocation patterns. To guarantee optimal resource utilization across various healthcare facilities or departments, it directs decisions on resource reallocation, such as redistributing funding, modifying staffing levels, or reallocating facilities. Furthermore, the evaluation of healthcare interventions and programs is made possible by DEA in healthcare through the use of DEAP. Researchers have access to input data (e.g., resources, staff) and results (e.g., health outcomes, and service provision) to evaluate the efficacy and efficiency of various interventions. This analysis offers empirically supported insights into the effects of interventions, guiding future resource allocation plans and policy choices.

Moreover, provider network analysis is supported by DEA in healthcare through DEAP. To increase productivity and care quality, DEA assesses the effectiveness of provider networks and healthcare delivery systems to find areas for cooperation, integration, or consolidation. It informs choices about the organization and management of a network by evaluating the combined effectiveness of linked providers. Finally, DEA in healthcare with DEAP is an important instrument for decision support and policy assessment. The results of the DEA can be used by policymakers to assess how incentives, rules, or policy interventions affect the effectiveness of healthcare. To improve patient outcomes and population health, efforts to increase the efficacy and efficiency of healthcare delivery are supported by this evidence-based approach, which guides policy development and implementation.

The Data Envelopment Analysis Program, or DEAP, is a useful tool for performing efficiency analysis in the healthcare industry. Data Envelopment Analysis (DEA) has many applications in this field.

Some key applications of DEA in healthcare using DEAP:

1. **Efficiency Assessment of Healthcare Providers:** DEAP can be used to evaluate the relative efficiency of healthcare providers, such as hospitals, clinics, or healthcare systems. By inputting data on inputs (e.g., financial resources, staff, facilities) and outputs (e.g., patient outcomes, quality of care), DEAP generates efficiency scores for each provider, allowing comparisons and identification of best practices.
2. **Resource Allocation Optimization:** DEA can help healthcare policymakers and administrators optimize resource allocation by identifying inefficient allocation patterns. DEAP enables users to assess how effectively resources are utilized across different healthcare facilities or departments, guiding decisions on resource reallocation to improve overall efficiency.
3. **Benchmarking and Performance Improvement:**

DEAP facilitates benchmarking exercises by allowing healthcare providers to compare their efficiency scores to those of their peers or best-practice standards. This comparative analysis can help identify areas for improvement and drive performance-enhancement efforts within the healthcare sector.

4. **Evaluation of Healthcare Interventions:** DEA can be used to evaluate the efficiency of specific healthcare interventions or programs. By inputting data on inputs (e.g., funding, personnel) and outputs (e.g., health outcomes, service delivery), DEAP enables researchers to assess the effectiveness and efficiency of different interventions, informing policy decisions and resource allocation.
5. **Provider Network Analysis:** DEAP can analyze the efficiency of provider networks or healthcare delivery systems. By inputting data on inputs and outputs for multiple interconnected providers, DEAP assesses the overall efficiency of the network and identifies opportunities for collaboration, integration, or consolidation to improve efficiency and quality of care.
6. **Policy Evaluation and Decision Support:** DEA can inform healthcare policy decisions by providing evidence-based insights into the efficiency and performance of healthcare providers or systems. DEAP enables policymakers to evaluate the impact of policy interventions, regulations, or incentives on healthcare efficiency, guiding future policy development and implementation.

All things considered, DEAP is a potent instrument for performing efficiency analyses in the healthcare industry, giving stakeholders the ability to appraise, standardize, and enhance the performance of healthcare providers, optimize resource distribution, assess interventions, and guide policy choices to raise the efficacy and efficiency of healthcare delivery (Aloh et al., 2020; Bem et al., 2014).

9.3. Clinical Efficiency

Clinical efficiency, which includes a range of tactics and procedures targeted at enhancing patient care procedures, raising standards, and making the most use of available resources in clinical settings, is a crucial component of healthcare delivery. It entails expediting procedures, cutting down on waste, cutting down on delays, and improving the caliber and efficacy of patient care. For healthcare organizations to provide high-quality care while controlling costs, raising patient satisfaction, and producing better health results, clinical efficiency is crucial.

The streamlining of clinical procedures and workflows is a crucial component of clinical efficiency. This entails locating and getting rid of bottlenecks, redundant processes, and inefficiencies in the healthcare delivery system. Healthcare providers can find ways to improve the flow of patients through different stages of care, standardize protocols, and streamline processes by examining every stage of the patient care journey. By guaranteeing that patients receive timely and appropriate interventions, standardizing order sets, protocols, and pathways for common procedures or conditions, for instance, can lower variation in care practices and increase efficiency.

The efficient use of resources, such as staff, tools, and supplies, is a crucial aspect of clinical efficiency. Healthcare providers must optimize resource allocation to address patient needs while reducing wastage and avoidable expenses. This could entail adjusting staffing levels to better meet patient demand, planning procedures and appointments to make the most use of available resources, and putting inventory control systems in place to avoid shortages or overstocking of necessary supplies. Additionally, by enhancing communication, supporting clinical decision-making, and streamlining documentation, utilizing technology like electronic health records (EHRs), telemedicine, and decision-support tools can increase efficiency.

Clinical efficiency also includes ways to shorten wait times and make care more accessible. Prolonged wait times for consultations, procedures, or appointments can result in unsatisfied patients, postponed diagnosis and treatment, and higher medical expenses. By using appointment scheduling software, cutting down on no-shows, streamlining clinic operations, and putting patient flow improvement techniques into place, healthcare providers can increase productivity. For instance, wait times can be shortened and access to care can be enhanced by employing predictive analytics to estimate patient demand and modify staffing levels appropriately.

Moreover, improving the standard and safety of patient care is a key component of clinical efficiency. Healthcare providers can guarantee that patients receive high-quality care that complies with established standards and best practices by embracing evidence-based practices, following clinical guidelines, and putting quality improvement initiatives into action. This could entail carrying out routine audits, keeping an eye on clinical results, and putting performance improvement initiatives into action to address problem areas and encourage ongoing learning and development. Furthermore, encouraging a culture of safety, cooperation, and teamwork among medical professionals can aid in lowering medical errors, averting unfavorable incidents, and enhancing patient outcomes.

Moreover, patient-centered care, which prioritizes attending to each patient's particular needs, preferences, and values, is strongly associated with clinical efficiency. Healthcare organizations can improve patient satisfaction, engagement, and treatment plan adherence by incorporating patients in decision-making, offering personalized care plans, and encouraging shared decision-making between patients and providers. Because care is customized to each patient's unique needs and circumstances, the patient-centered approach not only enhances the patient experience but also helps to improve health outcomes.

Clinical efficiency is a broad term that includes a range of tactics and approaches meant to enhance patient care procedures, improve results, and make the most of available resources in clinical settings. Healthcare providers can increase efficiency, improve patient satisfaction, and enhance patient outcomes by optimizing resource allocation, reducing wait times, improving quality and safety, and promoting patient-centered care.

9.3.1. Tips for Improving Clinical Efficiency

Without a doubt, clinical effectiveness is crucial, regardless of the size of the team or the organization. An operation that is not as efficient as it should be can cost the practice money and time, as well as the ability to serve the greatest number of patients.

Below is a look at how to increase clinical efficiency with a smaller staff in healthcare:

1. **Eliminate Paperwork:** Reducing paperwork is one of the easiest ways to increase practice efficiency with a smaller staff. The more time you free up to work on more crucial tasks, the more time you can spend scanning paper documents, sending faxes, and filing paper documents. For instance, capturing blood pressure, weight, and temperature readings automatically with smart devices cuts down on the amount of time spent on patient paperwork.
2. **Focus Physician Time on Patient Care:** In any clinical setting, the aim is for doctors to spend as much time as possible with their patients. Sadly, having too many responsibilities assigned to treating physicians when there aren't enough staff members can take away from their time spent with patients. Take all the necessary steps to stop this, including implementing new technology.
3. **Master Your EMR/ EHR Templates:** Gaining proficiency with your EMR/ EHR templates can improve clinical efficiency and save a significant amount of time. These templates can provide shortcut options, particularly useful for routine procedural tasks. During a patient interaction, for instance, "dot phrases" enable providers to type a few brief words or phrases, and those phrases automatically expand to a full block of text. Collaborate with the technology supplier, make the most of any provided training, and ensure that every employee understands how to maximize the functionality of the systems in use.
4. **Be Prudent When Hiring:** In the medical field, turnover rates increased as a result of the pandemic. In just a few months, the percentage of healthcare workers leaving their jobs rose from 31.2% to 50.6%. Even though those figures have begun to level off, a high turnover rate can seriously impair practice effectiveness. New hires always need time to get used to their jobs and receive the necessary training. If the employee leaves after receiving training, then there has been a waste of important funds. Thus, exercise extra caution when recruiting. Examine hiring practices, set strict hiring criteria, and, if necessary, enlist the assistance of a reputable staffing firm.
5. **Train Team Members to be Gatekeepers:** The outpatient team must serve as the physician's gatekeepers for them to commit time to their patients. To put it another way, a doctor should only be asked to perform a task after they can act on behalf of the

patient. As much as possible, the team should handle non-emergency tasks in the clinic. Having a well-trained and equipped team of professionals who recognize that the primary care provider's attention must be focused on patient interactions makes all of this possible.

6. **Use a Good Scheduling System:** Effective appointment scheduling is essential for a practice to run smoothly. The best EHRs integrate seamlessly with other patient scheduling software or have built-in patient scheduling features. Ensure that the equipment your clinic uses is optimized for its intended use, with minimal downtime, no problems with double booking or downtime, and integrated features to discourage no-shows.

7. **Maximize Appointments and Minimize Downtime Resulting from No-Shows:** When you are not seeing patients, this is known as downtime and cannot be billed. Consequently, it is pointless to pay the employees any money to fill this idle time. Making the most of appointments and putting a plan in place for dealing with no-shows are crucial to ensuring that as many minutes are profitable as possible. The healthcare sector loses $150 billion a year due to no-shows. Take all the necessary steps to prevent patients from missing their appointments, such as providing flexible scheduling and employing automated systems like texts to remind patients.

8. **Simplify Patient Check-In and Check-Out Processes:** Protracted check-in and check-out procedures can be time-consuming for staff and are inefficient. Improving front desk technology can have a significant impact on efforts to boost clinical productivity. For instance, patients can check themselves in using their mobile devices when they arrive for their appointments by substituting the manual check-in process with e-check-in options.

9. **Understand the Experience from the Patient's Perspective when Designing Clinical Workflows:** Think about inviting "secret shopper" patients. Typically, you hire these patients to assist you with scheduling appointments and provide input on waiting times and how well your time was spent with the doctor. The knowledge you gain from these encounters can be priceless and assist you in creating the most effective clinical workflow possible.

10. **Use Clinician-Centered Design with EHRs:** Clinician-centered EHRs are appropriate for use in clinical settings. The system should be made as efficient as possible, with the face sheet and dashboard arranged to meet the needs

of the clinician. This is one of the main reasons it's critical to select an EHR that can be easily customized to fit the unique workflow of the practice. There will be less of a learning curve and a chance of wasting time when using the program the more customized it is.

11. **Use the Right Technology Partners:** You will constantly work with different technology partners because modern medical practices rely heavily on technology for efficiency. Operational efficiency is genuinely impacted by something as basic as having a reliable EHR technology provider. For example, clinical workflow is hampered until you can speak with a technician for assistance if an EHR provider does not have a help desk available when needed.
12. **Eliminate Overtime:** Paying overtime regularly is often a sign that the staff-to-patient ratio is not optimal. Rather than regularly paying overtime, it might be more cost-effective to think about adding a staff member.
13. **Measure Performance and Identify Pain Points and Opportunities:** To maintain clinical efficiency over time, never stop tracking how the clinic is operating to identify any pain areas that require attention. Ask for input on areas where time and resources are being squandered by speaking with practice managers and employees. Evaluate overall no-show rates, wait times, and downtimes to determine areas for improvement.

9.3.2. Clinical Collaboration in Healthcare

To ensure effective collaboration among healthcare professionals, hospitals, and practices should invest in communication technology that facilitates easy access to patient information and keeps the team connected. Digitization allows providers to offer extremely individualized care.

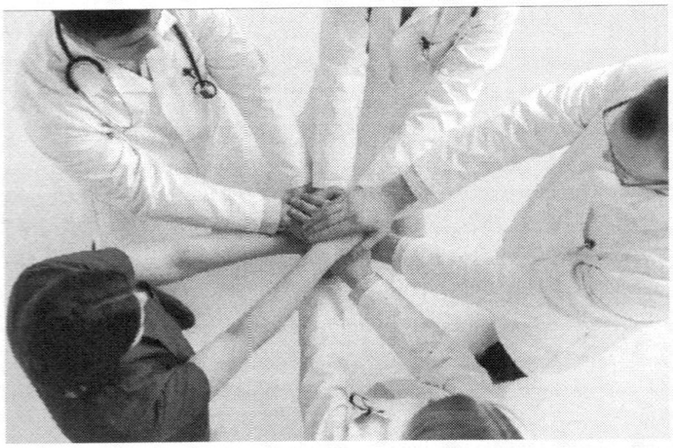

Source: https://prognocis.com/wp-content/uploads/2022/01/group-of-doctors-with-hands-together-at-hospital-1024x683.jpg.webp.

9.3.2.1. Emerging Digitalization Trends for Healthcare Collaboration

The value of funding at least one of these digital innovations is sufficiently demonstrated by the available data. Regardless of the practice or hospital size, they transform healthcare.

9.3.2.2. IoT and Wearable Devices

Both the patient and the healthcare provider may benefit from the use of wearable technology. This technology is revolutionizing patient diagnosis, disease management, and preventive care by fusing cutting-edge hardware, mobile apps, and predictive analytics. Healthcare practitioners can make better decisions by using the continuous flow of user data generated by these devices, which includes information on blood pressure, breathing patterns, and even sleep cycles for more accurate diagnosis.

9.3.2.3. Telemedicine

Even for the sick, elderly, and uninsured, telemedicine remains a popular substitute for in-person visits. Healthcare organizations and practitioners must make investments in digital technology and an EHR that supports it if they want telemedicine to realize its full potential. For telemedicine software to function, patients must have easy access to doctors and medical facilities on the Internet. Patients will find it easier to find practices and doctors when they are more visible online thanks to Omnicore's local SEO ultimate guide.

More people can now get accurate diagnoses without visiting a medical facility thanks to telemedicine. Collaboration among healthcare professionals facilitates communication, leading to improved treatment options and more efficient decision-making.

9.3.2.4. Big Data

Policymakers, organizations, and scientists can use big data to make precise recommendations and policy decisions that have the potential to change lives. When applied correctly, data analytics in healthcare can lower healthcare costs, help prevent avoidable diseases, and enhance patient quality of life. Healthcare providers can more easily provide better healthcare outcomes by using big data to analyze patient health conditions and self-care. Big data is the only tool available to the healthcare sector that can help find relevant data and apply it to predictive analysis for improved diagnosis and prevention.

9.3.2.5. Cloud Technology

Healthcare organizations are linked and have access to safe and secure digital data thanks to cloud computing. The medical industry constantly gathers patient data, research findings, and disease information from a variety of sources. Healthcare companies had to pay for pricey systems to store data and information before the advent of cloud computing. The medical industry's ability to store and retrieve data has evolved as a result of cloud storage. Because the information is accessible from any location at any time through a variety of devices, healthcare professionals are better able to collaborate. Since data is bounced off multiple servers instead of being in one location, storing it in a centralized cloud network is safer.

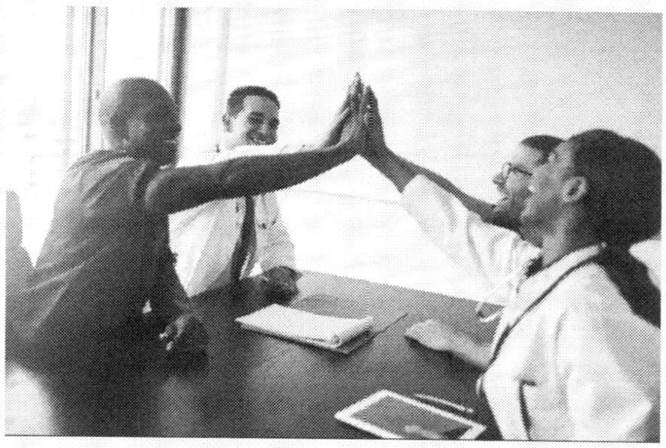

Source: https://prognocis.com/wp-content/uploads/2022/01/young-medical-specialists-high-five-1024x683.jpg.webp.

9.3.2.6. Ways to Conduct Clinical Collaboration

9.3.2.6.1. Define a Healthcare Collaborative Approach

A facility must create a clear collaborative strategy for healthcare collaboration to succeed. This entails assembling personnel and associates for the assignment and modeling the composition of a cooperative team. A collaborative team is made up of medical professionals from various fields who share similar objectives for patient care and are tasked with providing supplementary work to help achieve these objectives. This involves first-contact physicians and nurses for patients as well as inpatient hospital staff, as well as paramedics who transport patients to the emergency room.

To make sure they meet every requirement for patient care, the team should have a formal channel of communication with the patient and family. Mobile phones and other technological gadgets can improve communication between team members inside and outside. The use of the Situation-Background-Assessment-Recommendation (SBAR) is common among healthcare practitioners. The purpose of this communication program is to improve team and individual interactions in healthcare. By using standardized forms, checklists, and guides, this system enables healthcare professionals to communicate more accurately, consistently, and efficiently.

9.3.2.7. Delegate Team Member Roles

Depending on their profession and level of education, healthcare professionals differ in their abilities. Delegating roles is necessary because this restricts the knowledge and experience that various members of a collaborative health team can possess. Understanding the various roles and responsibilities in the various professions represented in the collaborative team is essential to successful collaboration. Every member of the team, from specialists to ambulatory care providers, should be aware of their own responsibilities as well as those of other healthcare professionals, such as nurses, doctors, social workers, and pharmacists. This information offers a starting point for productive teamwork.

9.3.2.8. Assign Tasks and Responsibilities

Members of the team need to be aware of their roles regarding patient care for collaboration to be effective. Meeting patient care objectives and attending to the patient's needs should be the team's main priorities. This outlines the composition of the team as well as the duties delegated to each member. Healthcare providers can achieve shared responsibility, coordination, and communication when they view one another as partners rather than rivals.

9.3.2.9. Practice Collaboration

Team members can only become flawless collaborators by continuously practicing together. Through practice, a team can come up with novel ideas and answers for various patient care requirements. Collaborating in a group setting brings about a diversity of perspectives that inevitably leads to disagreements and conflict. These are necessary components for the growth of cooperative efforts to continue, which is why team members must always be trained in problem-solving techniques. Working together is a continuous process that promotes learning and development.

9.3.2.10. Why Clinical Collaboration is Essential?

9.3.2.10.1. Automation

Clinical collaboration facilitates process automation in the healthcare industry, which streamlines the IT process. Delivery of medical services is accelerated through the automation of several healthcare processes. This makes it easier to manage patients and provide care more quickly.

9.3.2.10.2. Improved Patient Care

When a patient with back pain walks into an emergency room, a group of physicians, nurses, and specialists treat the patient and come up with workable answers for their needs. This is only feasible with cooperation. Greater health outcomes and patient-centered care are the results of this collaboration.

9.3.2.10.3. Fewer Medical Errors

In the healthcare industry, poor communication can lead to serious consequences such as misdiagnosis, incorrect treatment, and missed symptoms. According to statistics, medical errors rank third among the leading causes of death in the United States, resulting in over 2,50,000 deaths annually. Working together allows medical staff to communicate more effectively, which lowers the number of medical errors. By working together, healthcare professionals can guarantee that all the information they need to treat patients safely and accurately is available to all those involved in their care.

9.3.2.10.4. Reduced Inefficiencies and Costs

0Healthcare facilities stand to gain millions of dollars from fewer medical errors caused by incorrect diagnosis and treatment. Clinical collaboration also reduces operational inefficiencies and workflow redundancies, which saves money for healthcare organizations. A study found that 20 hospitals saw a 50% decrease in the fall rate after increasing nurse-physician collaboration. Additionally, the durations of stay were shortened by 0.6 days, and the annual bed turnover was raised by 20%. The rate of surgical start times has also increased due to clinical collaboration, saving over 700 hours that would have otherwise been lost over four years.

9.3.2.10.5. Higher Job Satisfaction

The knowledge base, philosophy, and culture of the hospital govern every department within the healthcare system. In the context of power dynamics, certain professionals' opinions are given greater weight than others. Both patient outcomes and some healthcare professionals' morale are negatively impacted by this. The greatest solutions come from clinical collaboration, in which each person involved in patient care plays a vital role. Working together fosters a feeling of community and camaraderie among healthcare professionals, which improves recruitment, retention, and job satisfaction.

9.3.3. Common Challenges in Clinical collaboration

9.3.3.1. Lack of Clinical Ownership and Engagement

Getting every healthcare employee in a company to participate in collaborative processes can be difficult at times. This causes gaps in the exchange of information, which impacts patient cooperation and care.

9.3.3.2. Lack of Board Support and Engagement

The failure of the health facility board to support collaboration efforts can deter the digitization process. This has an impact on the motivation of other willing players.

9.3.3.3. Failure to Embrace External Collaboration

While it is easy and safe to maintain internal collaboration efforts, external collaboration with other health professionals can better serve the industry.

9.3.3.4. Hierarchical Structure and Hospital Culture

The process of clinical collaboration may be slowed down by a department's or organization's lack of support. Because their suggestions and hard work are consistently disregarded, subordinates who don't feel like they are being heard are less willing to cooperate (Hafez et al., 2020; McGlynn et al., 2008).

A Closer Look

human Health system

The human health system is a complex network involving various interconnected components that work together to maintain and improve human health. At its core are healthcare providers such as doctors, nurses, and allied health professionals who deliver medical care and treatment. Supporting them are healthcare facilities ranging from hospitals and clinics to specialized treatment centers. Additionally, the health system includes public health agencies responsible for disease prevention, health promotion, and community health initiatives. Pharmaceutical companies play a crucial role in developing medications and therapies to treat illnesses and improve health outcomes. Health insurance providers and policymakers ensure access to healthcare services and shape healthcare policies.

Together, these components form a dynamic system aimed at addressing the diverse health needs of individuals and populations, continually evolving to meet new challenges and opportunities in healthcare delivery and public health management.

Summary

- Human health efficiency encompasses a multitude of factors that contribute to the overall well-being and functioning of the body. From the molecular level to the systemic, humans operate within a delicate balance of biological processes aimed at maintaining homeostasis.
- Productivity and efficiency are two fundamental concepts that play a crucial role in the success of individuals, organizations, and economies.
- Healthcare is a complex sector, subject to fast changes in medical practice as new treatments are developed as well as administrative bureaucracies and state involvement that can slow the adaptation of new technologies.
- The efficiency of health systems was also found to be affected by how users interacted with the health service providers. Health systems where patients exercised choice of health providers were associated with higher technical efficiency.
- Orchestration is the biggest lever to improving operational efficiency. Consolidating work, and an emphasis on streamlining and standardizing processes can remove bottlenecks and speed up productivity.
- Data Envelopment Analysis (DEA) is a widely used method in the field of health economics for evaluating the relative efficiency of healthcare providers, such as hospitals, clinics, or healthcare systems.
- Data Envelopment Analysis (DEA) is a powerful mathematical tool used in health economics to evaluate the efficiency of healthcare providers, such as hospitals, clinics, or healthcare systems.
- One of the key features of DEA is its ability to handle different types of DEA models, including input-oriented and output-oriented models, as well as models with variable returns to scale (VRS) or constant returns to scale (CRS).
- Data Envelopment Analysis (DEA) is a valuable methodology extensively applied in healthcare to assess the efficiency of healthcare providers, and DEAP (Data Envelopment Analysis Program) serves as an essential tool for conducting such analyses.
- Clinical efficiency is a critical aspect of healthcare delivery that encompasses various strategies and practices aimed at optimizing patient care processes, improving outcomes, and maximizing resource utilization within clinical settings.
- Efficient collaboration among healthcare workers, hospitals, and practices should invest in communication technology that keeps the team connected and makes patient information easily accessible.

References

1. Aloh, H. E., Onwujekwe, O. E., Aloh, O. G., & Nweke, C. J. (2020). Is bed turnover rate a good metric for hospital scale efficiency? A measure of resource utilization rate for hospitals in Southeast Nigeria. *Cost Effectiveness and Resource Allocation, 18*(1), 21.

2. Bem, A., Ucieklak-Jeż, P., & Prędkiewic, P. (2014). Measurement of health care system efficiency. *Management Theory and Studies for Rural Business and Infrastructure Development, 36*(1), 25–33.
3. Grieco, P. L. E., & McDevitt, R. C. (2017). Productivity and quality in health care: Evidence from the dialysis industry. *The Review of Economic Studies, 84*(3), 1071–1105.
4. Hafez, R. (Ed.). (2020). *Measuring Health System Efficiency in Low- and Middle-Income Countries: A Resource Guide*. Joint Learning Network for Universal Health Coverage, International Decision Support Initiative (iDSI), The World Bank Group.
5. McGlynn, E. A., Shekelle, P. G., Chen, S., Goldman, D. P., Romley, J. A., Hussey, P. S., de Vries, H., Wang, M. C., Timmer, M. J., Carter, J., Tringale, C., & Shanman, R. M. (2008). *Identifying, Categorizing, and Evaluating Health Care Efficiency Measures*. McGlynn.
6. Selvaraj, S., Mukhopadhyay, I., Kumar, P., Aisola, M., Datta, P., Bhatt, P., Mehta, A., Srivastava, S., & Pachauli, C. (2014). Universal access to medicines: Evidence from Rajasthan, India. *WHO South-East Asia Journal of Public Health, 3*, 3–4.
7. World Health Organization, Anand, S., & Fan, V. (2016). *The Health Workforce in India*. World Health Organization.
8. Yip, W., & Hafez, R. (2016). *Reforms for Improving the Efficiency of Health Systems: Lessons from 10 Country Cases*. World Health Organization.

Chapter

PUBLIC HEALTH AND POLICIES

10

Contents

Introduction

Public health and policies are intertwined elements crucial for safeguarding the well-being of communities and populations. Public health focuses on promoting and protecting the health of individuals and the broader society. It encompasses a wide range of activities, from disease prevention and health promotion to the surveillance of health trends and the development of policies aimed at improving population health outcomes. Public health initiatives address various factors influencing health, including environmental, social, economic, and behavioral determinants. By adopting a proactive approach, public health endeavors to prevent diseases, prolong life, and enhance the quality of life for all members of society.

Central to the effectiveness of public health efforts are policies that provide a framework for action and guide decision-making at local, national, and global levels. Public health policies encompass a diverse array of measures, from legislation and regulations governing healthcare delivery to initiatives promoting healthy behaviors and environmental sustainability. These policies are informed by scientific evidence, public health research, and input from various stakeholders, including healthcare professionals, policymakers, community leaders, and advocacy groups. Through the implementation of evidence-based policies, governments, and organizations seek to address health disparities, mitigate health risks, and create environments that support healthy living.

Together, public health and policies form a dynamic and interconnected system aimed at protecting and promoting the health and well-being of populations. By fostering collaboration among stakeholders, leveraging scientific research, and prioritizing prevention and equity, public health policies play a critical role in shaping healthier and more resilient communities. However, the effectiveness of these policies depends not only on their design and implementation but also on factors such as funding, political will, and public engagement. Therefore, fostering a supportive policy environment and advocating for policies that prioritize public health are essential steps in achieving the overarching goal of improving population health and ensuring health equity for all.

Orientation and Directional Terms:

Term	Definition	Illustration
Community medicine	Community medicine, also known as public health or preventive medicine, is a branch of medicine that focuses on the health of populations rather than individual patients. Community Medicine is concerned with the promotion, protection, and maintenance of the health and well-being of communities through the application of medical knowledge and skills.	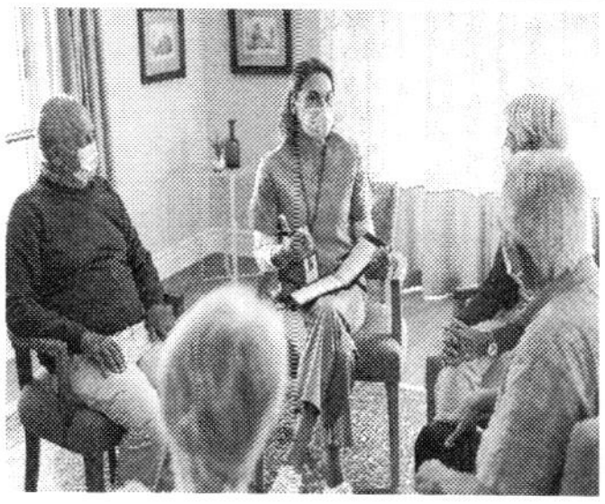
Health promotion	Health promotion is the process of enabling people to increase control over, and to improve, their health. It moves beyond a focus on individual behavior towards a wide range of social and environmental interventions.	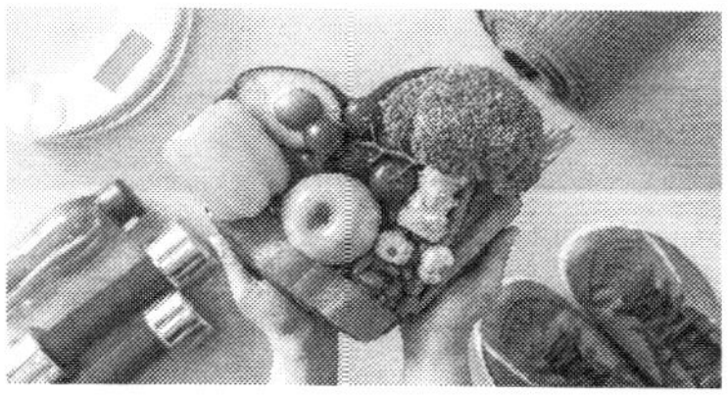
Environmental health	Environmental health examines the interaction between the environment and our health. We use the following definitions: Environmental health refers to aspects of human health (including quality of life) that are determined by physical, chemical, biological, social, and psychosocial factors in the environment.	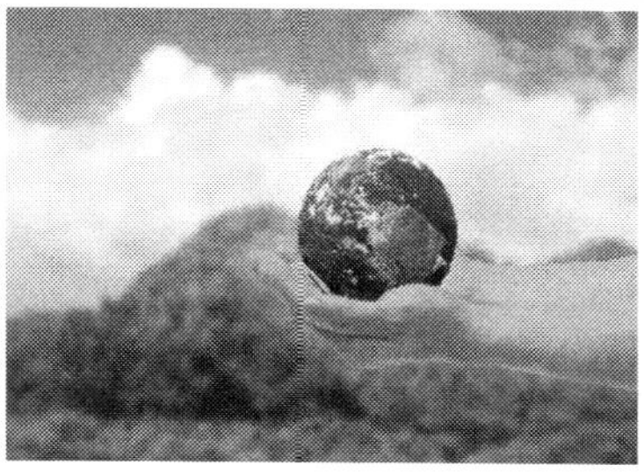
Public health administration	Public health administration professionals improve the health and well-being of the public at large by assessing their health needs, developing outreach programs, and managing public health facilities.	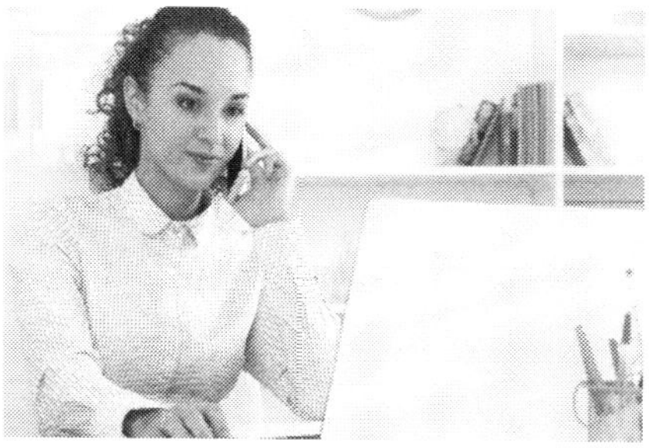
Health insurance	Health Insurance is a contract between the policyholder and the insurer where the health insurance company provides financial coverage to the insured up to the sum insured limit.	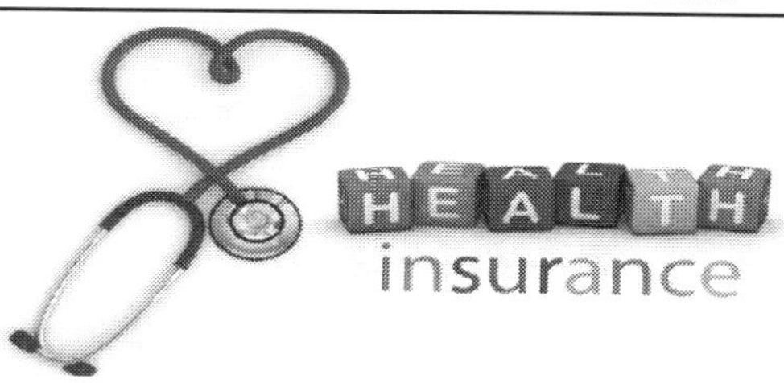

10.1. Public Health

Public health includes sanitation, personal hygiene, management of infectious diseases, the art and science of preventing disease, extending life, and promoting physical and mental health, as well as the coordination of health services. The concept of public health represents the understanding of the value of community action in the promotion of health and the prevention and treatment of disease that has arisen from everyday human interactions involved in addressing the myriad issues of social life.

The terms "social medicine" and "community medicine," which are synonymous with public health medicine and are commonly used in the UK, refer to the medical professionals who practice community medicine. The field of public health primarily focuses on influencing and managing the environment for the good of the general public, greatly drawing from medical science and philosophy. Thus, housing, water supplies, and food are its main concerns. Farming, fertilizers, poor drainage and sewage disposal, buildings, broken HVAC systems, machinery, and hazardous chemicals are some of the ways that these can become contaminated with harmful substances. The larger endeavor of maintaining and enhancing public health includes public health medicine. Community physicians collaborate with various professionals, such as architects, builders, chemists, physicists, toxicologists, and sanitary and HVAC engineers in addition to factory and food inspectors. The welfare, safety, and health of people at work are the main concerns of occupational medicine. Given that its goal is to lower the risks in the workplace, it could be seen as a subspecialty of public health medicine.

To preserve, maintain, and actively promote public health, specific information-gathering techniques (epidemiology) and corporate structures are needed to act upon and implement significant findings. By establishing a correlation between variables like nutrition, environment, radiation exposure, or cigarette smoking and the incidence and prevalence of disease, epidemiologists can use statistics to explain and characterize the occurrence of disease in a population. The government establishes agencies to formally inspect and monitor water supplies, food processing, sewage treatment, drains, and pollution through laws and regulations. The management of pandemic and epidemic diseases, developing protocols for suitable medical treatment and isolation measures, and releasing travel advisories to stop the spread of the disease outside of afflicted regions are other concerns of governments.

Numerous national and international public health agencies have been established to assist in the control and surveillance of disease within societies. For instance, a special public health ministry was established for England and Wales by the Public Health Act of 1848 in the United Kingdom. The Centers for Disease Control and Prevention (CDC) in the US conduct national research and oversee public health initiatives. The World Health Organization (WHO) has a similar function on a global scale. The World Health Organization (WHO) plays a critical role in supporting the adoption of administrative and organizational strategies to address health-related issues in developing nations across the globe. When building health service systems in these nations, considerations such as health issues, resource constraints, medical staff education, and others must be made.

The development of vaccines and antibiotics, among other scientific and medical advances in developed nations, has been essential in providing much-needed assistance to nations with high rates of illness. Still, the global incidence of preventable diseases and neglected tropical diseases is unusually high, even with the increase in resources and the enhancement of their mobilization to the most affected areas. One of the main objectives of global public health is to lessen the incidence and impact of these diseases. Nonetheless, the fact that these illnesses are still prevalent throughout the world is a crucial sign of the challenges that societies and health organizations face today.

10.1.1. History of Public Health

The history of public health is nearly as old as the history of humankind. Among the customs that may have developed during a civilization are taboos against disposing of waste in public spaces or close to sources of potable water; funeral customs; and group support for childbirth.

The history of the ancient societies (those existing before 500 BC) is based on archaeological discoveries made in the Indus Valley (North India) circa 2000 BC, which show evidence of home drains, bathrooms, and sewers beneath street level. Between 2700 and 2000 BC, there was evidence of drainage systems in the Middle Kingdom of ancient Egypt. Written records about public health existed 3,900 years ago, in the form of the Hammurabi codes of Babylon. Guidelines for personal hygiene, campsite sanitation, well disinfection, leper isolation, waste disposal, and maternity hygiene were found in the Book of Leviticus (1500 BC).

Public health was practiced in the Classical Cultures (500 BC–500 AD) as the Olympics for physical fitness, community sanitation, and water wells during the golden age of ancient Greece; and as aqueducts for water transportation, sewer systems, rules regarding street cleaning, and slave infirmaries by the Romans. Between 500 and 1500 AD, health issues were thought to have spiritual roots and remedies. To Pagans, they were powers beyond this world; to Christians, they were penalties for transgressions. Several of the deadliest epidemics, including syphilis, leprosy, and the plague (also known as the Black Death) in the 14th century, were caused by the disregard for biological and physical causes.

The era of renaissance and exploration (1500–1700 AD) was the rebirth of thinking about the nature of the world and humankind. There was a growing belief that diseases were caused by the environment, not by spirits and critical thinking about disease causation, e.g., "malaria" - bad air. In the 18th century, there were problems of industrialization, urban slums leading to unsanitary conditions, and unsafe workplaces. Edward Jenner (1796) demonstrated vaccination against smallpox.

Although industrialization remained a problem in the 19th century, advances in agriculture contributed to better nutrition and, in the final quarter of the century, significant progress was made in identifying the causes of communicable diseases. Notable advancements were the Koch Postulate (1876) and Louis Pasteur's germ theory (1862).

The 20th century saw the development of health resources (1900–1960), social engineering (1960–1973), health promotion (Primary Healthcare), and the market period (1985–and beyond). In the 21st century, the challenges are lowering the burden of excess morbidity and mortality among the impoverished, fending off threats from the economic crisis, creating healthier environments and lifestyles, creating more efficient health systems, and making investments in increasing knowledge bases.

10.1.1.1. Historical Markers in the Development of Public Health (Selected)

1700 BC	The Code of Hammurabi – Rules governing medical practice.
1500 BC	Mosaic Law – Personal, food, and camp hygiene, segregating lepers, overriding duty of saving of life (PikuahNefesh) as religious imperatives.
400 BC	Greece – Personal hygiene, fitness, nutrition, sanitation, municipal doctors, occupational health; Hippocrates – clinical and epidemic observation and environmental health.
500 BC to AD 500	Rome – aqueducts, baths, sanitation, municipal planning, and sanitation services, public baths, municipal doctors, military, and occupational health.
500–1000	Europe – the destruction of Roman society and the rise of Christianity; sickness as punishment for sin, mortification of the flesh, prayer, fasting, and faith as therapy; poor nutrition and hygiene pandemics; anti-science; care of the sick as religious duty.
1348–1350	Black Death – origins in Asia, spread by the armies of Genghis Khan, The world pandemic kills 60 million in the 14th century, 1/3 to 1/2 of the population of Europe.
1300	Pandemics – bubonic plague, smallpox, leprosy, diphtheria, typhoid, measles, influenza, tuberculosis, anthrax, trachoma, scabies, and others until the 18th century.
1673	Antony van Leeuwenhoek – microscope, observes sperm and bacteria.
1796	Edward Jenner – first vaccination against smallpox.
1830	Sanitary and social reform, growth of science.
1854	John Snow – waterborne cholera in London: The Broad Street Pump.
1854	Florence Nightingale, modern nursing and hospital reform – Crimean War.
1858	Louis Pasteur proves no spontaneous generation of life.
1859	Charles Darwin publishes on the origin of species.
1862	Louis Pasteur publishes findings on microbial causes of disease.
1876	Robert Koch discovers *anthrax bacillus*.
1879	Neisser discovers gonococcus organism.
1882	Robert Koch discovers the tuberculosis organism, *tubercle bacillus*.

1880	Typhoid bacillus was discovered (Laveran); leprosy organism (Hansen); malaria organism (Laveran).
1883	Robert Koch discovers the bacillus of cholera.
1883	Louis Pasteur vaccinates against anthrax.
1884	Diphtheria, *staphylococcus*, *streptococcus*, and *tetanus* organisms identified
1890	Anti-tetanus serum (ATS)
1892	Gas gangrene organism discovered by Welch and Nuttal
1894	Plague organism discovered (Yersin, Kitasato); botulism organism (Van Ermengem).
1923	Health Organization of League of Nations
1926	Pertussis vaccine developed
1928	Alexander Fleming discovers penicillin
1929–1936	The Great Depression – widespread economic collapse, unemployment, poverty, and social distress in industrialized countries.
1946	World Health Organization was founded.
1977	WHO adopts Health for all by the year 2000
1978	Alma-Ata Conference on Primary Healthcare
1979	WHO declares eradication of smallpox achieved
1981	First recognition of cases of acquired immune deficiency syndrome (AIDS).
1989	International Convention on the Rights of the Child.
1990	W. F. Anderson performs the first successful gene therapy.
1992	United Nations Conference on Environmental and Development, Rio de Janeiro
1992	International Conference on Nutrition.
1993	World Conference on Human Rights, Vienna.
1994	International Conference on Population and Development, Cairo.
1998	WHO Health for All in the 21st Century adopted.

The new public health has a narrow focus. It is related to or includes all public and private initiatives aimed at lowering the disease and promoting actions that directly lead to better health. Its initiatives cover everything from child care and nutrition labeling to immunizations, health promotion, and ensuring that healthcare is easily accessible and well-managed. In a world with scarce resources and high standards, the planning, management, and monitoring functions of a health system are essential. To provide the feedback and control data required for effective management, this calls for a well-developed health information system. Together with participation from nongovernmental organizations (NGOs), knowledgeable media, and powerful professional and consumer organizations, it involves duties and coordination at all governmental levels. Clearly defining a person's obligations for their health and that of the healthcare provider for human, superior care are equally crucial.

10.1.2. Health Promotion

The goal of health promotion is to improve the well-being of both the individual and the community through various activities. It aims to give the community and the individual more influence and ownership over their health. By reducing certain risk factors and disease determinants that negatively impact a person's health, well-being, and ability to contribute to society, it works to improve social welfare and health. It does this by setting cost-effective goals that take into account both the scope of the issue and the likelihood of successful interventions.

A vital component of public health, health promotion can be implemented in clinics, hospitals, and other service settings in addition to the community. Teaching is necessary to increase awareness and inform people about lifestyle and health factors that may put them at risk.

The elements of health promotion comprise of:

1. Addressing the population as a whole in health-related issues, in everyday life as well as people at risk for specific diseases.
2. Directing action to risk factors or causes of illness or death;
3. Undertaking activities approach to seek out and remedy risk factors in the community that adversely affect health;
4. Promoting factors that contribute to a better condition of health of the population;
5. Initiating actions against health hazards, including communication, education, legislation, fiscal measures, organizational change, community development, and spontaneous local activities;
6. Involving public participation in defining problems, and deciding on action;
7. Advocating relevant environmental, health, and social policy;
8. Encouraging health professionals' participation in health education and health policy.

10.1.3. Major Disciplines in Public Health

- Nutrition is the science of food, the nutrients and other substances therein, their action, interaction, and balance concerning health and disease.
- Reproductive health is a state of complete physical, mental, and social well-being, not only the absence of disease or infirmity, in all matters relating to the reproductive system and its functions and processes.
- Environmental Health: The basic approach to environmental control is first to identify specific biological, chemical, social, and physical factors that represent hazards to health or well-being and to modify the environment in a manner that protects people from harmful exposures. The principal components of environmental health are water sanitation, waste disposal, etc.

- Health Education is defined as a combination of learning experiences designed to facilitate voluntary actions conducive to health. It is an essential part of health promotion.
- Epidemiology is the study of the frequency, distribution, and determinants of diseases and other related states or events in specified populations. The application of this study to the promotion of health and the prevention and control of health problems is evident.
- Health Economics is concerned with the alternative uses of resources in the health services sector and with the efficient utilization of economic resources such as manpower, material, and financial resources.
- Biostatistics is the application of statistics to biological problems; application of statistics especially to medical problems, but its real meaning is broader.
- Health Service Management is getting people to work harmoniously together and to make efficient use of resources in order to achieve objectives.
- Ecology: is the study of relationships among living organisms and their environment. It is the science, which deals with the inter-relationships between the various organisms living in an area and their relationship with the physical environment. Human ecology means the study of human groups as influenced by environmental factors, including social and behavioral factors.
- Research is a conscious action to acquire deeper knowledge or new facts about scientific or technical subjects. It is a systematic investigation towards increasing knowledge. It aims at the discovery and interpretation of facts, revision of accepted theories, or laws in the light of new facts or practical application of such new theories or laws.
- Demography is the study of population, especially concerning size and density, fertility, mortality, growth, age distribution, migration, and the interaction of all those with social and economic conditions.

10.2. Modern Organizational and Administrative Patterns

10.2.1. International Organizations

The need for international cooperation in the protection of health has been demonstrated by the spread of epidemic diseases since ancient times. National quarantines in Europe and the Middle East were among the first attempts at global disease control. Several related conferences aimed at drafting international quarantine regulations took place after the first official international health conference, which took place in Paris in 1851. In 1907, the International Office of Public Health (L'Office International d'Hygiène Publique) was founded in Paris as a permanent health organization. Its duties include receiving notifications of serious communicable diseases from participating nations, relaying this information to its member nations, and researching and creating sanitary conventions and quarantine laws about rail and shipping travel. In 1948, the World Health Organization (WHO) finally took over this organization. The organization of international health in the Americas most likely got its start in 1887 with a regional health conference held in Rio de Janeiro. Following a series of conferences between American nations starting in 1889, the Pan-American Sanitary Bureau was established. In 1949, it changed its name to the Pan-American Health Organization and became a regional office of the World Health Organization.

The aftermath and emergence of health organizations have been impacted by war. The League of Nations established a Health Section in 1923 following World War I, and it operated until the Second World War. Following the conflict, the United Nations Relief and Rehabilitation Administration (UNRRA) was established to mitigate the spread of disease by organizing and processing displaced people. It was in charge of the preparations that resulted in the UN special agency, WHO, being established. WHO is focused on social, mental, and physical well-being rather than just the absence of disease.

The World Health Assembly, which is made up of representatives from the member states, is in charge of overseeing WHO's operations. Diseases and issues that are widespread worldwide and call for international response were discussed at the first assembly. Priorities were set for sexually transmitted diseases, malaria, tuberculosis, the promotion of health, environmental factors that contribute significantly to mortality, and nutrition. Since then, more need areas have been added.

One of the organization's primary responsibilities is providing governments with advisory services via its regional staff. WHO can stay in touch with sources of financial aid and needs by using local representatives in many less developed countries as well as regional offices in several industrialized and developing nations. Many expert committees examine particular issues in specialized fields.

WHO has tight ties to international labor unions and other United Nations organizations, including the Food and Agriculture Organization (FAO) and the United Nations Children's Fund (UNICEF). UNICEF has concentrated its assistance on maternity and child health services and the prevention of infections, particularly in young people, since its founding in 1946. The development of vaccines, the establishment of environmental sanitation, the supply of clean water, and the training of domestic staff in their home nations—particularly in rural areas—have all been given top priority. In underdeveloped nations, organized health services are the conduit for aid. Persuading governments to conduct nationwide surveys to determine the fundamental needs of their children and to develop suitable national policies has been the focus of recent efforts.

There are three primary categories of activities that make up WHO's work. In the first place, it serves as a global clearinghouse for disease-related information and has established a standard procedure for reporting illnesses and fatalities. It has created globally recognized drug standards and compiled a list of "essential" medications that are safe, affordable, and work well. It has provided funding and sponsorship for numerous research initiatives around the globe. Second, the World Health Organization has supported widespread efforts to combat endemic and epidemic diseases, many of which have proven to be highly effective. Third, through offering technical assistance, expert teams to conduct surveys and showcase projects, and support for regional and national health development initiatives, WHO aims to enhance and broaden the public health administration and services of member nations.

10.2.2. Developed Countries

Health administration techniques differ between nations. A department that oversees both health and related functions often groups together major health functions. In the US, the Department of Health and Human Services is in charge of the programs covered by national legislation; in the UK, the Department of Health and Social Security is in charge of them.

There aren't many comprehensive central health departments; other departments also run some kind of medical program. No nation subordinates the medical care provided to its armed forces to the national health authority. Coordination is crucial since it is impractical to have unity of control at the center. Federal systems further complicate central administration. There are 50 states in the union, and no two have the same organizational structures for healthcare.

10.2.2.1. Patterns Shared Among Developed Countries

The individual in charge of overseeing national health affairs is typically a cabinet member. Advisory councils are widely employed to address significant national health issues by incorporating the opinions of eminent scientists, medical professionals, and local leaders.

A local health unit is an institution that works under the supervision of a medical officer and offers fundamental community health services. Usually, a local government is in charge of it. Maternal and child health, infectious disease prevention, environmental sanitation, keeping statistics up to date, public health nursing, medical care, and frequent school health services are among its programs. Care for the elderly, the physically disabled, the chronically ill, and mental health services are just a few of the community health services for which the local health unit can offer the administrative framework. Due to the correlation between social problems and health issues within a family, there are benefits to combining welfare and health services, even though social welfare services may be offered by a different organization.

A local health unit may serve a few thousand people or several hundred thousand people. Providing healthcare to a large, sparsely populated rural area and a municipality with a population of 1 or 2 million presents very different challenges. One issue with managing local health services is deciding whether to organize them regionally or under independent local authorities to prevent service duplication, promote coordination, and make effective referrals.

Most nations offer some form of public healthcare as a service. It might only apply to those who are hospitalized for specific conditions, such as acute infections, mental illness, TB, and chronic illnesses. For some particular population groups, such as Indians and Eskimos in the United States and Canada, where the federal government provides healthcare, comprehensive health services may be offered. Medical insurance is required in many nations, and in some—like Denmark—medical insurance also covers general medical care in addition to hospitalization. There are a few nations that have fully socialized their health services, such as the UK and NZ. Another way to refer to these socialized health services is as public or universal healthcare systems.

Health administration is pluralistic in nations like the U.S. and the Netherlands, where voluntary and nonprofit organizations run the majority of general hospitals and fund a sizable portion of healthcare services. This complicates coordination, but voluntary work offers the benefits of encouraging administrative experimentation and directly involving citizens in the creation of health services.

Regional health service planning for specific populations is becoming more popular. In an ideal scenario, health professionals who work in community health centers and who go beyond the centers into the communities and homes with preventive, promotional, and educational services provide the first level of contact between the population and the system, which can be called primary care. Patients referred from primary care centers receive secondary care at the next level of care from specialists in community hospitals. Lastly, a major medical center offers tertiary, or super-specialty, care. Patients, medical records, and healthcare professionals are exchanged back and forth between the different levels of this regional program. In North America, where volunteer hospitals handle the majority of the short-term general services and maintain administrative autonomy, regionalization has been less successful than in Europe.

10.2.2.2. Variations Among Developed Countries

The way health services are organized and managed varies significantly among developed nations. For instance, the National Health Service in the United Kingdom is implemented with significant autonomy delegated to local government. The United States approaches health services in a pluralistic manner, with the private sector playing a major role and local, state, and federal governments having different areas of responsibility.

The focus in the United Kingdom gradually shifted from environmental to personal public health during the first half of the 20th century. A series of laws, the most significant of which was likely the Maternity and Child Welfare Act (1918), gave county governments primary authority over the majority of the work. Around 16 million workers received benefits from National Health Insurance (1911), which also started a process that resulted in the National Health Service Act (1946). Hospitals, general practitioners, and public health were among the health services that were fully covered by the National Health Service Act. Nonetheless, the service continued to be on the outskirts in three categories of care: (i) General practitioners or family doctors provide primary medical care. Locally, this service is run by an executive council. A group of individuals on a specific registry must receive primary care from each general practitioner. (ii) Hospitals are run by regional authorities and offer both inpatient and outpatient care as well as specialist consultation. A later idea assigns hospital services to a specific population to each district general hospital. And (iii) local governments are in charge of providing services like health centers, domiciliary midwifery, home nursing, home assistance, health visiting, and illness prevention.

The state was in charge of preserving and advancing public health in the Soviet Union. All medical services were available to the general public for free. The full integration of curative and preventive services, medicine as a social service, preventive programs, health centers or polyclinics (clinics that handled a variety of diseases), and community involvement were the guiding principles of the health services.

The public health services for the Soviet Union were directed by the Ministry of Health. Each of the 15 republics of the union had its ministry. Each republic was divided into *oblasti* (provinces), which in turn were divided into *rayony* (municipalities) and finally into *uchastoki* (districts). Each subdivision had its health department accountable to the next highest division.

There were established protocols for referring patients from the polyclinics and smaller hospitals in the uchastoki to the larger hospitals in Rayon; additionally, feldshers, or medical personnel trained in medical care, and other medical personnel were referred to internists, pediatricians, and, if required, more highly specialized personnel. The health services of the United States can be considered at three levels: local, state, and federal.

Locally, within broad guidelines created by the state, there is significant autonomy in cities or counties. The management of communicable diseases, clinics for mothers and children, especially for specific preventive and diagnostic services, public health nursing services, environmental health services, health education, vital statistics, community health centers, hospitals, and other medical care facilities, as well as community health planning and coordination, are some of the roles played by local programs, which vary in size and scope.

Although multiple agencies may be involved, the state's Department of Health is ultimately in charge of health policy. The state Department of Health typically performs the following five duties: licensing individuals, organizations, and businesses that serve the public for health purposes; providing financial and technical support to local governments so they can run health programs; expanding and improving hospitals, medical facilities, and health centers; and providing medical and custodial care, such as running hospitals for mental illness.

The Department of Health and Human Services Public Health Service is the main federal health agency, although several other departments have roles and interests in health as well. Federal health agencies are in charge of enhancing state and local services, managing interstate health risks, and collaborating with other nations on global health issues. Additionally, the federal government is responsible for the following specific duties: (i) guarding the country against infectious diseases imported from overseas; (ii) meeting the medical needs of American Indians, veterans, merchant seamen, and military personnel; (iii) defending consumers against tainted or mislabeled food, medications, and cosmetics; and (iv) controlling the production of biological products like vaccines. The federal government also funds and encourages health services, medical research, and educational initiatives across the nation.

In the United States, a large portion of health work is done voluntarily. While they may also be active at the state and federal levels, voluntary organizations in the health sector primarily operate at the local level. These organizations, which receive the majority of their funding from private sources, support initiatives in the fields of health services, education, and research.

There are numerous ways to receive and pay for medical care. These include public institutions like hospitals, clinics, state, county, and federal health centers, as well as private hospitals and doctors who either work alone or increasingly in groups. Medical expenses are typically covered by voluntary health insurance, public monies, or private funds. As a result, the range, content, and caliber of health services vary greatly in the United States. Several separate organizations offer these services. Nonetheless, they essentially form a cooperative alliance for safeguarding and advancing human health.

Changes in the direction of health services in the United States have been influenced by the realization that, although many people receive excellent care from the current system, there are others for whom it is either insufficient or inadequate. Similar to this, the rapidly increasing costs of healthcare prompted proposals for new models of healthcare delivery and financing as well as a reevaluation of the personal medical care system as a whole.

10.2.3. Developing Countries

Developing nations have occasionally taken inspiration from developed nations that have contributed to their history when addressing healthcare issues. For instance, though there have been modifications to meet local needs, the educational and healthcare systems in the former British colonies in Africa and Asia still follow British models. Countries impacted by Belgium, the Netherlands, and France may see comparable results.

Though some less developed nations exhibit distinct patterns in the organization of healthcare, other less developed nations also exhibit significant differences and gaps in the administration and availability of health resources. These differences and disparities are more noticeable in less developed than in developed areas because in the former there are complex factors (like social or political instability) that can make the delivery of healthcare more difficult or even completely unworkable. Nations with such erratic healthcare systems frequently rely on aid from international agencies.

10.2.3.1. Patterns Shared Among Less-Developed Countries

Even though each nation is different, less developed nations can be categorized according to a common, if somewhat idealized, administrative pattern. A Ministry of Health oversees all health services, except a tiny amount of private practice. It is divided into approximately five bureaus or departments: hospital services, health services, education and training, personnel, and research and planning. The nation is home to numerous hospitals and health facilities. Dispensaries, or health outposts, are located at the edge of the system and are typically manned by one or two untrained employees. The dispensaries are frequently ineffective and, when feasible, are converted into full-fledged health centers. The cornerstone of the system is health centers and the things they do. Auxiliaries with four to 10 years of basic education and one to four years of technical training typically work in health centers. A midwife, a medical assistant, a sanitarian, and an auxiliary nurse may be among the staff members. Trained in illness diagnosis and treatment, the assistants refer patients with conditions beyond their scope of practice to a physician. For a population of 10,000–25,000, these auxiliaries collectively offer complete healthcare. A district with between 1,00,000 and 2,00,000 residents is served by multiple health centers, a district hospital, and other facilities. The district medical officer is in charge of all health services and, with the help of other professionals and support staff, combines the health initiatives into an all-encompassing program.

The allocation of duties between professionals and auxiliary personnel is crucial. By taking care of a lot of relatively easy problems, the auxiliaries free up the professionals to handle more difficult issues, supervise and train the auxiliaries, and plan and run the programs.

Patients with complex issues may be referred to a regional hospital for more specialized care, as the district hospital depends on it. At this level, regional medical officers can oversee both regional hospital services and regional health services administratively. In certain cases, the Ministry of Health's central administration also acts as a central planning unit in addition to providing policies and direction for the whole health system.

System failures are frequently caused by issues with long-distance communication and transportation, manpower and resource shortages, and inadequate staff training and motivation. However, the public health systems established in Asian and African nations have generally offered a solid foundation for further advancement within the context of national development.

10.2.3.2. Variations Among Less-Developed Countries

Latin American nations' public health systems are very different from those in Africa and Asia in terms of structure. These variations reflect the various historical contexts of the different areas. In general, the nations of Latin America are wealthier than those of Asia and Africa. Both private practice and private or volunteer organizations are more common. Local and federal governments are primarily responsible for providing health services. Additionally, many Latin American nations have worker-financed healthcare systems, including hospitals and clinics. Regarding health centers, hospitals, and preventive services, the distribution of health services is comparable to that of Asia and Africa. Compared to Asian and African nations, Latin America has utilized auxiliary resources less frequently. Health planning techniques have been developed at a leading edge in Latin America. One of the world's most sophisticated methods of health planning is used in Chile.

Thailand has never been colonized, so it has no historical precedent supporting a specific delivery system for healthcare. For the benefit of both rural and urban residents, the Thai Ministry of Health operates a sophisticated network of hospitals and health facilities throughout the nation. The nation enacted a universal healthcare program in 2001, with private funding augmenting government funding for the most part. There are several distinct divisions within Thailand's public health services—e.g., for nutrition, sexually transmitted infections, and tuberculosis.

10.2.3.3. Health Problems and Obstacles

Several interconnected issues make it challenging to provide healthcare to the citizens of less developed nations. These are brought on by the types of diseases and health risks, the distribution and scarcity of resources, the structure of healthcare systems, and the training of medical professionals working within them. The pressures of rapidly expanding populations are woven throughout the health programs of the less developed countries, complicating them at the national and family levels.

The types of diseases in various nations vary, as do the ages at which they affect people and the rates at which they occur. Some nations have shorter life expectancies than others, primarily as a result of the high mortality rates among young children in the less developed nations. For instance, the risk of death for children under five in Southeast Asia is three to four times higher than that of children in the Americas. In Africa, the death rate for infants (those under one year old) is roughly six times higher than in Europe, and the under-five mortality rate is more than eight times higher.

In the less developed world, respiratory infections, malnutrition, and diarrhea are the main causes of illness and mortality among young children. These three factors are closely linked to economic status, customs, and culture. Food customs that cause children to be deprived due to taboos and simple oversight can result in malnutrition. Respiratory infections and gastroenteritis, an inflammation of the stomach and intestinal lining that typically comes with diarrhea, are frequently caused by infectious organisms, some of which may be resistant to antimicrobial medications. Treatment for these illnesses is made more difficult by their interactions with one another. The root cause is frequently malnutrition. It seems to set the stage for other illnesses in addition to causing harm to the body and mind, such as retarding development. When a child is malnourished, they get diarrhea, become too weak to eat, become dehydrated, and so on. A deadly infection like pneumonia could strike the weaker child. Alternatively, infection can hurt protein metabolism, which exacerbates malnutrition, to complete the vicious cycle.

The size of the family is another element that influences this. Children born into large, poorly spaced families are most likely to suffer from malnutrition, which can lead to death and disability. The high death rate among young children that follows frequently serves to reinforce parents' propensity to have more children. Families are not likely to have fewer members until it is clear that the children have a good chance of surviving. There is thus a cycle of fertility and mortality where high fertility causes high childhood mortality, which in turn promotes high fertility. High fertility is reflected in a large number of small children crammed into a poor home. This is the rationale behind the idea that effective strategies for lowering preventable child fatalities should be a part of population-control initiatives.

One of the most significant resource constraints is the lack of qualified workers. Population-to-nursing, bed, and physician ratios show the severity of these shortcomings and the stark variations found across nations. Thus, in less developed nations, the population-to-physician ratio varies greatly.

The amount of money available determines how many health professionals can be trained, how many can be kept in the field, and what resources they will have available to them while they are on the job. The amount that each nation spends on healthcare varies substantially. A nation must have sufficient resources in place to handle complicated and urgent issues, like obstetric and surgical emergencies that require hospital care, to attempt to provide healthcare for its citizens. In addition, it needs to actively search homes and communities for people who need care but are not seeking it, as well as identify the underlying causes of illnesses like gastroenteritis and malnutrition.

10.2.3.4. Education of Health Personnel

A specific set of issues arises in the training of health professionals. Perhaps because auxiliaries were not developed in more developed nations, their educational programs are tailored to the local environment. On the other hand, medical and nursing education is more akin to that of the more developed nations, better-equipping students for employment in industrialized nations than in their own. The incompatibility of education and job requirements has likely played a significant role in the inefficiency of healthcare systems as well as the exodus of professionals to more developed nations (Albert et al., 2001; Austin et al., 1995).

10.3. Progress in Public Health

10.3.1. Developed Countries

Among the more-developed countries, the following trends are apparent.

1. **Increasing Interest in National Governments:** In the past, governments were mostly focused on basic health issues like environmental sanitation, impoverished people's healthcare, quarantine, and communicable disease control. With time, a lot of them expanded into the realm of in-home, clinic, and hospital medical care services in order to offer complete healthcare to entire communities. This trend has been driven by three factors: (i) rising healthcare costs; (ii) growing recognition

of the economic damage that illness causes to a nation; and (iii) growing public interest in social services. Social legislation typically covers both health and social welfare, as health and welfare are seen as complementary in many regions, which promotes close collaboration between the two services.

2. **Changing Concepts of Preventable Disease:** Historically, a specific set of infectious diseases was included in the term "preventable disease." Nonetheless, because many common noninfectious diseases can also be prevented, the term has taken on a broader meaning. Preventive health services address a broad spectrum of health risks in the modern era, including cancer, rheumatism, cardiovascular disease, other chronic and degenerative diseases, and even injuries.
3. **Integration of Preventive and Medical Care Services:** Preventive health services emerged from the need to shield a healthy environment from epidemic diseases, whereas medical care was initially motivated by the humanitarian goal of healing the sick. Although they drifted apart, it became popular to incorporate them into an all-inclusive health service. In the Soviet Union, the centralization of all local health services under a single administration at the district hospital was a fundamental principle of public health. Today, local medical practitioners bring the two branches together in European countries and other places, particularly rural areas.
4. **Provisions Directed Toward Better Mental Health:** Preventive services should include mental health services. The availability of outpatient clinics and inpatient beds at general hospitals for early mental cases, the expansion of clinics offering child and marriage counseling, and programs for the treatment of alcoholics and drug addicts are some examples of improvements in mental health arrangements. Not insignificant advancements have also been made for socially maladjusted individuals. Notable developments include the expansion of research facilities and the general practitioners' growing comprehension of psychoneuroses.
5. **Growing Emphasis on Health Education:** Numerous nations have increased their funding for health education, typically in conjunction with nonprofit organizations. Local efforts are the most successful, particularly those conducted in schools. Health education is becoming more widely recognized as a vital preventive health service.
6. **The Bio-Statistical, Epidemiological Approach:** Planning, executing, and

assessing health services all depend on statistical services. The significance of data on the prevalence of illnesses and other issues, as well as the epidemiology required to address them, has grown due to the interest of public authorities in healthcare programs. Both are essential for the development, administration, and assessment of healthcare plans. The epidemiological method was originally developed to study infectious diseases, but it is now being used more and more to study noninfectious diseases and issues with medical care.

7. **Changes Resulting from an Aging Population:** An increase in older age groups in more developed nations necessitates the provision of specialized services by public health facilities. The treatment of the elderly involves addressing psychological issues brought on by inactivity and loneliness as well as taking steps to prevent chronic and degenerative diseases and premature aging. The rising incidence of dementia in senior populations in the 21st century presented serious problems for public health. Senior living communities and geriatric clinics have been established to address these demands and carry out studies on the senescence process.

8. **Concern Regarding the Quality of the Environment:** Increased industrial and commercial activity brought on by a growing population increases the amount of pollutants endangering the atmosphere, rivers, lakes, and oceans, as well as having detrimental effects on natural ecosystems. These impacts may result in deteriorations in the quality of the air, water, and species that provide food and medicine, all of which may have an impact on human health. Numerous nations have taken action to stop environmental degradation, and methods of international regulation have also been suggested and, in certain cases, put into practice.

10.3.2. Less-Developed Countries

Significant advancement is frequently accompanied by some degree of stagnation or even regression, given the abundance of severe health issues that people in less developed nations face and the scarcity of resources available to address those issues.

10.3.2.1. Infectious Disease Control

Examples of infectious diseases that have been tightly controlled globally are polio and measles. Once a terrifying infectious disease that affected children, smallpox was formally declared extinct in 1980. Considerable progress has been made in our understanding of other diseases, like meningitis and cholera, which may eventually lead to their control. Similarly, in the early 21st century, increased access to medication therapies and increased awareness of prevention measures led to a decrease in both new cases and deaths from acquired immunodeficiency syndrome (AIDS), which was initially identified in 1981. As humans altered their surroundings, some parasitic diseases proliferated. Schistosomiasis, which is caused by blood fluke infestations using snails as intermediate hosts, increased in areas with irrigation and man-made lakes, for example. Research has shed light on recently discovered mosquito-borne illnesses like chikungunya and Zika fever, as well as ways to stop the spread of extremely contagious illnesses like Ebola.

10.3.2.2. Malnutrition

Malnutrition on a large scale is still an issue, especially in small children who are malnourished in protein and calories. Undernutrition and malnutrition are targets for the development of more efficient educational programs and protein-rich food supplements in developing nations.

10.3.2.3. Family Health

Population growth issues have significant ramifications for both the family and the country. Issues related to human reproduction, human genetics, and maternal and child health are subsets of the larger issue of the health of the family as a fundamental and cohesive social unit. As a result, family planning and other aspects of family health are crucial to public health services.

10.3.2.4. Health Personnel

The deficiencies in the quantity and quality of health personnel are widely acknowledged. Health professionals' education is increasingly being matched to the specific health service they will work in. Close ties between academic institutions and the organizations in charge of providing health services are necessary to keep up with this trend.

10.3.2.5. Comprehensive Community Health Services

Community health is significantly impacted by the integration of curative and preventive services in comprehensive health organizational patterns. A community-wide network of integrated services that includes disease prevention, health promotion, and the treatment and rehabilitation of the sick is created.

10.3.2.6. National Health Planning

Allocating scarce health service resources to a large number of individuals involves complex decision-making, which highlights the importance of health planning and necessitates efficient health service systems. Numerous nations have set up health planning divisions within their national planning organizations or ministries of health. The close coordination of program planning, budgeting, implementation, and evaluation is a crucial component of national health planning.

10.4. Law and Public Health Policy

States are required by law and morality to defend their citizens' health from harm. Public health law and policy are two of the most significant tools that help states with this task. Law and policy have distinct but connected functions in preserving the general public's health.

Public health law is defined as the state's obligation and authority to guarantee the conditions necessary for people to be healthy as well as the restrictions placed on the state's ability to restrict people's freedom, privacy, autonomy, and proprietary rights. This definition includes the state's functional policies outlining the interventions it is willing to implement in order to carry out its strategy, as well as its strategic public health policy regarding its role and responsibilities with regard to population health.

10.4.1. Definition and Boundaries of Policy and Law

10.4.1.1. Public Health Policy

A process of research, negotiation, and consultation results in a plan of action that outlines a vision of the goals that have been identified for public health. Although private public health organizations may also develop policies about their public health objectives, the political or executive branch of the state typically determines policy in the context of public health. For instance, the Terrence Higgins Trust (THT), a British AIDS charity, has created a corporate strategy outlining the goals, parameters, and approaches of its AIDS services. Similar to THT, the goal of private agency policy is frequently to have an impact on how government policy is formulated.

A policy is a declaration of values regarding the significance of stated objectives and the suitability of methods for accomplishing them. States have created and improved public health policies that offer a coordinated and targeted set of solutions to specific public health issues. To varying degrees of complexity, the majority of states have policies in place to handle risks like food contamination, smoking-related illnesses, infectious diseases, and environmental damage. New policies are created or modified to address emerging threats to public health, such as the obesity epidemic.

A policy can be prescriptive, meaning it calls for certain actions to be taken after it, or descriptive, outlining a method to address a public health concern. The Philippine government will implement a balanced policy that regulates the use, sale, and advertising of tobacco products to promote a healthy environment. This is known as the prescriptive policy. The descriptive policy reads, "It is the policy of the State to protect the populace from hazardous products and to protect the right to health." A policy may be published for public consumption or kept private from the policymaker. Policymaking is an ongoing process. The principles guiding policy are constantly under review and may be contested by interest groups as well as advancements in the field of public health science. Political objections have undermined scientifically supported policies in the United States regarding needle exchange programs aimed at reducing HIV cases. Similarly, in Latin America, the tobacco industry's focused strategies have impeded the development of policies protecting people from secondhand smoking.

Policy may be decided after a long period of consultation or hurriedly in response to a new threat, and can be flexible in its response to new knowledge. Policies may be designed to be short-term or longer-term in their application, but the shelf life of government policy is likely to be limited to the government's term of office.

10.4.1.2. Public Health Law

Public health law is made up of legislative (enacted by parliament) and judicial (court rulings) declarations of norms or regulations controlling health interventions or health-related behaviors. Law is inherently a public domain.

Legislation is composed of written documents that outline the rights of those who are subject to certain powers, as well as the conduct expectations for the public and private sectors. Such a written document will be referred to as a code in some legal systems and as a statute, act of parliament, or ordinance in others. There may be "secondary" legislation in addition to the statute, act, ordinance, or code. This type of legislation has less authority and specifies more precisely how it is to be applied. This secondary legislation may be referred to as a code of practice, circular, decree, or regulation. The process by which these written documents are created and the state's jurisdiction to impose their provisions are what distinguish these documents from policies.

In a democracy, laws are made through a legislative process that allows public representatives to participate in the process of creating laws. There will be a clear definition of the legislative process, meaning that any flaw in it will make the legislation void and unenforceable. The legitimacy of the law-making body and the public's belief that the legislation has been decided in compliance with the legislative process are the sources of legislation's authority. Legislation made by state rulers in a nondemocratic setting may be made without public input or adherence to procedural laws; in these situations, the enforceability of the legislation comes from military might rather than the rule of law.

In certain legal systems, particularly those based on the Napoleonic Code, the written documents that comprise legislation contain the entire body of law. Common law systems, which are based on the British legal system and are found in other nations like the United States, Canada, Australia, New Zealand, and India, supplement legislation through judicially determined case law after interested parties are given a chance to present their case. In a common law system, parliamentary passed legislation supersedes judge-made law; however, in cases where parliamentary passed legislation is either nonexistent or unclear, judge-made law may take precedence. For instance, in England and Wales, a statute governs the age at which a minor may consent to sexual activity. However, there is no statute governing the age at which a minor may consent to medical treatment; instead, court rulings control this. Case law is the result of a synthesis of court decisions that give rise to legal principles rather than being found in a definitive legal document.

Policy informs and shapes law, at least good law, which is typically formulated after the policy debate is over. The parliamentary and judicial systems are intended to work toward a balanced reflection of views, even though it would be naive to suggest that the content of laws is impervious to vested interests and even though laws may be based on policies that have been appropriated by political or economic factions. Law will reflect values, but it will not explicitly state them. Any legal challenge in the courts should only target the legal system itself, not the values it is founded upon. If a law is opposed on the basis of its underlying values, the policy that underpins the law must be contested rather than the law itself.

It is both a good and a bad thing that the process of drafting new legislation, whether it comes from the courts or parliament, is slow and frequently tedious. Law may be ineffective if the public threat is novel in nature because of how rigid and powerless laws become when faced with unanticipated consequences due to the intricacy of the legislative process. However, once a law is in place, it cannot be changed or repealed without following a new procedure, and new governments may find it challenging to summarily overturn laws that were created in response to policies decided upon by previous administrations. The benefit of law is found in its weight. It is hard to dispute, has the ability to be enforced by state authority or custom, and has a significant impact on citizens' attitudes and behavior. Law should be upheld, and it usually is, even though many policies will never be put into practice. Indeed, one key distinction between law and policy is that the former can be enforced while the latter cannot.

10.4.2. The Relationship Between Public Health Law and Public Health Policy

10.4.2.1. Law and Strategic Public Health Policy

Law is not always a useful tool for expressing strategic policy and intangible concepts. Law, however, does play a part in educating the public about the significance of policy and the seriousness with which the government plans to carry it out. Additionally, it can help get the populace ready for the eventual implementation of useful policy measures. Instead of focusing on the actions of private organizations and individuals, laws outlining strategic policy will address the actions of public bodies, including political bodies. Such laws typically don't offer enforcement mechanisms, though public law may make it possible to challenge illegal activity. In the context of strategic policy, one of law's more significant functions is to clearly state the government's position on a matter of policy and, in doing so, to offer a vocabulary and instruments for discussion regarding the best ways to carry out government policy. Legislation enacting strategic policies can be used to create public entities and define their goals, principles, and roles.

The Hong Kong Council on Smoking and Health was established by the Hong Kong Legislative Council as part of its initial efforts to prevent the negative effects of smoking. This was accomplished through a statute that articulated a broad mission statement outlining the government's strategic policy goals regarding the negative effects of smoking, including public education and awareness campaigns, research coordination, and the provision of advice to bodies and agencies regarding health protection measures. The statute clarified government intentions and offered a forum for a more focused discussion on the types of powers and interventions that could be used to prevent tobacco-related harms, but it did not provide any explicit duties, powers, or enforcement mechanisms. Following discussions and deliberation regarding the means of achieving these strategic objectives, the Legislative Council enacted laws enacting the functional policy interventions the government planned to take to guarantee the accomplishment of these objectives. Examples of these interventions included the regulation of tobacco advertising and the specification of the information that must be included on cigarette packets. The regulations that followed supported this legislation in detail, including the government chemist's authority to ascertain the nicotine and tar content of cigarettes.

10.4.2.2. Law and Functional Public Health Policy

Strategic policy cannot be expressed through the use of law as effectively and efficiently as it can be used to enforce adherence to precise, functional, and functional norms of behavior. The acts of individuals, businesses, and public executive bodies may all be covered by laws enacting functional policy. In addition to prescribing and outlawing specific acts and conduct, they also set the parameters for how the law is to be applied. They enlist the assistance of other legal disciplines, including tort, criminal, public, and licensing law (especially judicial review). Establishing and upholding sound public health policy is a major focus of public health law.

In a unique way, law can impose enforceable obligations on people and public entities alike. The best way to ensure that an action or activity has been carried out when implementing a public health strategy is through the legal system. For instance, the prevention of communicable diseases depends on data on the prevalence and incidence of diseases, and many states have laws requiring disease notification as part of their public health arsenal.

Laws can grant authority to take actions that would otherwise be illegal or violate human rights. If a public health official must take action to prevent an infectious diseased person from being exposed to others, the state must establish legal grounds for detention or isolation so that the official can act without being rebutted. If not, the use of force to detain someone could be considered a criminal trespass or a violation of their right to liberty. The European Court of Human Rights ruled that the Swedish government had overreached itself in detaining an HIV-positive man because it believed his health-related behaviors posed a risk to the public's health. The detainee's rights to liberty, privacy, and family life were found to have been violated by the detention, and he was given compensation for this violation.

Law also acts as a constraint on the use of authority. The balance between the public interest and individual rights, as well as the relationship between the state and the individual, will be decided at the strategy level by government policy. These kinds of relationships will require legal expression in a non-authoritarian state. Each state, in light of its political, historical, and social environment, will have developed formal or informal policy on the extent to which interference with individual autonomy and privacy may be justified in the name of the public good. For example, mandatory vaccination and medical treatment may serve the utilitarian and communitarian objectives of reducing disease threat, but do these measures align with the state's strategic policy? Without legal expression for that policy, people won't have a way to legally challenge abuses of power, and public health officials won't know exactly when their authority to act in the interest of public health will be curtailed. The majority of states will have laws that define individual rights and offer remedies for those rights being violated. These laws may be expressed through legislation, customs, or the legal process.

An additional, more widespread function of law is to carry out functional policy. Beyond the mere formulation of policy, law has authority due to its status, integrity, and sanctity—values that should never be compromised. In a legal society, morality and wrongdoing are determined by the law, which is regarded as acceptable or unacceptable behavior. Law is customarily obeyed not because of its content but rather because it is a product of a legitimate act of the state's government or sovereign. Because they believe that the law expresses standards that warrant criticism and punishment for deviating from them, citizens obey the law. According to this perspective, citizens will follow the law despite their disagreements with its morality or soundness because it is the law. People adjust their behavior to comply with the law regardless of the possibility of enforcement or penalty because they view the law as a dictator of right or proper behavior.

Law has had a significant influence on how public health practices are developed. Seat belt and child safety seat requirements have resulted in a significant decrease in road traffic fatalities in numerous states. Although it was once believed that people bought safety seats or buckled up their seat belts out of fear of going to jail, it was soon realized that a good citizen saw these actions as proof of good behavior. Similar perspectives regarding behavior acceptance have been noted following the implementation of smoking laws. While it used to be possible for a nonsmoker to object to a smoker on the grounds that smoking infringed on the nonsmoker's right to clean air, after legislation intervened, the perception of a smoker in a regulated nonsmoking zone is now one of offense against society rather than the individual nonsmoker. The smoker's actions turn from being a personal annoyance to a public offense that includes a moral assessment of the smoker's behavior's social acceptability.

The implementation of effective public health policy is significantly influenced by the law's function as a social norm-setter. Even with strong public health advocacy and education, public health policies regarding tobacco smoke did little to lower the rate of smoking. Codes of conduct that are voluntary have not been effective. It's too soon to say whether or not laws have been successful in lowering smoking rates, but some evidence points to decreased cigarette sales in areas with smoke-free policies, improved worker health due to protection from secondhand smoke, and altered attitudes toward smoking habits. Research also indicates that residents of states without smoking bans may become suspicious of their own state's lack of legislation as a result of legal developments in other states.

10.4.3. The Limits of Law in the Implementation of Public Health Policy

While legislation can accomplish a lot to carry out policy, there are situations in which the measures it can take are ineffective or inappropriate, and policy is a more useful instrument than legislation. Laws that impose definite duties on state entities—like the duty to safeguard the right to health—are not very helpful. The South African Constitution attempted to guarantee that every person has the right to obtain healthcare services, and it required the state to take reasonable legislative and other actions to make this right a reality. The South African Constitutional Court acknowledged that the reality of these rights was that they were constrained by resources when people came to contest denials of healthcare services. It was determined that the principles of rationing healthcare provision were essential to a human rights approach to healthcare in an open and democratic society founded on the principles of equality, freedom, and dignity. The state could not be held accountable for any individual citizen's complete health.

Furthermore, the law is not very good at forcing people to take proactive steps to safeguard the interests of others. The law can control deliberate, careless, or negligent behavior. Some examples of this include making it illegal to spread disease carelessly, offering compensation to victims of careless radiation exposure, or making clear the limitations placed on doctors when treating patients. However, problems arise when a law tries to compel someone to fulfill a duty, like rescuing an accident victim or abstaining from work if an employee shows signs of influenza. The issue is how far the law can force someone to give up something important to benefit someone else. The law tends to operate under the assumption that individuals have responsibility for their safety outside of the deliberate, reckless, or negligent actions of others. Should an individual be required to put himself or herself at risk of physical harm to rescue another from drowning or from a violent attack? Should an individual be legally obligated to forgo earnings so that others can work without fear of infection? Employees who want to avoid the risk of infection must pay the price by avoiding areas that are contaminated. Nonetheless, policy easily accommodates the duty to act in others' best interests. The immunization policy, for instance, promotes vaccination even in cases where it serves the purpose of protecting the herd rather than the individual receiving the vaccination. Based on the idea that people may have to make some sacrifices for the greater good, the majority of states have developed vaccination policies that include advocacy programs to promote vaccination. States rarely impose vaccination requirements on their citizens, but legal challenges to such mandates have not always been successful, suggesting that the state may have a valid reason to use its authority to compel people to act in the public interest. Historically, however, forced vaccination campaigns have not worked, as seen with smallpox vaccination programs in South Asia, the United States, and England. Public health agencies experienced administrative and financial difficulties as a result of these programs, which also incited violent resistance and noncooperation and reduced the efficacy of emergency measures.

A more useful tool in these situations is policy. If the government were to adopt the stance that, in specifically defined situations, such as when a pandemic of human influenza was imminent, all afflicted or exposed individuals should be placed under isolation or vaccinated, then functional policies could be developed quickly, flexibly, and with a time constraint to address the issue at hand. Legal enforcement is not as likely to result in compliance as other strategies. Examples of these include offering free medical care or providing state compensation for lost wages. Some states, like the United States and France, have achieved something akin to a vaccination mandate by administrative means by making childhood vaccination a requirement for state-provided services like schooling.

Law is also a poor tool for compelling public entities to exercise any authority they may possess. For instance, it is typical for public health officials to be able to separate individuals who have infectious diseases. Very rarely does the law provide others a way to force the official to use their power if they refuse to do so and others are in danger. This is because legal power inherently includes the ability to act or not act, and it is the person bestowed with the power to decide whether to exercise that discretion. Legal systems rarely allow for the coercion of an official to take action, even in cases where doing so would turn that official's power into a duty and cause grave harm. The legislation would have stated so if the legislature had intended for there to be a duty to act. In exceptional cases, such as when the failure to exercise the power was wholly unreasonable or the failure was to stop a violation of a legally protected human right, there may be a remedy available. The Indian Supreme Court has ruled that water is a communal resource that the state holds in public trust and that the right to life includes the right to the basic needs of life. According to this interpretation, the state has a legal obligation to safeguard water sources, and any inaction on its part—such as failing to clean up rivers and wells—could result in legal action. Nonetheless, policies are typically more appropriate than laws for controlling the use of authority, and they may even impose on public bodies a social or political duty to use their authority under specific conditions. Policies can adapt to the needs of society and changing conditions. The law is an ineffective and crude tool for this.

Another drawback of the law is that it is an ineffective instrument in situations where compromise or discussion are required. Due to the adversarial nature of law, it is not a flexible enough tool to serve as a framework for negotiation or mediation. However, it can be used to establish and authorize mediation bodies and may even provide leverage to persuade individuals or bodies to engage in these processes. Once more, policy is a better means of establishing the parameters of negotiations and is better suited to adjust those parameters when doing so is desirable from a political or practical standpoint.

The last restriction on law is that since national legislatures and courts typically enact laws, laws seldom have any effect outside of state borders. Threats to public health, however, know no geographical boundaries. States have very little extraterritorial authority, though it has occasionally been used to prosecute foreign pedophiles by Section 34 of the United Nations Convention on the Rights of the Child, which obliges states to take national, international, and bilateral action to stop the exploitation of children for sexual purposes.

Law made by a supranational organization, like the European Union, which has the authority to issue directives with which member states are required to comply, is an exception to the domestic character of law. Through the imposition of coordinated frameworks for protection against global public health threats, such as contaminated food or environmental harms, supranational law-making powers may promote public health in member states. However, a nation-state may be prevented from shielding its citizens from health risks by supranational legislation that is designed to serve an objective other than public health. For example, the European Common Agricultural Policy is credited with driving up the cost of nutritious fruits and vegetables by mandating that produce be destroyed to keep prices stable. However, the fact that processed food is less expensive than fresh food is a concern in the fight against the obesity epidemic.

States are likewise subject to international conventions, agreements, strategies, and laws. These international agreements regulate state behavior and have the power to establish strategic policy. While they typically do not directly address private sector or individual behavior or establish matters of functional policy, they can be a valuable tool for public health. National laws then implement the functional policies that are derived from the strategically agreed-upon international framework. Aiming to strike a balance between technological innovation and the social and economic welfare of consumers, the World Trade Organization (WTO) oversees the TRIPS agreement (Trade-related Aspects of Intellectual Property Rights), which lays out strategic policy on the patenting of pharmaceutical products. The Doha Declaration amended it in 2003 to permit developed states to export pharmaceuticals to other states where a recognized national health concern existed, provided that the exports were made independently of any commercial agreement. The agreement permits states to enact laws that infringe on patent holders' rights under certain conditions, such as national emergencies, and it depends on the signatory states to do so. Standardized TB treatment procedures are outlined in the WHO DOTS (Directly Observed Therapy) strategy for tuberculosis control; some of these procedures may need legislative support. To address the serious threat of tuberculosis, Russia, for instance, has passed regulations to support TB control in line with the DOTS strategy.

International conventions primarily address the state's duty to safeguard the rights of its citizens. The strongest expressions of obligation can be found in documents like the International Declaration of Human Rights which include civil and political rights like the right to life and the right not to be subjected to torture. Signatory states to the Convention are obliged to incorporate these safeguards into their national laws. A more "progressive" realization of rights within national law is the foundation of instruments that aim to protect economic and social rights, such as the right to work, the right to education, and the right to be free from discrimination in the provision of public goods like health services. These instruments recognize that the social and economic environments of some states may make it more difficult to implement these rights. Implementation, however, is contingent upon the state's desire to pass legislation that reflects established international policy about all rights conventions.

The WHO Framework Convention on Tobacco Control is a more inventive application of the convention instrument, as it promotes the use of law at the national and international levels to support tobacco-related policies. A unique application of WHO's international treaty-making authority, the Convention addresses a worldwide public health issue in light of the prevalence of tobacco addiction and related diseases in both developed and developing nations. In contrast to alcohol and obesity, the tobacco industry actively targets poorer nations, which has resulted in a disproportionate amount of harm from tobacco use. The application of international law to address an international health concern is a novel approach, even though it has long been acknowledged that the implementation of tobacco control strategies can help to avert the health costs of tobacco use and that legislation is a crucial vehicle for such strategies.

The WHO has the authority to enact regulations on public health, but it has seldom done so. To establish an international legal framework for the control of communicable diseases, the World Health Organization (WHO) updated its antiquated and ineffective International Health Regulations in 2005. This was done in response to the SARS pandemic and the growing threat of infectious diseases. National laws must be drafted to reflect international control measures, according to the TRIPS agreement, the DOTS strategy, human rights conventions, the Tobacco Convention, and international health regulations. National laws will be used to implement functional strategies targeted at specific public health interventions or specific health harms. International documents contain global policy strategies in legislative form.

10.4.4. Law and Policy as Dual Mechanisms in Public Health

Policies and laws by themselves are insufficient to address today's pressing public health issues. When policy is codified in legislation, it functions as a dual mechanism, with policy being more effective than law alone. A combination of purpose-driven functional policies—some of which are incorporated into laws to provide duties, powers, and enforcement provisions—and strategic public health policy, which may be expressed in legislation to demonstrate political will, could make up such an approach.

The topic of bicycle road safety illustrates how the law may be utilized as a tool to carry out policy. Bicycle accidents are the main cause of brain injury in China, and cyclists make up 45% of traffic fatalities in Wuhan, China. As in many other states, China acknowledges the critical public health concern of bicycle and motorcycle safety. The Helmet Initiative is one part of a policy strategy the WHO has developed to reduce motorcycle and bicycle fatalities. The WHO has addressed the issue of cycle safety. The availability and cost of safety helmets, as well as social attitudes, have hindered policy implementation in numerous countries. In China and other similar states like Vietnam, Thailand, and the Philippines, bicycle helmets might only be found in upscale stores at premium prices. However, a large number of helmets sold today are produced in these states.

It has been demonstrated elsewhere—in Sweden, for instance—that mandatory helmet wear is one of the best ways to lower the death and injury rates from bicycle accidents, while public health education initiatives do not considerably lower cycling fatalities. Following the introduction of helmet-wearing laws in Thailand by WHO policy, there was a 56% decrease in fatalities. In addition to providing tools for enforcement, such as fines and license suspensions, the law also serves to inform drivers and riders about appropriate and inappropriate driving practices. The law may also control the built environment to create bike lanes or set speed limits for two-wheeled vehicles. Laws that require helmet-producing factories to use excess plant capacity to produce helmets for local consumption at a reduced or subsidized cost could also help to increase access to helmets in lower-income countries like China.

The best way to address the negative effects of alcohol abuse on public health has been demonstrated to be policy supported by legislation. It is commonly known that alcohol use contributes to both mortality and morbidity. Several states, especially those in northern and English-speaking Europe, have created functional policies to address specific issues like alcohol-related psychiatric disorders, alcohol-induced physical disease, alcohol-fueled violence, and alcohol-related motor accidents. One such strategy is the Alcohol Harm Reduction Strategy for England. These laws encourage initiatives, such as public awareness campaigns and education programs, but they have not been very successful in lowering alcohol consumption. The strong interests of the alcohol industry have played a significant role in impeding the execution of policy-driven initiatives.

Conversely, legislative actions that uphold policy have proven successful. The implementation of driving laws that set maximum alcohol levels, the taxation of alcohol to drive up its price, the imposition of license requirements on bars and restaurants, and the civil liability of those who serve alcohol to unsuitable individuals have all been effective in lowering alcohol consumption or its negative effects. In a similar vein, it's now acknowledged that legislative backing is necessary for policy approaches to combat the obesity epidemic. The goals of strategic policy have not been met by voluntary agreements for broadcasters to refrain from advertising foods high in fat, salt, and sugar (HFSS) that are targeted toward children, voluntary codes of practice on the nutritional standards of school food, voluntary codes on the inclusion of nutritional information in food labeling, and voluntary agreements within the retail trade on the pricing of healthy foods. Food manufacturers contend that it is inappropriate to regulate food products because, in contrast to alcohol and tobacco, HFSS foods are not inherently harmful if consumed in moderation. Due to the economic might of the food lobby and the possibility of losing money from food marketing and advertising, policy strategy compliance has been discouraged. Around the world, governments are looking to the law to give them more effective tools in the fight against obesity, and some states (like Sweden and Quebec) have started enacting laws to limit the activities of food manufacturers in the area of obesity prevention (Fichtenberg et al., 2002; Francis et al., 1981).

10.5. Public Policy and Health Economics

10.5.1. The Market-Based System

The fundamental difference between the approach to the provision of healthcare in the United States and most other industrialized nations is that the United States is more market-oriented, and insurance coverage is less inclusive. When health insurance is offered to workers as part of their compensation package, it is a tradeoff for higher cash wages, and it is not a "right." In most states, employers are not required to offer health insurance to employees. Whether they do so depends on the labor regulations between workers and employers. In other industrialized nations, people generally contribute to a system of social insurance, either through general income tax or payroll taxes. This is true in the United States only of the Medicare contribution, although personal income taxes also support Medicaid, the State Children's Health Insurance Program (SCHIP), the National Institutes of Health, and the healthcare infrastructure, including subsidies to hospitals and medical schools.

All societies ration scarce resources. Therefore, the question is what basis should be used to ration access to healthcare. A market-based system relies more heavily on the price mechanism as a rationing device. The U.S. healthcare system is a mixture of a market system and a system in which services are allocated on other bases. For example, Medicaid and SCHIP do not use the price mechanism to allocate healthcare resources. Medicare relies less on it because services are so heavily subsidized.

10.5.1.1. Demand versus Need

The greater reliance in the United States on the market and rationing by price, rather than by the government, is paralleled by an approach in healthcare economics that focuses on supply and demand. Thomas Rice is critical of a demand-driven system. He questions the concept of consumer sovereignty in a situation where demand determines the direction of technology development in healthcare. These criticisms rely on the assumption that nonmarket-based methods can and should be used to prioritize and determine the distribution of the resources a society decides to devote to healthcare. This approach requires faith that there is a way of determining an objective standard of health needs and an appropriate distribution of care.

10.5.1.2. Evaluating Efficiency versus Equity

Critics of a healthcare system usually evaluate it based on two criteria: efficiency and fairness (or equity). In most economic decisions, there is some degree of tradeoff between the two criteria. To use a previous example, pricing insurance using experience rating is more efficient than broad-based community rating because it relates the marginal cost of insuring the individual to the price of the insurance policy. However, risk sharing through community rating is thought to be more equitable because consumers are not penalized for poor health.

In the case of healthcare, equity and efficiency may also be complementary. It is widely believed that the social costs of healthcare for the uninsured are higher than if they were insured, given that our society does not generally refuse to provide healthcare to the sick, even if they cannot pay. It is argued that the uninsured do not receive healthcare until illnesses are more advanced and that this results in higher treatment costs than if they had access to preventive care or earlier treatment. Moreover, people without health insurance tend to overuse hospital emergency room services, which are more expensive than physician office visits for non-emergent cases.

A good deal of research has provided estimates of the incremental costs associated with insuring the uninsured. A 1993 study by Long and Marquis provides an estimate of $28.6 billion. Adjusting for increases in the number of uninsured from 1993–2001 raised the estimate to $35 billion. A more recent study by Miller et al. provides 2002 estimates ranging from

$44.9 billion to $57.4 billion, assuming the spending of the currently uninsured mirrors that of the privately insured. If we assume that the healthcare utilization and spending are comparable to those of the Medicaid population, the range is from $35.1 to $38.1 billion. Both sets of estimates deduct the value of in-kind uncompensated care that this group would receive if uninsured.

The health status of the community also has public good aspects because poor health is associated with lower labor force participation, poverty, and homelessness. Low health status is also associated with increased risks of spreading transferable diseases to other members of the community. The reduction in these indirect social costs that would be accomplished by insuring the uninsured should be subtracted from the increase in direct healthcare costs. A full cost analysis of the lack of access to healthcare also needs to take into account the losses due to shorter lives or a lower quality of remaining life years (QALYs).

10.5.1.3. The Rising Cost of Healthcare

Increases in healthcare costs are an international problem. David Cutler pointed out that social insurance systems were originally more concerned with equity and provided most of what people wanted without a great deal of concern with efficiency. Today, this is no longer possible. The common problem facing all industrialized nations is how to pay for the level of healthcare that their citizens want. Given the dramatic improvements in medical technology, people everywhere have rising expectations about what can be done to improve their health. The public healthcare systems are finding it necessary to cut back on coverage by limiting emergency care, and/or requiring higher copayments for services. With this trend, satisfaction surveys with health systems are much lower in most countries than a decade ago.

10.5.1.4. Technology Change and the Cost of Healthcare

A number of economists have demonstrated that the largest contributor to rising healthcare costs is advances in technology. Although the cost of healthcare is worth it, it is important to develop strategies to identify particular components of healthcare expenditures that have low marginal benefits. Technological change shifts the production function for health in favor of more healthcare versus other inputs. This has been the story of healthcare in the United States during much of the second half of the 20th century. Therefore, there is no mystery as to why the total amount of medical spending is rising. A projection made in 2002 estimated that medical care would comprise 16.8% of the U.S. GDP by the year 2010.

10.5.1.5. The Role of Market Imperfections

The contribution of market imperfections to the cost of healthcare has been a constant concern in health economics. Critics have often associated a combination of fee-for-service payment and the lack of price competition with monopoly rents to providers. The healthcare market does not consist of small, perfectly competitive firms subject to long-run zero profit competitive equilibrium. Instead, the markets for goods and services provided by physicians, hospitals, and pharmaceuticals are at best monopolistically competitive. However, price competition has increased greatly and was introduced largely because of the active role of third-party payers, both private and public. Managed care has also provided a mechanism for negotiating fees with hospitals, physicians, and pharmaceutical manufacturers.

10.5.1.6. Imperfect Information

Problems associated with imperfect information occur not only in the insurance markets but also in the provision of healthcare. Integrated delivery systems may contribute to this because managed care subscribers often have little knowledge of the costs of the different services that they consume. One way to improve efficiency is for health plans to provide information about the costs of particular services. This is likely to be more helpful in decisions about non-acute care.

Another area of imperfect information that affects both costs and quality of care is the lack of systemization of medical records of patients. There is a lack of formally articulated instructions from patients about their desires for end-of-life treatment. A nontrivial proportion of the total expenditure of healthcare in the United States is devoted to keeping very sick and terminally ill people alive by artificial means that are frequently counter to their wishes, which can no longer be expressed. In many cases, the treatment is not regarded by the medical community, family members, or most members of society as humane.

10.5.1.7. Inefficiency of Insurance Markets

Advocates of a single-payer system often point to the costs of administering an insurance system that consists of insurance contracts with such a confusing array of technicalities about coverage. A system of multiple insurers is administratively more expensive than a single-payer system. However, it provides more choice to consumers, as well as more problems of adverse selection. It is unclear whether streamlining and standardizing insurance coverage (which would require additional regulatory costs and limit consumers' options) would bring about a net improvement in social welfare.

A lower deductible on an insurance policy is inefficient when its marginal cost is greater than the marginal benefit of additional coverage. The load or loading fee is a much higher proportion of the insurance premium in low deductible policies. This is one of the reasons why some economists have advocated a combination of high-deductible insurance policies (usually called catastrophic coverage) and personal medical savings accounts.

Experience rating is a well-known form of achieving greater efficiency in insurance markets. Price discrimination is based on differences in the costs of insuring different individuals, promoting efficiency by relating marginal costs and price. It is a common practice in the homeowners,' life insurance, and automobile insurance markets. Experience rating also removes the incentive to cream skim, the practice whereby insurance companies purposely select healthier clients. The argument for community rating is that risk sharing among members of the community is more equitable. It is thought to be unfair to charge people more for insurance because they experience unavoidable bouts of illness or deterioration of health. Because the purpose of insurance is to pool risks, experience rating, if carried to an extreme, undermines the goal of insurance (Ham et al., 1990).

There is considerable evidence that medical malpractice law in many states does not promote higher quality care, but contributes substantially to the costs of medical practice and encourages the practice of defensive medicine (Gostin et al., 2000).

A Closer Look

Public Health Development

Public health is an evolving field that constantly adapts to new challenges and discoveries. In recent years, there has been a closer look at various aspects of public health development, highlighting achievements and areas needing improvement.

One significant aspect receiving increased attention is preventative healthcare. Governments and health organizations are increasingly emphasizing the importance of preventing diseases rather than just treating them. This shift in focus involves promoting healthy lifestyles, implementing vaccination programs, and conducting screenings for early detection of illnesses. By prioritizing prevention, public health initiatives aim to reduce the burden on healthcare systems and improve overall population health outcomes.

Another area of scrutiny is health equity. Disparities in healthcare access and outcomes based on factors such as race, ethnicity, socioeconomic status, and geography continue to persist in many parts of the world. Addressing these inequities requires targeted interventions, including increasing access to healthcare services in underserved communities, promoting culturally competent care, and tackling social determinants of health such as poverty and discrimination. Achieving health equity is not only a matter of social justice but also essential for achieving optimal public health outcomes for all.

Furthermore, there is a growing recognition of the interconnectedness between various domains of public health. Issues such as climate change, urbanization, and globalization have significant health implications, requiring interdisciplinary approaches for effective solutions. For example, climate change contributes to the spread of vector-borne diseases and exacerbates air pollution, leading to respiratory illnesses. Addressing these challenges necessitates collaboration between environmental scientists, policymakers, and healthcare professionals to develop strategies that mitigate environmental risks and protect public health.

In addition, advancements in technology are reshaping the landscape of public health. From the use of big data and artificial intelligence for disease surveillance to telemedicine for remote healthcare delivery, technology can revolutionize how public health interventions are designed and implemented. However, ensuring equitable access to these technological innovations and addressing concerns related to data privacy and security are critical considerations in harnessing the full potential of technology in public health.

Overall, taking a closer look at public health development involves examining not only the progress made in addressing existing health challenges but also identifying emerging threats and opportunities for innovation. By prioritizing prevention, promoting health equity, fostering interdisciplinary collaboration, and leveraging technology, we can work towards building healthier and more resilient communities.

Summary

- Public health is the art and science of preventing disease, prolonging life, and promoting physical and mental health, sanitation, personal hygiene, control of infectious diseases, and organization of health services. From the normal human interactions involved in dealing with the many problems of social life, there has emerged a recognition of the importance of community action in the promotion of health and the prevention and treatment of disease, and this is expressed in the concept of public health.
- Health promotion is a guiding concept involving activities intended to enhance individual and community health well-being. It seeks to increase involvement and control of the individual and the community in their health. It acts to improve health and social welfare and to reduce specific determinants of diseases and risk factors that adversely affect the health, well-being, and productive capacities of an individual or society, setting targets based on the size of the problem but also the feasibility of successful interventions, in a cost-effective way.
- The official responsible for the administration of national health affairs is, in most cases, a member of the cabinet. Advisory councils are frequently used to bring the ideas of leading scientists, health experts, and community leaders to bear on major national health problems.
- Medical care is a public service to some degree in most countries. It may be limited to the hospitalization of persons afflicted with certain ailments—for example, mental disease, tuberculosis, chronic illness, and acute infections.
- Developing countries have sometimes been influenced in their approaches to healthcare problems by the developed countries that have had a role in their history. For example, the countries in Africa and Asia that were once colonies of Britain have educational programs and healthcare systems that reflect British patterns, though there have been adaptations to local needs. Similar effects may be observed in countries influenced by France, the Netherlands, and Belgium.
- Public health law has been defined as the power and duty of the state to ensure the conditions for people to be healthy and the limitations on the state's power to constrain autonomy, privacy, liberty, and proprietary interests of individuals and businesses.
- Public health policy is determined by a process of consultation, negotiation, and research, which leads to a plan of action that sets out a vision of identified public health goals. In the context of public health, the policy is usually determined by the political or executive arm of the state, although private-public health agencies may also formulate policy about their public health objectives.

References

1. Albert, M., Ostheimer, K., & Breman, J. (2001). The last smallpox epidemic in Boston and the vaccination controversy 1901–1903. *New England Journal of Medicine, 344*, 375–379.
2. Allwright, S., Paul, G., & Bernie, J. M. (2005). Legislation for smoke-free workplaces and health of bar work before and after study. *British Medical Journal, 331*, 1117–1126.

3. Austin, J. (1995). *The Province of Jurisprudence Determined*. Cambridge University Press.
4. Barnoya, J., & Glantz, S. (2002). Tobacco industry success in preventing regulation of secondhand smoke in Latin America: The 'Latin project.' *Tobacco Control, 11*, 305–314.
5. Chinkin, C. (2006). Health and human rights. *Public Health, 120*(Supplement 1), 61–70.
6. Department of Health, Western Australia. (2005). *New Public Health Act for Western Australia: A Discussion Paper*. Government of Western Australia.
7. Euromonitor International. (2006). *NRT Smoking Cessation Aids in Ireland*. Euromonitor International.
8. Fichtenberg, C. M., & Glantz, S. A. (2002). Effect of smoke-free workplaces on smoking behavior: Systematic review. *British Medical Journal, 325*, 188–194.
9. Gostin, L. O. (2000). Public health law in a new century. *Journal of the American Medical Association, 283*, 2837–2841.
10. Ham, C. (1990). Analysis of health policy–Principles and practice. *Scandinavian Journal of Social Medicine* (Supplement 46), 62–66.
11. Hart, H. L. (1994). *The Concept of Law* (2nd ed.). Clarendon Press.
12. Hendrie, D., Miller, T., & Orlando, M. (2004). Child and family safety device affordability by country income level: An 18-country comparison. *Injury Prevention, 10*, 338–343.
13. Jones, K., Wakefield, M., & Turnbull, D. (1999). Attitudes and experiences of restauranteurs regarding smoking bans in Adelaide, South Australia. *Tobacco Control, 8*, 62–66.
14. Li, G., & Baker, S. (1997). Injuries to bicyclists in Wuhan, People's Republic of China. *American Journal of Public Health, 87*, 1049–1052.
15. Martin, R. (2006). The limits of law in the protection of public health and the role of public health ethics. *Public Health, 120*(Supplement 1), 71–77.
16. Marx, F., Atun, R., Jakubowiak, W., McKee, M., & Coker, R. (2007). Reform of TB control and DOTS within Russian public health systems: An ecological study. *The European Journal of Public Health, 17*(1), 98–103.
17. Ministry of Health, New Zealand. (2002). *Promoting Public Health, Preventing Ill Health and Managing Communicable Diseases: Public Health Legislation Discussion Paper*. Ministry of Health.
18. Pilkington, P. A., Gray, S., Gilmore, A., & Daykin, N. (2006). Attitudes towards secondhand smoke amongst a highly exposed workforce: A survey of London's casino workers. *Journal of Public Health, 28*, 104–110.
19. Room, R., Babor, T., & Rehm, J. (2005). Alcohol and public health. *Lancet, 365*, 519–530.
20. Rosenstock, L., & Lee, J. L. (2002). Attacks on science: The risks to evidence-based policy. *American Journal of Public Health, 92*, 14–18.

INDEX

D

E

F

G

H

I

ABOUT THE AUTHOR

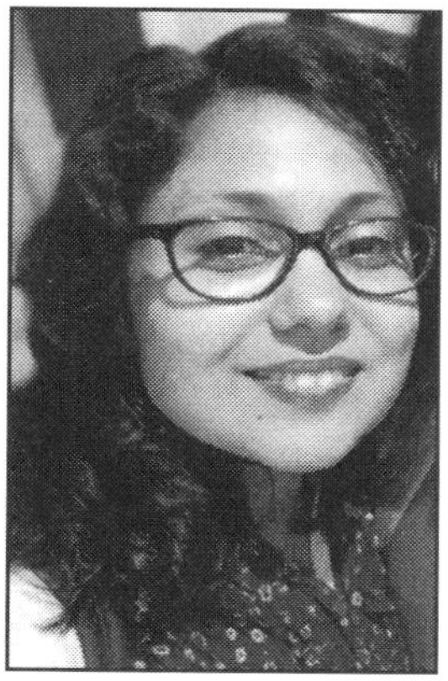

Dr Kavita Ramanathan is an accomplished medical professional with experience working through the length and breadth of India. With 16+ years in clinical and anatomic pathology, she understands the normal and abnormal functioning of the human body in depth. Also, she held positions in the senior management for 8+ years and designed business strategies. She successfully helped organisations attain profitability while maintaining quality and service standards. Additionally, during the COVID-19 pandemic, she contributed significantly by aligning operations to support government initiatives. She earned her undergraduate and graduate medical degrees from reputed institutions under the University of Mumbai, India, and she also holds an MBA in Finance. Dr Kavita volunteers with a non-profit organisation where she tutors students from low-income schools for over two decades. Post-pandemic, she quit her corporate job to pursue her passion of teaching and writing. Currently, she tutors high school and university students in biology, psychology, and medical sciences. Additionally, she authors books, articles, and blogs on topics related to health and well-being. Her strong academic background, enriched with a vast and varied experience, shapes her into a mature and sensible professional.

FSC
www.fsc.org
MIX
Papier | Fördert
gute Waldnutzung
FSC® C083411

Kolibri 360 GmbH
Ferdinand-Jühlke-Straße 7
99095 Erfurt, Deutschland
produktsicherheit@kolibri360.de